A TEXTBOOK OF GENERAL PRACTICE

Third edition

Edited by

Anne Stephenson
MBChB MRCGP Dip. Obst. PhD (Medicine) FHEA
Senior Lecturer in General Practice & Director of Community Education,
Department of Primary Care and Public Health Sciences,
King's College London School of Medicine,
King's College London, London, UK

HODDER

First published in Great Britain in 1998 by Hodder Arnold
Second edition published in 2004
This third edition published in 2011 by
Hodder Arnold, an imprint of Hodder Education, a division of Hachette UK,
338 Euston Road, London NW1 3BH

http://www.hodderarnold.com

Hachette UK's policy is to use papers that are natural, renewable and recyclable
products and made from wood grown in sustainable forests. The logging
and manufacturing processes are expected to conform to the environmental
regulations of the country of origin.

Whilst the advice and information in this book are believed to be true and
accurate at the date of going to press, neither the author[s] nor the publisher
can accept any legal responsibility or liability for any errors or omissions that
may be made. In particular (but without limiting the generality of the preceding
disclaimer) every effort has been made to check drug dosages; however it is
still possible that errors have been missed. Furthermore, dosage schedules are
constantly being revised and new side-effects recognized. For these reasons the
reader is strongly urged to consult the drug companies' printed instructions
before administering any of the drugs recommended in this book.

British Library Cataloguing in Publication Data
A catalogue record for this book is available from the British Library

Library of Congress Cataloging-in-Publication Data
A catalog record for this book is available from the Library of Congress

ISBN-13 978 1 444 120 646

1 2 3 4 5 6 7 8 9 10

Commissioning Editor:	Joanna Koster
Project Editor:	Stephen Clausard
Production Controller:	Jonathan Williams
Cover Design:	Amina Dudhia
Indexer:	Lisa Footitt

Cover image © designer_things – Fotolia

Typeset in 9.5pt Minion by Phoenix Photosetting, Chatham, Kent
Printed and bound in Spain by GraphyCems

What do you think about this book? Or any other Hodder Arnold title?
Please visit our website: www.hodderarnold.com

CONTENTS

CONTRIBUTORS

Mark Ashworth BM MRCP DTM&H DM FRCGP Clinical Senior Lecturer, Department of Primary Care and Public Health Sciences, Guy's Campus, King's College London, London, UK

Paul Booton BSc (Hons) MB BS MRCP MRCGP Department of Primary Care and Public Health Sciences, King's College London School of Medicine, King's College, London, UK

Joanna Collerton BM BCh MRCP MRCGP Senior Research Fellow, The Institute for Ageing and Health, University of Newcastle, Newcastle upon Tyne, UK

Helen J. Graham DCH FRCGP FHEA Senior Lecturer and Learning and Teaching Co-ordinator, Department of Medical Education, Guy's Campus, King's College London School of Medicine, London, UK

Graham Hewett MSc BA (Hons) Clinical Governance Development Manager, South East London Shared Services Partnership, London, UK

Roger Higgs MBE MA FRCP FRCGP General Practitioner and Professor of General Practice and Primary Care, Department of Primary Care and Public Health Sciences, King's College London, London, UK

Mary Lawson BSc (Hons) Director of Education, Australasian College of Emergency Medicine, Melbourne, Victoria, Australia

Gael Ogunyemi Department of Primary Care and Public Health Sciences, King's College London School of Medicine, King's College London, London, UK

Richard Phillips MA MRCP ILTM Senior Lecturer, Department of Primary Care and Public Health Sciences, King's College London School of Medicine, King's College London, London, UK

Maggie Rose MBBS BSc Paediatric Trainee Doctor, London Deanery. Junior doctor observer, The Institute of Medical Ethics

Mary Seabrook BEd DMS PhD (Education) Freelance Education and Training Consultant and Professional Life Coach, London, UK

Anne Stephenson MBChB MRCGP Dip. Obst. PhD (Medicine) FHEA Senior Lecturer in General Practice and Director of Community Education, King's College London Undergraduate Medical Education Team, Department of Primary Care and Public Health Sciences, King's College London School of Medicine, London, UK

Ruth Sugden RGN DN Cert FPN MSc (Health Sciences) Senior Teaching Fellow and Phase 5 Lead for General Practice, King's College London Undergraduate Medical Education Team, Department of Primary Care and Public Health Sciences, King's College London School of Medicine, London, UK

Jackie Tavabie MSc MBBS FRCGP DRCOG ILTN General Practitioner and GP Trainer, Ballater Surgery, Orpington, Kent, UK

Patrick White MD MRCP FRCGP Senior Lecturer, Department of Primary Care and Public Health Sciences, King's College London School of Medicine, King's College London, London, UK

Ann Wylie PhD MA FRSPH FAcadMEd FHEA Deputy Director of Community Education, King's Undergraduate Medical Education in the Community Team (KUMEC), Senior Teaching Fellow, Phase 4, Health Promotion and SSC Lead and Head of Phase 4 SSC Sub-Committee, Department of Primary Care and Public Health Sciences, King's College London School of Medicine, London, UK

PREFACE

This third edition is primarily intended for undergraduate medical students. However, it will also be useful for new doctors, general practitioners (especially teachers) and other health professionals. As a medical student 35 years ago, I was very keen to meet patients and experience the full range of conditions that I would face as a medical practitioner. I was also aware that my time as an undergraduate was limited. It was therefore important for me to gather a kernel of knowledge, skills and professional behaviour to allow me to be a good and safe-enough doctor. However, at that time, either in the way that I perceived it or in the way that it was presented to me, general practice seemed to be such a vast and loosely determined discipline as to be too difficult to be used in this process. On the other hand, it also appeared to have the dimensions and potential that I needed to explore the realms of health, illness and healing. Now, as a teacher and practitioner of general practice, I have been able to revisit the discipline from a new perspective and in a much more productive way.

Over the past 35 years the discipline of general practice has been greatly developed and refined so that departments of general practice are now in the forefront of medical education. The broad base of knowledge and wide range of skills that general practitioners (GPs) hold and the opportunities that primary care affords in terms of an understanding of health and illness, together with the great organizational advancements that have occurred in primary care, are now widely recognized to offer a rich learning resource for budding clinicians. Undergraduate education, generally, also continues to be in a phase of rapid development. In Britain this is being promoted by the General Medical Council, which has outlined recommendations most recently revised in 2009 in *Tomorrow's Doctors*. It sees the development of personal and professional values as being as important as the acquisition of knowledge, understanding and skills. It encourages clinical experience, opportunities to learn from patients from a range of backgrounds, learning from other health professionals, and the promotion of small-group and self-directed learning, with regular information about progress. Departments of general practice have been prime movers in these directions.

This book reflects this development. It is a distillation of what is necessary for a medical student and a new doctor to know and understand about general practice and being a GP. The chapters from the second edition have been updated, some quite substantially. The book is designed to encourage deep learning – a clearly presented and interesting text with a core of important information, and opportunities to reflect and experiment with the ideas in order to integrate and commit them to memory. In this edition single best answer questions at the end of most chapters help this process, as do red flags, which mark essential information. It is left to your GP teachers and other specialists to provide the detail with which you can build on what is presented here.

The book ends with two chapters about your intended life as a doctor, included to emphasize the fact that all the clinical knowledge and skills in the world do not, on their own, lead to a healthy and fulfilling life. In the demanding world of medicine, this can be easily forgotten. It is with this sentiment that I present this book, as well as with the wish that, as lifelong learners, we continue to experience the fulfilment that a life in medicine can provide.

Anne Stephenson

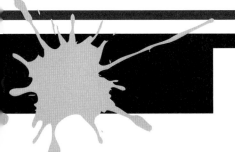

ACKNOWLEDGEMENTS

Editing the third edition of this book has, once again, been a good process. My thanks go to the contributors and the publishers for their hard work and patience.

I also acknowledge and value the help the following people gave to me and the contributors in writing this book.

- The undergraduate general practice teachers at what was the King's College School of Medicine and Dentistry and The United Medical and Dental School and is now, after merger, the King's College London School of Medicine. They have, over the years, developed the teaching philosophy and skills that are reflected in this text.

- The students who, through their feedback, encourage us to provide the best learning environment possible.
- The patients who were patient with us when we were student learners and who teach us.
- The various authors and publishers for permission to reproduce material.
- Ms Karen Fuchs who took the photographs and the medical students, general practice staff and patients who allowed the photographs to be taken.

I am grateful to Amadis and Meera for being so generous in their support.

Finally, I dedicate this book to Mum and Dad.

Anne Stephenson, 2011

INTRODUCTION

General practice is an important place for the education and training of medical students. Not only does it offer a large number of training opportunities in which medical knowledge can be applied, basic clinical skills acquired and attitudinal and ethical concerns explored, it also provides a wide variety of learning situations in which sound management decisions can only be made when this knowledge and skill are integrated with the experience and understanding of the practitioner, the patient and the community in which they reside. This textbook seeks to support and reflect this process.

The information that this textbook provides is largely generic in that it can be applied to all areas of medicine. In fact, general practice is a good teacher of the basic principles without which the more in-depth information provided by other specialisms cannot be understood. Although the book is largely based on the British experience, it is recognized that readers will be drawn from other countries and so the contents are relevant to any medical system.

The learning style of the book is based on experiential and reflective principles, cornerstones of modern educative theory and practice. Most medical teachers are now aware of the 'experiential learning cycle' (Figure I.1) and use it in their teaching. Students learn by doing: active learning experiences are provided for the student and time is given for reflection on what actually happened. The student is then encouraged to think about and make sense of the experience, identifying principles and generalizations that can be taken forward into new situations. Other experiences can then be planned to support and further explore insights around these topics. Although this approach appears obvious, it is not always followed or valued. However, experiential and reflective learning is profound. Students who are encouraged to learn in this way have the potential to understand that every patient encounter is unique and that their education cannot provide definite answers to every question, only ways of approaching patients and clinical situations. In this process, the individual student's experiences and insights are valued and can be developed through self-directed learning, essential for ongoing professional development.

Tutor quote

I shall tell you about these American students. I think it is about my own hang-up about using certain new words and trying new skills. You have got to try them and this applies to other tutors. This situation was after the course that we attended. The homework was to try to use reflection in your practice when you are teaching. I had these American students who had been with me all day and there were two of them and maybe it was because there were two of them I didn't particularly talk with them. It seemed quite difficult to do and I was sitting in the car with them after the surgery and I wondered whether I should use the word 'reflection' or should I say, 'Can you first remember what happened and then can you remember what was in it that you learnt?' . . . something like that. Then I debated that briefly

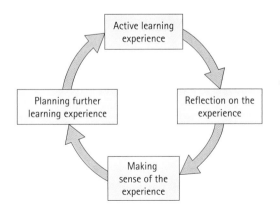

Figure I.1 The experiential learning cycle.

and then I thought, 'No, let us just throw it in', and I said, 'Could you reflect on what we did today?,' and that was it, and for the whole journey there was all this information coming through. I was amazed at the detail and the maturity and that that word was enough. There was no need to dress it up, no need to assume that they wouldn't understand. We sometimes do not give them the credit they deserve. So I think for me what there is to learn is to try new things, techniques; some might fail, some might succeed spectacularly and that one was a very good one. I enjoyed that.

(It should be noted that the tutor quotes that appear throughout the book have not been quoted from the authors of the chapters.)

Ways of using this book

For the reasons explained above, this book is a mixture of textbook and workbook. It is not necessary to work through the book from the first to the last page. Rather, we encourage you to work with the chapters that are relevant to your course and stage of development and of interest to you and your tutor. However, as each chapter works as a unit, it may be of greatest use to you if you read the chapter as a whole before you decide how to use it to structure your learning experiences.

Hints for conducting the exercises

The exercises are of two main types: Thinking and Discussion Points and Practical Exercises. The *Thinking and Discussion Points* encourage you, on your own or with your tutor and colleagues, to reflect on your knowledge and experiences around a particular topic. Examples are: 'What has influenced your views on general practice?' or 'What questions would you like to ask a patient before you decide whether or not to visit them at home?' This type of exercise is generally used to introduce a topic. It values your personal insights and past experience as highly relevant to your understanding of the topic and to how you might approach further learning around the topic. The text often gives you pointers to help you in your thinking.

The *Practical Exercises* give you a structure with which to investigate further a particular topic. Examples here are: 'A way of evaluating the effectiveness of a consultation' or 'How to find out more about a particular medical condition'. These need to be carried out in tandem with your tutor, and some exercises have extra guidance for your tutor so that they can run more smoothly. Once again, the text often gives extra help in what you might get out of the exercise.

Case studies

Case studies have been included to make the information more real. All of these are based on real experiences or an amalgam of real experiences. Where the stories are about people, many identifying characteristics have been changed to protect confidentiality.

References and further reading

As mentioned previously, the factual content of the book has been kept to a minimum. The focus has been placed on you experiencing and researching relevant clinical areas. To this end, references and further reading have been placed at the end of each chapter. We strongly encourage you to spend time capitalizing on your practical learning by reading around the topics that have been thrown up by clinical situations.

As with other medical teaching, there are times when your tutor is unable to take much of an active role in your learning. You may sometimes feel at a loss to know how to use your session in general practice most wisely. If this happens, flick through the book and pick out an area that interests you. Read through the chapter and the exercises. You may be able to go to the practice library or online to research a subject, interview a member of the practice staff about a topic that interests you, discuss one of the thinking points with a colleague, prepare a presentation for your next seminar, or just have a cup of tea and relax until your tutor returns. We hope that this book can be a companion to you in such situations.

The chapters

This book celebrates the differences and variety in the way that general practitioners (GPs) and general practices work. Thus every chapter, although structured along the same lines, is presented in a slightly different way, dependent on the topic and the writers' approach. Chapters are of different lengths and some are more discursive and philosophical, others more practical and factual. In the development of the book the writers frequently shared their ideas on what each chapter might contain, so we hope that the book appears cohesive and that links between chapters are evident.

The book opens with a chapter on learning in general practice that is a useful starting point for all readers as it outlines the learning opportunities that may be offered in the general practice setting as well as some of the challenges that may present. Chapter 2 provides a brief overview of the place of general practice in the wider primary healthcare system, particularly with reference to Britain, but with some reference to other countries.

The next four chapters outline the basic skills of a GP. Chapter 3 introduces the central activity of a GP, the consultation. To have some understanding of what happens when a patient and a doctor meet is essential to an effective outcome. The earlier a student can understand the basic principles behind such professional communications, the easier it will be to develop this most important skill. The most frequent practical skills required of a GP and useful for any doctor are described, in detail, in Chapter 4. These descriptions are often missed out of medical texts and should provide a helpful introduction to the supervised practice of these skills. Chapter 5 explores the diagnostic and acute management processes on which a GP's work is based. Chapter 6 discusses the topic of prescribing, such an important area of a doctor's work both in terms of patient well-being and economic burden. The information and exercises contained in these chapters can be generalized to any clinical situation and so have relevance to other medical disciplines.

One of the commonest questions that students ask when they enter general practice is how the presentation of illness differs from that of hospital medicine. Undergraduate medical curricula have often omitted teaching around illnesses that are perceived as not important by virtue of being either minor or self-limiting. However, the bulk of illnesses presenting to the healthcare system are of these types. Chapter 7 describes the common illnesses that people present to general practice, many of which will never need hospital care and yet are important for any doctor to know about. This chapter also gives guidance to students on how to access information on these illnesses.

Psychological issues are given a special chapter, Chapter 8, as they are of particular relevance in a general practice setting where knowledge of patients and their inner and outer environment provides insights into the nature of all patient presentations.

Chapter 9 addresses the management of the chronically ill. This essential clinical subject may be seen as not as exciting or as fulfilling as areas of acute medicine, and the mention of long-term illness may even lead to a feeling of hopelessness or failure on the part of the clinician. However, chronic illness has a profound effect on the lives of patients and their families. Structured care in such situations is now being seen to provide great advantage, and general practice is at the forefront of these developments.

Treating people at home can provide unique insights into their illness and treatment. General practice can provide such opportunities and Chapter 10 gives an introduction to how a medical student can best benefit from such an experience.

Health promotion is discussed in Chapter 11. This is an area of clinical work – logically more important than treating illness once it has occurred – often cited as important by medical teachers and yet very often, in practice, ignored or approached badly with poor outcomes.

Chapter 12, 'Healthcare ethics and law', is included because the 'broader questions about what is best for patients or staff, what it is right to do, or whether we are acting within the law commonly arise in practice for anyone who reflects on their work.' This chapter suggests ways of approaching ethical and legal issues and reaching conclusions that are satisfactory for all concerned.

Medical knowledge is increasing at a rapid rate and, looking from the outside, it must sometimes seem to medical students that the task of becoming a competent doctor in a few short years is impossible. Where does one begin? We hope, in this textbook, not to alarm you further. We have deliberately kept facts to a minimum and concentrated on important principles rather than dazzle you (or frighten you) with detail. Actually, you will get there, and much more easily if you start with the basics, fully understand them and have carefully structured experiences on which to hang them. But how do we keep up with research evidence and relating this to improvements in patient care? Chapter 13, on quality assurance, examines ways in which you can cope with change and the acquisition of knowledge and skills and ensure that new treatments are instituted effectively with risks to patients kept to a minimum.

The business side of medicine has long been seen as perhaps necessary but not relevant to a medical student's education. With the recent increase in the complexity of health service delivery, a working knowledge of medical management is no longer an option but an essential part of every medical student's training. Chapter 14 provides an introduction to this subject using 'the general practice' as a manageable unit with which to explore this area.

Chapter 15, 'Preparing to practise', is aimed at the later years of a medical student's progression to becoming a doctor. Nine learning objectives, around clinical reasoning, written communication skills, teamwork, organizational skills, uncertainty and personal limitation, working with constructive criticism, professional conduct and lifelong learning, explore areas of professional development that are essential for the safety of a new doctor.

Finally, whether or not you are an aspiring GP, Chapter 16 talks about the life of a GP to remind us that a personal and a professional life are inextricably intertwined and to concentrate on one without regard for the other will only lead to discontent. Whatever branch of medicine you enter, we hope that, by reading this chapter, you will be encouraged to consider how you live your life so that you experience fulfilment both professionally and personally.

We have put red flags against some points in the text which we judge to be essential to be aware of in terms of patient or practitioner safety.

Most chapters end with five Single Best Answer questions to test your understanding. These questions may need extra 'research' if your subject-specific learning is so far incomplete. We have chosen what we think are the best answers (see the Appendix) – for some of the questions you may argue them with your tutor and peers.

Finally a glossary has been added to help with the definitions of terms common to the work of GPs.

CHAPTER

1

LEARNING IN GENERAL PRACTICE: WHY AND HOW?

- Introduction
- Frequently asked questions about learning in general practice
- Suggested preparation/early orientation
- Ten tips for learning in general practice
- Common problems and dilemmas for students in general practice
- Summary points

The structure, culture, atmosphere and pace of general practice are different from those of other healthcare settings. General practice provides an opportunity to learn new things and to compare different approaches to healthcare. This chapter will help you to plan how to get the most out of general practice.

LEARNING OBJECTIVES

By the end of this chapter you will be able to:
- identify what can best, or only, be learnt in general practice;
- compare the hospital and general practice settings from the perspective of doctors, patients and students;
- plan ways of learning effectively in general practice.

Introduction

Students often have preconceptions about what they are going to learn in general practice. The following expectations were expressed by students preparing for their attachments.

Student quotes

'It will be nice to see a broader spectrum of the community – in hospital it's mostly older people. I'm looking forward to seeing children and babies.'
'Seeing a wide spectrum of people and problems, not knowing what sort of problem is going to present next. Being able to use all your medical knowledge.'
'Improving my interviewing and diagnostic skills.'
'Experience to observe some more social skills, e.g. breaking bad or unwelcome news.'
'Seeing what a GP's life is like. Good to check out career options.'

Others commented on aspects of the learning process they thought they would enjoy.

Student quotes

'It will be good to have a bit of independence rather than six or so students stood around one patient and being questioned.'
'Patients may actually like to talk to us. In hospital they get a bit sick of seeing students.'
'Being involved at a more personal level with the patients, e.g. many GPs seem to know their patients and families very well and the GP is someone seen as a friend too.'

Students can also have concerns about learning in general practice. Here are some of the common concerns.

Student quotes

'I might get a GP who's not keen on teaching and just leaves you sitting there.'
'Dealing with ailments that are mundane and medically uninspiring.'
'Feeling isolated or not liking the GP with whom I am spending my time.'

'The fact that the problem presenting can be almost anything – how do you come to a diagnosis in such a short amount of time?'

'I am worried about the level of knowledge that is required and the degree of autonomy given.'

'Difficulty in getting to the place as I don't have any transport.'

To address these points, we include below a list of frequently asked questions.

Frequently asked questions about learning in general practice

Why learn in general practice?

In recent years, major components of healthcare have been transferred out of the hospital and are now only found in the community. For example, community rehabilitation has increased enormously as patients often leave hospital shortly after their operations or treatment. Chronic or long-term diseases, such as hypertension, asthma and diabetes, are managed primarily in the community, as is much terminal care. Hospitals are offering increasingly specialized care, and patients are often only in hospital during particular, critical stages of their illness. Without community experience, students would see little of many common conditions and snapshots of disease and treatment rather than natural progression and long-term management. General practice also provides a good context for learning particular skills and aspects of medicine (see 'What will I learn in general practice?').

Is general practice relevant for those going into hospital careers?

Many factors influence a medical student's choice of specialty, but more graduates will eventually enter general practice than any other specialty. Some decide early that they want to take this option; others plan a career in hospital medicine but find, for various reasons, that they switch to general practice at a later stage. Before deciding on a career path, it is important to explore all the options, and general practice attachments will give insight into this branch of medicine.

Whatever your choice of specialty, it will be important that you have a good understanding of all the services available in primary care and how to access them. Without a detailed knowledge of what is available within your area, you will not be able to refer patients appropriately, and thus provide the best care for them.

How will it help when I start work?

Many Foundation Year 2 doctors (pre-specialty training) do a three or four month placement in general practice and there are plans for all FY2 doctors to do so. Studies of general practice teaching suggest that it promotes a patient-centred approach to medicine which will be useful in any specialty. It should help doctors to acquire knowledge of primary and community services, enabling hospital patients to be discharged effectively and receive the appropriate care in the community, and should reduce unnecessary readmission.

How will it help to pass examinations?

This depends on individual medical schools and the nature of their assessments. General practice provides the opportunity to experience a lot of common illnesses. These will be central to the core curricula which medical schools assess. In addition, general practice commonly provides one-to-one or small group teaching, which allows for the possibility of teaching tailored to particular learning needs. Thus it is a good opportunity to ask for help and experience in the areas you find most difficult. It is also a good environment in which to get supervised practice of the sort of clinical skills that are tested in Objective Structured Clinical Examinations (OSCEs) and other clinical examinations.

What will I learn in general practice?

Key areas for learning in general practice include the following:

1. The range of statutory and voluntary services which contribute to health and well-being, and how to access them:
   - the structure, functioning and funding of community health and social services,
   - when, how and to whom to refer patients, and who can refer to whom,

- understanding of what voluntary sector services offer patients and how this contributes to health.

2. The effects of beliefs and lifestyle factors on health:
   - how patients' beliefs, understanding and attitudes towards health affect their use of services, e.g. why people don't take medication, the impact of religious and cultural beliefs, attitudes towards complementary therapies,
   - how to involve patients in decision making, e.g. healthy lifestyle choices,
   - health promotion and disease prevention skills and strategies.

3. Environmental, social and psychological factors affecting health:
   - reasons for the differential morbidity and mortality rates in different geographical areas,
   - causes of health inequalities between different groups of people, e.g. reasons for differential rates of mental illness diagnoses among different cultural/gender groups,
   - learning to recognize and explore the impact of psychological as well as physical causes of illness, e.g. social isolation, stress in the workplace, unemployment and family dynamics.

4. The management of common conditions:
   - diagnosis and ongoing management of common conditions, e.g. depression, hypertension, diabetes,
   - detecting and preventing long-term complications,
   - experience of the progression of illness and its impact on the lives of patients and their families,
   - the differing roles of the general practitioner (GP) and other members of the practice team, hospital team and social services,
   - practical ways of supporting patients and carers,
   - ongoing monitoring and screening of patients.

5. Specific skills:
   - the skills required to distinguish between serious and non-serious conditions, e.g. whether a depressed patient is at risk of suicide or self-harm, whether a methadone patient is at risk of relapse, monitoring a pregnancy for signs of risk such as pre-eclampsia, deciding whether a rash on a child is due to measles, meningitis or an allergy,
   - practical skills, such as measuring blood pressure, giving an injection, examining an ear and immunization regimes.

6. A different model of healthcare practice:
   - a different approach to patients and their healthcare needs,
   - a different model of inter-professional working,
   - a different organizational structure,
   - learning to function in a primary care team.

Below, students describe some of the things they have learned in general practice.

Student quotes

'You got more of a view of the whole patient – the GP tends to know the whole family.'

'You learn to rely less on investigations.'

'They let you go and clerk and examine and they come in and you present, and that was excellent because it gets your clerking and examining skills up to scratch and it's a different type of clerking than in the hospital. It's got to be done in about a minute or two. It makes you learn hopefully to home-in on something. You learn to sort what is most important.'

'Dealing with a wide variety of cases and a wide range of patient groups.'

'You don't actually understand what other people in the team do until you see it and how useful it is. . . it opens your eyes and you realise medicine is not the be-all and end-all of the thing.'

'It changed the way I take histories quite dramatically – you learn to always have a hypothesis in your head and always be thinking, formulating differential diagnoses earlier basically, and taking a more directed and useful history.'

In general then, we suggest that general practice is the best place to learn about:

- the range of primary care services and how to access them,
- the effects of patient beliefs and lifestyle factors on health,
- environmental, social and psychological factors affecting health,
- the management of common conditions,

■ the skills required to distinguish between serious and non-serious conditions.

Why can't I stick to 'real' medicine?

By 'real' medicine, students usually mean patients with good signs and symptoms, with an acute illness that can be cured by the doctor, often by some 'high-tech' intervention. In fact, only a tiny proportion of healthcare actually takes place in the hospital, and teaching hospitals in particular are very specialized, often taking very rare cases. Despite advances in technology and treatment, many conditions cannot be cured, and the doctor's role is often one of providing long-term care, support and symptomatic relief. Spending time in general practice provides a more realistic picture of the healthcare required to manage conditions with high mortality and morbidity rates. It is also a myth that there is no acute medicine in general practice. For example, most heart attacks and acute psychiatric crises occur outside the hospital. Traditionally, medical education was based almost exclusively in hospitals. This is changing to reflect current patterns of care, and to provide a better balance of experience.

What will I do in general practice?

General practice attachments at different stages of the medical course may be designed to fulfil different purposes, for example learning about general practice as a potential career, learning specific skills, accessing a wide range of patients or facilitating the long-term follow-up of an individual patient or family. The purpose of the attachment will dictate to a large extent whether you spend your time observing practice, practising skills, interviewing patients, collecting information for a project (e.g. audit data) or doing other activities.

The quotes below reflect the variety of learning a student may experience at different times within the medical course in general practice.

Student quotes

'It was good for learning a lot of specific procedures like taking blood pressure, looking in ears and eyes, giving injections.'
'You can see how the team work, how they interact. It gives you more understanding of their role and what actually the patients go through. I saw a

suspected case of meningitis, and I'm not sure if it was or not, but that was interesting.'
'The best thing was going to visit patients in their own homes. Patients behave differently in their own homes than in surgery.'
'I saw a patient at home with classic signs of asthma attack.'
'I was actually being helpful. I wasn't in the way. I was doing stuff that other people couldn't do and that was really nice. People were listening to you.'
'As we got to know the patients, they came back and made appointments to see me especially and so I sort of built up a relationship with them in a short time.'

How can I make the most of my time in general practice?

In most jobs, you become more proficient with experience. Many students enjoy learning in general practice because they get more direct supervision (often one-to-one teaching), which can be closely tailored to their individual learning requirements.

Students in general practice have to accept the limitations of the clinical environment, and recognize that their learning cannot always be a priority. For example, teachers may be called away at short notice or there may be no diabetic patients available on the day students plan to examine or interview them. Students have to find ways to gain the experience they need within the existing structures. This section looks at what you can do to make the most of your time in general practice and to cope with any problems that may arise.

Suggested preparation/early orientation

Before the placement starts, you will need to consider practical issues, such as transport, access, security and personal safety, particularly if you are on an individual placement. There are many resources on which you can draw within a general practice. At the start of your attachment, we suggest that you undertake the following.

■ *Introductions*: Introduce yourself to everyone for courtesy and security reasons, and so that you can return when you need help. Remember to include part-time and non-clinical staff, such as visiting or associated counsellors, health visitors, midwives, hospital consultants providing outreach clinics, child psychologists, complementary therapists, behavioural therapists, community pharmacists or community psychiatric nurses.

- *Staff in the practice*: Find out what their roles and responsibilities are, when they work and what training and experience they have.
- *Patient notes*: Find out where these are stored, in what format (paper or electronic) and how to access specific sorts of information. Remember to consider issues of confidentiality. Check the practice guidelines on this.
- *Patients*: There are opportunities for meeting patients outside the actual consultation, e.g. in the waiting room, patients coming in to collect prescriptions, make appointments or see other members of the practice team. Be careful not to upset the appointments system, so make sure that the relevant staff know what you are doing, where you will be and how long it will take. Some practices may have a spare room. Remember to consider issues of confidentiality, informed consent and privacy.
- *Relatives and friends*: A patient's relative or friend may also provide useful opportunities for finding out about the impact of illness, use of services, etc.
- *Clinics and other activities*: Find out what else happens in your general practice and when. For example, there may be special health promotion or disease-related clinics, meetings of patients' or carers' support groups, staff meetings or voluntary groups which you can ask to attend.
- *Other resources*: Find out what other resources are available. These may include health education leaflets for patients, clinical books and journals for staff, videos or computer programs and postgraduate learning events.

Ten tips for learning in general practice

In general practice, as in many other situations, how people present and conduct themselves will affect how they are treated. Below are listed ten

tips for having a successful attachment in general practice; these have been devised by teachers and students. Most will also be applicable in other clinical settings.

1. *Attend*: There is, unsurprisingly, a high correlation between students who attend regularly and those who do well in finals and other examinations. Arrive punctually and let the practice know if, for any reason, you cannot attend.
2. *Set yourself clear and realistic goals*: Try to identify specific objectives for your time in general practice, in consultation with your GP and the medical school. Clarify at the beginning what you should have achieved by the end, and keep your goals under review. Mark off items you have achieved and add new ideas as you go along.
3. *Base your reading around the patients you see*: Many doctors vividly remember patients they met as students and what they learnt from them. The patient provides a hook on which you can hang your knowledge and will help you to relate theory to practice.
4. *Say hello to everyone every day*: This may sound silly, but a little goodwill goes a long way and will help you to fit in. Also think about how you present yourself, e.g. dressing in a way that patients and GPs will find acceptable.
5. *Ask questions*: Teachers often say that they wish students would ask more questions as it helps them to teach at the right level. It also shows that you are interested and enthusiastic.
6. *Ask for teaching, supervision and feedback*: In the rush to get things done, teachers may overlook opportunities for you to practise skills or learn about something new. If you see such opportunities, ask if you can gain experience and then ask for feedback on how you did.
7. *Choose your timing and don't react personally*: Most people are willing to help and will often go out of their way to do so. However, certain times are better than others. Don't ask for things when people are obviously rushed off their feet. Try to help out wherever possible.

If someone appears unhelpful, it may be because they are under stress, so don't take it personally. Choose your timing and, if there is someone who always seems busy, ask when would be the best time for you to talk to them.

8. *Recognize the potential of those around you to teach*: The GP is an obvious source of help, but many other people have expertise which may not be immediately obvious. Look on everyone you meet in the practice as a potential teacher. Receptionists, for example, may be skilled in communicating with angry patients. Patients and their relatives may be enormously knowledgeable about their particular conditions and the local services available.

9. *Thank people when they devote their time to teaching you.*

10. *See the wood and the trees*: During your time in general practice, you will probably meet many patients and hear lots of individual stories. While it is important to see and respect each person as an individual, you also need to relate your experience to more general principles and concepts you have learnt in other parts of the course. Think about how the basic science, sociology, psychology, communication, public health medicine, ethics and law, etc. which you have covered apply to each patient you meet.

Common problems and dilemmas for students in general practice

General practices vary greatly, for example in size, style, provision, ethos and staffing. There is probably no such thing as a 'typical' general practice. Equally, undergraduate courses vary in terms of the amount of time you will spend in general practice, what you are expected to learn, who teaches you and how well it integrates with the rest of your studies.

In this section we look at some difficulties encountered by students in general practice and how you could deal with them if they happened to you.

Student quote
'The patient refused to see me so I had to leave.'

In general practice, patients often feel able to say 'no' to things which they might not in hospital. Don't take it personally. Make sure your GP knows if you need experience in a particular area so that he or she can try to identify another opportunity.

Student quote
'The worst thing was meeting angry patients. One patient was really annoyed by my presence out of no reason.'

There may be a reason that you're not aware of – again, don't take it personally unless you know that you have contributed to the situation, perhaps inadvertently. Some patients may feel inhibited or embarrassed or unwilling to have a student present, particularly for personal worries or intimate examinations.

Student quote
'It was the same patients every time with trivial complaints, much less exciting than in hospital.'

Learning to distinguish the genuinely trivial from early signs of something more serious is an important skill to develop, as described above. Is a headache a sign of stress, period pains or an incipient brain tumour? Sometimes patients present with a seemingly trivial symptom as a cover for something that is really worrying them. When you see patients with trivial complaints, think about what would signal to you that this could be something more serious? Draw up a differential diagnosis and rank in terms of likelihood. Also consider what has motivated the patient to bring this complaint to the GP and how this need could be addressed.

Student quote
'The GP couldn't be bothered. I just had to sit in the corner and listen.'

In these situations, it is a good idea to have some activities in mind which you can use to fill this time. Throughout this book there are various exercises that you could use in this way, or you

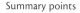

may think of your own. However, your tutor should also guide and facilitate your learning. If you are not satisfied, you should first make an attempt to improve things for yourself. For example you could:

- ask questions of the GP following the consultations,
- tell your GP that you're not clear what you should be getting out of the sessions and ask for clarification,
- ask the GP how he or she feels you are getting on,
- tell the GP you're worried that you're not learning enough and ask for suggestions as to what you should do,

- ask if you can clerk and present some patients,
- ask if you could gain some practical experience as you feel you learn better that way,
- read up about certain areas the previous evening and then look out for these in the consultations,
- approach another member of the practice team and ask for help.

If you have made efforts to improve the situation and are still feeling unhappy, you should probably now approach the course organizer for help. You are entitled to expect a certain minimum standard of teaching from your GP.

SUMMARY POINTS

To conclude, the most important messages of this chapter are as follows:

- General practice provides an opportunity to see a large volume of undifferentiated patient problems, which will give you a broader overview of illness patterns and allow you to develop your diagnostic and 'sifting' skills. About half of medical students eventually practise as a GP.
- General practice provides the best opportunity to see the progression and management of disease, to study common illnesses and to practise many clinical skills. It provides insight into environmental, social and psychological factors which contribute to ill-health, and represents a different model of care from that of hospital medicine.
- Students can take steps to make their time in general practice productive.

CHAPTER

2

GENERAL PRACTICE AND ITS PLACE IN PRIMARY HEALTHCARE

- What is primary healthcare and what is it aiming to achieve?
- Who are the principal members of the primary healthcare team?
- How do general practice and the GP contribute to primary healthcare?
- How do we ensure that the patient receives most benefit from general practice and the primary healthcare service?

- What is the future for general practice and primary healthcare?
- Summary points
- References
- Further reading
- Single best answer questions

The work of the general practitioner (GP) and the general practice team takes place within the context of the primary healthcare setting. To make sense of general practice, the student needs to understand something of its relationship to the primary healthcare system. The central figure in regard to care within the system must be the patient.

LEARNING OBJECTIVES

By the end of this chapter you will be able to:
- define primary healthcare and list what it is broadly aiming to achieve;
- name a few of the principal members of the primary healthcare team and briefly describe their roles and training;
- place general practice in the context of the primary care service;
- describe the role of the GP in the functioning of general practice;
- list the kinds of things that a patient requires of general practice and the primary care service in order to receive most benefit from it;
- consider the possible future of general practice and primary care.

What is primary healthcare and what is it aiming to achieve?

Primary healthcare – that which provides healthcare in the first instance – is present in one form or another for all peoples in the world. Whether it be for someone who needs antenatal care, an immunization, a dressing for a minor injury, a blood pressure check or an immediate assessment and referral for suspected appendicitis, primary care systems are an essential part of any health service. In some countries primary healthcare systems look after the great majority of most people's health issues. In other, more affluent, countries, secondary and tertiary services play a larger part in the delivery of healthcare. However, it is widely recognized that a substantial and effective primary healthcare service is the cornerstone of a healthy population and that, without this, the provision of healthcare is an expensive and ineffectual exercise (Rawaf *et al.*, 2008).

What is the definition of primary care?

It is not something that is done in one place or by one type of health professional. It is a network of community-based healthcare services, supported by a network of social services that provides over 90 per cent of healthcare in the UK. In its most restricted sense, it means 'first contact care' and this can be provided by any number of different healthcare workers. However, primary health services have a much wider role than this. Their role includes health maintenance, illness prevention, diagnosis, treatment and management of acute and chronic illness, rehabilitation, the support of those who are frail or disabled, pastoral care and terminal care.

What is primary healthcare aiming to achieve?

There are four main objectives of a primary healthcare service (Marson *et al.*, 1973):

- It must be accessible to the whole population.
- It must be acceptable to the population.
- It must be able to identify the health needs of a population.
- It must make the most cost-effective use of its resources.

Obviously, given that resources are limited, all these objectives cannot be perfectly met. However, these are goals that we can aim towards.

People need to be able to see their doctor (or another health professional) when necessary without having to wait unduly for an appointment. The distance between the patient's home and the healthcare centre should be as short as possible. Where the patient has difficulty in getting to the healthcare centre, a home-visiting service should be provided. All efforts should be made to enable the patient and professional staff to communicate effectively.

In terms of acceptability, regular reviews of services must include a measure of patient and professional satisfaction. The rights and responsibilities of both patient and health professional need to be considered and made clear to both parties. This process is a constant and developing one.

In setting up mechanisms to identify a population's health needs, we get away from just responding to demand to a position where we can start properly to distinguish priorities in the services we provide. Strategic planning based on need rather than demand will make the best use of limited resources.

Given that we (as provider and user) have decided on the minimum standards we wish to uphold and the priorities for service provision and development, we then need to determine the resources that are available for healthcare and decide how to apportion them. To provide all desirable services would be impossible, so judgements need to be made as to the most cost-effective use of limited person-power, money and effort. This kind of decision is bound to be made partly on guesswork, as it is rare that all the information required to make such decisions is available.

Who are the principal members of the primary healthcare team?

In the UK National Health Service (NHS), there are two main providers of primary care: *general practice* and *community health services*. Other providers, such as accident and emergency departments, dentists, pharmacists, opticians and optometrists, will not be mentioned here. In addition, out-of-hours services offer general practice care; UK NHS Direct, which opened in 1998, offers 24-hour advice about personal healthcare; and NHS walk-in centres, the first of which opened in 2000, offer free health advice and treatment for minor injuries and illnesses and are open and available for anyone.

General practice (family practice) provides first contact, patient-centred, comprehensive and continuing care to a patient population. The general practice tasks are to promote health and well-being; treat illness in the context of the patient's life, belief systems and community; and work with other healthcare professionals to coordinate care and make efficient use of health resources. It has responsibility for a population of people and is activated by patient choice.

Community health services are provided by a variety of generalist and specialist staff who have particular functions, such as the multidisciplinary care of the long-term ill, continuing care for those discharged from hospital, services for well people (including school health, child health and sexual health/family planning), care for particular groups of the population at risk (for example the homeless, refugees) and the provision of such things as training or equipment on a wide scale.

They also provide support to general practices with all these activities, as well as providing staff such as health visitors, district nurses, community midwives and community psychiatric nurses who work with general practices.

Principal members: who they are and what they do

Members of the primary healthcare team are many and various. Table 2.1 lists some of the more well-known UK professionals, particularly those who work with general practice. The role of the GP is discussed later in this chapter.

Boundaries

In the UK, as in many other countries, increased importance (and thus resource) is being placed on the primary care sector of the health service. With this has come the realization that we must become much clearer about the responsibilities of each of its professional groups. Within the primary care service there are many health professions, often with very different ways of working. Their connection with secondary health services may also become troublesome if communication is not very clear. A 'seamless service' is a concept often mentioned, but we are in danger of ever-increasing fragmentation if we do not respect and know about each other's skills, and work together in developing and delivering services.

Table 2.1 A selection of the members of the UK general practice team

Name	Employed by	Role includes	Training
Receptionist	General practice	Reception and telephone duties, filing	Various
Practice manager	General practice	Planning, organizing, managing a general practice	Various
Practice nurse	General practice	Assessment, diagnosis, treatments, health promotion, special extended roles	Registered General Nurse (RGN), nursing experience
District nurse	Primary care trust	Assessment, dressings, stoma care, arranging services, support	RGN, nursing experience, specialist training
Health visitor	Primary care trust	Antenatal, 'under 5' care, sometimes elderly care	RGN, nursing experience, specialist training
Community psychiatric nurse	Primary care trust	Assessment, management and support of the mentally ill	RGN, nursing experience, specialist training

Case Study 2.1

Mrs C, a 95-year-old woman, lives with her daughter. She wakes one morning and finds herself unable to talk properly or move her right arm. Her daughter, on finding her like this, rings their general practice and speaks to the receptionist, who arranges for their GP to visit. The GP visits and finds Mrs C peaceful and adamant that she does not want to be hospitalized. The daughter agrees with this and is willing, with support, to care for her mother at home. The GP contacts the district nurse for an assessment of the nursing needs.

Many situations like this occur in general practice and require the cooperation of patients, their informal carers and several members of the healthcare team.

Case Study 2.2

Ms F, a 28-year-old woman on medication for schizophrenia, presents to her GP pregnant. She wishes to keep the baby. With the woman's consent, the GP contacts her psychiatrist and community psychiatric team, who make arrangements to see her, check her medication and arrange for close follow-up. The GP also makes an appointment for her with the hospital antenatal services. The woman offers to come back and see the GP the next week with her partner, the father of the baby, to talk about the pregnancy further.

Sometimes, the kind of care required can be very resource intensive. What do you think enabled this woman to obtain such integrated care so quickly and efficiently?

How do general practice and the GP contribute to primary healthcare?

Traditionally, general practice, with its central figure, the GP, and its central activity, the consultation, has been the cornerstone of primary healthcare. Historically, this has developed from 'the doctor working alone' to 'the practice as an organization'. As this model of healthcare has been widened to include consideration of such things as population-based health promotion (as well as diagnosis and treatment) and care of populations (as well as individuals), the role of general practice has changed and that of the GP has become less clear. (See more in Chapter 16, 'Being a general practitioner'.)

Thinking and Discussion Point

- What do you see your GP doing?
- What connections does he or she make?
- What do you see as the advantages and disadvantages of your GP's role?

Core values of GPs

The majority of GPs would see their central activity as the consultation in which doctor and patient meet and work together to make decisions regarding the patient's health and life plan (see Chapter 3). However, with the mounting complexity of health service provision, this role is increasingly in conflict with other administrative and population-based responsibilities. The same can be said of the role of other primary care practitioners, for example the practice nurse, the speech therapist or the audiologist.

Practical Exercise

Spend 10 minutes discussing with your GP tutor what areas of his or her work are most important and/or satisfying. Pick the top three and list them in order of priority.

Core values of the practice

The major responsibility of the general practice, on the other hand, is to its practice population as a whole, ensuring that its patient population obtains the best service possible and that the general practice is organized and managed to meet this responsibility (see Chapter 14).

Is personal care compatible with teamwork?

As GPs have traditionally been the leaders in their general practices, the new and more time-consuming responsibilities of running a practice have often resulted in confusion and dissatisfaction amongst GPs and other practice staff. Is the traditional role of a GP compatible with the more population-based role of 'new' general practice? Increasingly, other professionals, such as practice managers, are being brought in to complement the GP's work and deal with areas of work not directly connected with the consultation (see Chapter 14).

Power, ethics, accountability

Difficulties in working relationships may arise because of the differences in power structures, ethical considerations and accountability between the practitioner and the practice. Practitioners usually see their major responsibility as being 'their' patients and, in theory at least, aim to empower patients as much as possible. They are mainly accountable to their patients and to their peers. The practice, on the other hand, is mainly responsible for the practice population and may need to have 'power over' the decisions of a few to benefit the whole. Accountability for the practice is to the practice population and, in Britain, nationally to the Secretary of State for Health for General Medical Services (GMS) practices and locally to the Primary Healthcare Trusts for Personal Medical Services (PMS) practices. (See more about these arrangements, and possible changes in contracts with the changes to the NHS, in Chapters 14 and 16.)

How do we ensure that the patient receives most benefit from general practice and the primary healthcare service?

'Patients as experts'

For a consultation to work, doctors and patients need to see themselves as experts in their own right, meeting to share ideas and come to an understanding of what is happening and what needs to be done in a particular situation (more on this in Chapter 3). The patient comes to a consultation with knowledge of the nature of the presenting issue and the historical and psychosocial context in which it is embedded. The patient also has the power to decide, ultimately, what the outcome will be. The doctor, on the other hand, has access to specialist biomedical information and to services. Without a sharing of these pieces of information, the course of action that is best for the patient, and most cost effective, may not be followed.

Case Study 2.3

Mr S, a 69-year-old man, has been taken to hospital by ambulance, very frightened, after suffering a sudden attack of light-headedness. This clears before the doctor has seen him, enabling him to be sent home. He is later told that this symptom is a side effect of the anti-hypertensive drug on which he has recently been started. Once he knows this, he deals effectively with the symptom, which, after a little time, becomes much less of a problem.

The importance of communication

An explanation of the possible side effects of his medication on initiation of treatment would have prevented unnecessary distress and an expensive trip to hospital for this man.

What patients can teach practitioners

It is important for doctors and students to listen and learn from patients and to understand illness as a human experience rather than just a cluster of symptoms and signs.

Case Study 2.4

Mr G, an 84-year-old widower who lived alone, had mild non-insulin-dependent diabetes mellitus. His GP was constantly frustrated by the man's refusal to adjust his diet. One day Mr G asked the GP to visit him at home. He spoke with the GP about his life and the few pleasures left to him, of which sweets and biscuits were one. The GP was able to see that the problem was her inability to accept the more limited but possible and reasonable goals of the patient.

Consulting the patient

An encouraging sign in the development of primary care services has been the inclusion of 'patients' in the development process. User and community participation at all levels of practice development has led to the setting up of patient-participation groups and dialogue between service providers and 'users'; self-help and community groups which provide information and support for those with particular conditions or in particular situations; and government-funded Local Involvement Networks that provide the public with an opportunity to become involved in improving health and social services.

What is the future for general practice and primary healthcare?

The British situation

In Britain, since the beginning of the 1990s, the pace of primary care development has been extremely rapid and, since April 1996, the development of the NHS has been led by primary care. The central place of general practice in the provision of primary healthcare services has not been challenged. However, there has been an increasing reliance on general practice to continue to develop and provide free and equal access to healthcare in the face of greater restraints on resources. This has placed an enormous strain on general practice providers. In spite of this, a large range of primary care activities and organizations has been developed and introduced to meet the challenges and to support general practice. These have included a move towards integrating health and social services in primary care; primary care-led purchasing; a greater accountability of general practice to the NHS; general practice fund-holding; the development of paperless general practice systems, morbidity databases and audit; the development of general practice management; the introduction of the nurse practitioner; and experimentation with different types of integrated community care centres. In the UK, with the increasing demand for primary care, government plans are to increase the proportion of GPs from one third, as it is now, to at least half of all graduates (Department of Health, 2008). A new scheme is currently (2011) being introduced which will involve GPs, in groups or consortia, in commissioning care. GPs are being asked to prioritize NHS services and apportion NHS funds (Department of Health, 2010). How successful this will be is yet to be ascertained.

The international situation

All around the world primary care is being increasingly recognized as central to a good health service, needing to be supported by secondary and tertiary services rather than being dominated by them. The WHO–UNICEF meeting in Alma-Ata in 1978 (World Health Organization, 1978) underlined this principle, and the Alma-Ata Declaration, in which many countries including Britain committed themselves to raising the profile of primary care, was an important catalyst in the development of primary care.

The international exchange of ideas in this field has been very active since then, and shared challenges and responses to these challenges are evident. Particular demographic developments are common shared problems internationally, such as an increasingly ageing population; escalating costs of healthcare, particularly with new technologies; greater restraints on spending; an over-supply and/or a maldistribution of doctors; a devaluing of the primary care generalist and a greater administrative burden on healthcare workers. The WHO 2003 International Conference on Primary Healthcare in Alma-Ata, the twenty-fifth anniversary of the 1978 meeting at which the Alma-Ata Declaration was presented, requested member states to continue to work towards providing adequate resources for primary healthcare; tackling the rising burden of chronic conditions; supporting the active involvement of local communities and voluntary groups in primary healthcare; and supporting

research in order to identify effective methods for strengthening primary healthcare and linking it to overall improvement of the healthcare system. Of particular importance is whether or not the role of the primary care practitioner as gatekeeper is supported. In European countries such as Britain or Denmark where this is so, there is generally control of the geographical distribution of doctors, registration of patients, paying of GPs by capitation and salary, and essential 24-hour patient-care coverage. In European countries where the primary care doctor is not a gatekeeper, such as Germany and Sweden, these characteristics commonly do not exist, and the role of the primary care generalist is not as developed or valued. Outside Europe, for example in Canada and Australasia, these grouped correlations are not as evident. In the USA, a useful distinction exists between the gatekeeping role of the practitioner within a health maintenance organization (HMO) and the non-gatekeeping role of the private primary care practitioner. It has been shown that fee-for-service practitioners have a 40 per cent excess of hospital admissions over HMO practitioners. However, the relationship between different systems and quality of care is extremely difficult to measure past very crude parameters such as life expectation. Assessing quality is the present-day task.

SUMMARY POINTS

To conclude, the most important messages of this chapter are as follows:

- A primary healthcare system provides healthcare in the first instance.
- A primary healthcare system aims to be accessible, acceptable, cost effective and responsive to health needs.
- The GP works as a member of a general practice and of the primary healthcare team that has responsibilities both to the individual and to the community as a whole.
- The patient and the health practitioner need to work together to ensure that health-related decisions are optimal.

References

Department of Health 2008: *A high quality workforce: NHS next stage review*. London: Department of Health.

Department of Health 2010: *Equity and excellence: liberating the NHS*. London: The Stationery Office.

Marson, W.S., Morrell, D.C., Watkins, C.J. and Zander, L.J. 1973: Measuring the quality of general practice. *Journal of the Royal College of General Practitioners* 23, 23–31.

Rawaf, S., De Maesseneer, J. and Starfield, B. 2008: From Alma-Ata to Almaty: a new start for primary health care. *The Lancet* 372(9647), 1365–7.

World Health Organization 1978: *Primary health care*. Geneva: WHO.

Further reading

Gregory, S. 2009: *General practice in England: an overview*. London: The King's Fund.

Meads, G. (ed.) 1996: *Future options for general practice*. Oxford: Radcliffe Medical Press.

Pratt, J. 1995: *Practitioners and practices – a conflict of values?* Oxford: Radcliffe Medical Press.

The above two books from the Primary Care Development Series, published in association with King's Fund, London, focus on the development of general practice within the British primary healthcare service. The discussions also include the international context.

With the constant development of primary care around the world, the following websites give some of the most up-to-date information:

www.nhshistory.com/

www.nhs.uk/

www.who.int/

The following references are also worth reading:

Mathers, N. and Hodgkin, P. 1989: The gatekeeper and the wizard: a fairy tale. *British Medical Journal* 298, 172–4.

WONCA Europe 2002: The European definition of general practice/family medicine. www.globalfamilydoctor.com/publications/Euro-Def.pdf

SINGLE BEST ANSWER QUESTIONS

2.1 Primary healthcare is:

a) A network of community and hospital services that provide essential care to patients
b) Healthcare provided by general practitioners (family physicians)
c) The treatment of acute illness
d) Healthcare provided in the first instance by a variety of community-based services
e) That which provides about 50 per cent of healthcare in the UK.

2.2 Primary healthcare aims to provide:

a) Healthcare to whoever needs it at whatever cost
b) Healthcare to those who can afford it
c) Healthcare based on demand
d) Healthcare to those who can access it
e) A service that is able to identify and prioritize a population's health needs.

2.3 The UK primary healthcare team includes:

a) General practitioners whose core role is to manage a practice
b) Hospital outpatient staff who make appointments for patients from the community
c) Health visitors who look after the families of children under 5
d) Practice nurses who have to have achieved a degree-level practice nurse training programme
e) District nurses who manage all nursing services in their area.

2.4 Power, ethics and accountability

a) In the UK, as at April 2011, accountability of the practice is to the British Medical Association
b) The route to patient participation is through practice-based patient groups
c) Practices are mainly responsible for their patient population rather than individual patients

SINGLE BEST ANSWER QUESTIONS CONTINUED

d) GMS and PMS contracts are between a GP and their PCT (as at April 2011)

e) GPs are mainly accountable to their practice staff.

2.5 Mr G makes abusive remarks to a receptionist. He has no mental illness. On witnessing this, and as the doctor seeing Mr G for a routine appointment, do you:

a) Quickly consult with Mr G without referring to what has gone on to save any more trouble?

b) Discuss the situation with the patient, explain to Mr G that the practice does not accept this type of behaviour, ask him to apologize to the receptionist, and explain that if this happens again he is at risk of being removed from the practice list?

c) Apologize to the receptionist and explain that it is the practice's responsibility to care for all patients whatever their behaviour?

d) Agree to Mr G relating to receptionist staff of his choice?

e) Allow reception to sort the problem out?

3

THE GENERAL PRACTICE CONSULTATION

- The general practice consultation
- The content and process of the consultation
- Roles within the consultation
- The doctor- and patient-centredness of the consultation
- The patient's tasks in the consultation
- The doctor's tasks in the consultation

- The formal staging of a consultation
- Behaviours that help or hinder a consultation
- The narrative approach to the consultation
- Summary points
- References
- Further reading
- Single best answer questions

The central event in the general practitioner's professional life is the consultation. There are a number of perspectives and frameworks that you can employ to assess the effectiveness of consultations. From observing others' consultations, you can begin to reflect upon how to make your own consultations more effective.

LEARNING OBJECTIVES

By the end of this chapter you will be able to:
- understand the qualities of the general practice consultation;
- define and view the content and process of a consultation, the roles within it and doctor-centred and patient-centred approaches;
- view, document and reflect upon the patient's and doctor's tasks in the consultation;
- formally stage a consultation by using three given frameworks;
- consider behaviours that help or hinder a consultation;
- consider the narrative approach to the consultation.

The general practice consultation

About one million general practitioner (GP) consultations take place in the UK each working day (Gregory, 2009). The meeting between a GP and a patient, at which health-related issues are presented and explored and management decisions made, provides the material with which general practice works.

Understanding what happens in a consultation is key to understanding the role of the GP. To focus on the consultation is a valuable and manageable task from which further exploration of primary care medicine can follow.

The general practice consultation has a set of particular qualities that set it apart from other types of consultation:

- The patient makes the decision to consult with the GP. This is an important difference from, for example, the hospital-based consultation, in which patient contact is, in the UK, generally initiated by referral from another doctor. Patients in primary care thus come with their own agenda, often unknown by their GPs until presentation. Effective communication between GP and patient is the key to accurate identification and discussion of the pertinent issues. The idea of the patient-centred consultation, in which the practitioner works with the person rather than the illness or the presenting issue, is explored further later in this chapter.

■ The general practice consultation is well situated for what is called 'whole-person medicine'. The GP is often the first and frequently the only medical port-of-call for the patient, who might present for a variety of reasons repeatedly and over a long period of time. The family, friends and community of the patient are also often known by the GP in a similar way. The GP can therefore often understand the patient and the presentation in the context of the fullness of the patient's life. A great understanding of who the patient is and the meaning of the presentations can thus be achieved.

■ GPs and their patients are readily accessible to one another, often over many years. This results in the opportunity for a kind of medicine that allows for a developing professional relationship between patient and doctor and provides for:
   – an extended type of patient and doctor observation, allowing the collection and processing of information over a period of time;
   – an extended type of diagnostic process which can be developed and altered over time and which can incorporate many levels of information, including physical, psychological and social aspects;
   – comprehensive care, which considers the physical, psychological and social needs of patient, family, carers and community;
   – continuing care, which can be initiated by the patient and flexibly adapt to unforeseen as well as foreseen needs;
   – preventive care, where every presentation is an opportunity for health promotion.

■ The general practice consultation is a central activity within the UK health service, as it is in the main through the GP that the patient gains access to the more specialized and usually more expensive health services. The GP thus has a central role in the proper use and containment of limited health resources.

It is important to recognize these qualities and to realize that to be party to a single consultation and fail to see this in the context of many such consultations over time leads to a limited understanding of the process of general practice.

Thinking and Discussion Point

Consider a type of consultation other than a general practice consultation (e.g. a hospital-based consultation).
- What are its particular qualities?
- How does it compare with the GP consultation?
- What are the perceived strengths and weaknesses of each type of consultation?

As part of your training, especially initially, you will do some 'sitting in' on GP consultations (although we encourage you also to 'sit in the doctor's chair' and interview patients under close supervision as early as possible). It is useful to have some frameworks with which to view and experience this event. In this way, you will become a more active observer and your observations will be of greater value to yourself, your tutor and, ultimately, the patient. Observing and reflecting upon your tutor's consultations will be a good introduction to your own consulting and provide a template for thinking about consultations you observe in other parts of your course.

There have been many frameworks set up for describing a consultation; a few of the major ones are outlined below.

Before we look at some observation frameworks, there are three concepts with which you need to be conversant in order to understand more fully what is going on.

1. The difference between content and process in the consultation.
2. Roles within the consultation.
3. The doctor-centred and the patient-centred approach to the consultation.

The content and process of the consultation

There is a basic distinction between the tasks that are focused upon in a consultation (the content) and the behaviours that go on in the consultation (the process). Obviously there are certain tasks that are accomplished within a consultation. Examples are defining the reason for the patient's attendance and arriving at a management plan. This is the content of the consultation. However, the way that the consultation is conducted (the process) is also very important and directly determines the effectiveness of the encounter. The process describes the way that the doctor and the patient behave towards each other, verbally and non-verbally.

Let me put it another way. The content and process have parallels in both music and theatre. In music the content would be the score and the process the dynamics. In theatre the content would be the script and the process the stage directions. You will probably need to observe

Practical Exercise

Sit in on two to four consultations. It would be useful if you could observe in pairs for this particular task so that you can take turns to record either process or content in successive consultations and put your findings together afterwards. Otherwise you will need to concentrate on content for one consultation (or part of a consultation) and process for another. Either way, compare notes with your tutor afterwards. You may wish to report on just part of a consultation, as reporting on the whole may prove to be too big a task.

quite a few consultations and discuss with your tutor these concepts in the context of what happens before you fully understand the difference. An example is provided in Figure 3.1.

The preceding exercise will help you to understand the concepts of process and content.

Roles within the consultation

Traditionally, society has assigned to doctors and patients certain roles or ways of behaving. Doctors have been given the power, authority and respect to attend to a patient's needs and make certain decisions on behalf of the patient. The patient has been encouraged to give this responsibility to the doctor and to enter into the 'sick' or 'dependent' role, at least temporarily or partially. The tendency is for doctors and patients to accept these behaviours and expectations and invite them from the other party. These assumptions are increasingly being challenged, with many doctors working towards becoming less autocratic and patients working towards retaining their autonomy. However, it is essential that we, when we are in the doctor role, become aware of these roles and tendencies and, for each patient encounter, determine how much they are in the best interests of patient well-being and when they are detrimental. At times, for example when a patient is very acutely and seriously ill, we may need to assume total responsibility for their care. However, in most situations, seeing the consultation as a meeting of two individuals, each with his or her own areas

Content	Process
Doctor: Are you sure of your dates?	Patient: Pregnant, little anxious.
Patient: Yes, I am 26 weeks.	Doctor: Busy, but interested; trying to establish how many weeks pregnant the patient is. *(leans forward)*
Doctor: You can't be!	Patient: Very sure of dates.
Patient: Yes I am. Look at the ultrasound report.	Doctor: Querying dates.
Doctor: When was the last one done?	Patient: Slightly interested and tells doctor about ultrasound.
Patient: Today.	Doctor: Relieved, slightly embarrassed. *(sits back)*

Figure 3.1 What happens in a consultation: an example of a recording sheet.

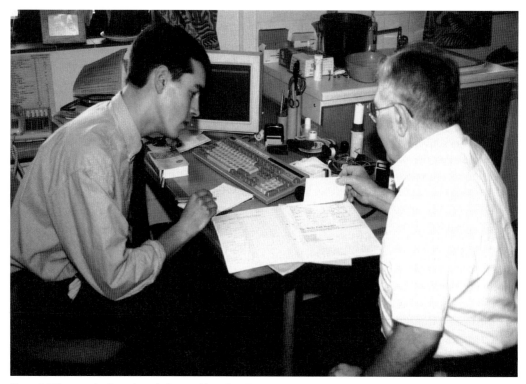

Figure 3.2 The consultation – but who's consulting whom?

of expertise, and focusing the consultation on the patient's ideas, concerns and expectations, seems the healthiest option. Of course we are all, at times, patients, so it is also helpful to reflect upon any changes in behaviour that might occur when we are in the patient role and how this impacts on the satisfaction, process and outcome of the consultation.

The doctor- and patient-centredness of the consultation

The degree to which a consultation is doctor-centred or patient-centred is related to the roles that the patient and doctor adopt in their interchange. It is measured by the extent to which the consultation agenda, process and outcome are determined by the doctor or the patient.

Obviously, the doctor has expert knowledge diagnostically and therapeutically. However, patients are also experts in that they bring with them the information and experience with which the consultation primarily works. At times,

patients are, in fact, much more knowledgeable about their illness or presenting issue than their doctor, for example when they have a rare medical condition or a condition that requires ongoing self-management. For a consultation to be successful, the doctor and patient must work together to agree on the issues that they are dealing with and to share information about the issues and possible explanations and consequences (Figure 3.2).

That the patient plays an active role in the consultation and that the patient and doctor have a dialogue and work together to come to a satisfactory conclusion are the aims of a consultation. Of most importance is the idea that the consultation is there to focus on patients and their ideas, concerns and expectations about what is happening to them. This is what is termed a *patient-centred consultation*.

Tutor quote

I had a female student here a year ago and I had an unusual experience with her. She was sitting here in this chair and I asked her to interview this guy who was 60, 65 perhaps … an alcoholic with TB … very nice quiet man who had not been attending for his treatment. He was always drunk and if you looked at him, you would think what a waste … you know … you could see that he was trying to be a nice man but he came over as a bit of a funny sort of chap … very sad case. I asked this student to take a history and I sat down there. She couldn't keep a straight face … she was actually laughing or smiling … she couldn't concentrate on what she was asking this man … it was really uncomfortable for me and for the patient. The patient suddenly stopped and said, 'Look young lady, you are laughing, you shouldn't laugh', and the odd thing was that I could see there was a problem and I couldn't cope with it, yet this man coped with it so well. Honestly it was so awkward. Then she said, 'I am not laughing', and then she became very serious because she realized there was something going on and there was a breakdown. He looked at me so all I could do was take over. I talked to him and I didn't know how I was going to take things forward and then, again, he saved us. He said, 'I am sorry young lady but I had to tell you. Somebody has to tell you. You can't laugh at patients. You have to be serious.' Then he carried on talking to her for a while and they had a conversation.

When he had finished, I mean, I was a bit shaken by the whole thing, I felt very angry, sorry for him. I felt sorry for her but I didn't know how to actually tackle her. So many issues. How do I tell her? Why was she laughing? Did I do that when I was young? That is where it is unresolved in my mind. I actually think she really did learn something from it and I definitely learnt something from it. I thought how graceful the patients are and how wonderful despite being alcoholic and how wise he was, you know, the way he dealt with it. I felt it was brilliant. She didn't really put herself in his shoes. Maybe if I could have told her that every time a patient comes in she needed to try to see if she could put herself in their shoes, she wouldn't actually have that problem, but it was too late.

The consultation in which the doctor interrogates the patient and determines diagnosis and further management without involving the patient in the process is a doctor-centred consultation. Most consultations lie somewhere on

the continuum between doctor-centredness and patient-centredness. Research shows that patients do want patient-centred care where doctors take into account 'the patient's desire for information and for sharing decision making and responding appropriately' (Stewart, 2001).

Given this background, and that you now have a basic understanding of the concepts of content, process, roles and patient- and doctor-centredness within a consultation, let us move on and look at a few of the common ways of viewing, documenting, reflecting upon and learning from the tasks and stages of a particular consultation.

Practical Exercise

Read through the rest of this chapter and pick out the framework that most appeals to you to begin with. Perhaps talk with your tutor before you sit in on a surgery, and discuss how you might like to start to focus on the consultations. Once you have looked at what goes on using one perspective, you might like to try some different ways of looking at the consultation. There may well be others that you discover or that your tutor suggests you explore further.

We will first look at the patient's task in a consultation and compare this with the doctor's task in ensuring that the patient's needs, perceived and real, are met. Remember that, from both the patient's and the GP's perspective, the real and the perceived needs of the patient may not always be the same. From here we will go on to consider a way of looking at a more formal staging of a consultation. The final framework that will be presented combines both the tasks and the formal staging of a consultation.

The patient's tasks in the consultation

Cecil Helman (1981), a medical anthropologist, suggested that patients come to the doctor to answer six questions.

1. What has happened?
2. Why has it happened?

3. Why to me?

4. Why now?

5. What would happen if nothing were done about it?

6. What should I do about it or who should I consult for further help?

The patient may not always ask all of these questions in every case. For example, not everyone would consider 'why to me?' and 'why now?' after falling down stairs and spraining their ankle (although they might be useful questions in such cases). Also, some consultations are about health promotion issues, for example pregnancy, contraception, well-man or well-woman care or immunization. However, particularly with more serious or long-term illnesses or when illnesses or accidents happen at inconvenient times, such as just before a wedding or in the midst of an important time of work, they may well be asked. It is important that the doctor is aware that the patient may be considering them, as sometimes they loom large in a patient's mind but may need a bit of sensitive probing by the doctor to bring out into the open. On the other hand, the patient may prefer to discuss such issues with another person such as a close friend or mentor, and the doctor also needs to be sensitive to this option. Here is an example to illustrate the patient's task.

Case Study 3.1

Mrs G, a 56-year-old woman, had come to see her GP two weeks earlier with a lump in her right breast which had been present for some time and which had been getting larger and more irregular. She had also noticed some similar, smaller lumps in her right axilla. It was obvious at this time that she was extremely worried, as both her mother and her sister had suffered from breast cancer. She was also just entering into a new and very promising relationship after being divorced 10 years previously, and her life otherwise was flourishing. Her GP referred her, urgently, to a specialist for assessment and it was discovered that she did indeed have breast cancer. Together, the GP and the patient made a long appointment to talk about what all this meant. Indeed, she did wish to talk around all of Helman's six questions. A very moving and intense consultation took place. Not

all the questions could be answered by patient or doctor and some of the others could be answered only partially. However, the opportunity to air these most important issues with someone she trusted went a little way towards relieving some of the profound anger and fear that she was experiencing.

This is a rather extreme example, the like of which, I expect, your tutor will not ask you to consider at this stage of your training. However, it illustrates the depth into which consultations, at times, enter. An exercise will be suggested to explore this further, in a simpler way, after the doctor's task in the consultation has been considered.

The doctor's tasks in the consultation

Perhaps the simplest model, used in medical schools for all types of 'medical encounters', is the 'three function' model (Gask and Usherwood, 2002). The three parallel functions are to build the relationship (with the patient), collect data and agree a management plan.

Roger Neighbour (2004), a GP, has looked at the tasks of a consultation purely from a doctor's viewpoint and has listed them as follows.

1. To connect with the patient: does this consultation feel comfortable?

2. To summarize and verbally check with the patient that the reasons for the attendance are clear: my understanding is . . .

3. To hand over and bring the consultation to a close, checking out with the patient: does that cover it?

4. To ensure that a safety net exists in that no serious possibilities have been missed: what if . . . ?

5. To deal with the housekeeping of recovery and reflection: am I okay to start another consultation?

Case study 3.2 is another example that illustrates this way of looking at a consultation.

Case Study 3.2

Mr D went to see a GP with a two-week history of lethargy, associated with an extremely sore throat and slight diarrhoea. The GP had not seen him before, although he had been a patient at the surgery for some time. Mr D's usual doctor was on holiday. He was anxious as he told the GP that his partner had similar symptoms that had been tentatively diagnosed as glandular fever. Mr D had also recently started an exciting new job and did not want to have to take time off.

It was important for the GP first to connect in some way with Mr D, as this was a first meeting and the patient was obviously worried about his condition and needed to trust that the GP was competent and had his best interests at heart. The patient talked a little about his new job and the good relationship that he had with the surgery and his usual doctor. The GP told him about other work that he was involved in at the hospital and how much time he spent doing sessions at the surgery. The GP then moved on to Mr D's reasons for coming to see him, first checking that he was clear about the presenting symptoms and anxieties. This checking out continued, at times, throughout the consultation.

As the consultation moved on, the GP discovered that Mr D was concerned about the slight possibility that he might have contracted HIV and they discussed this. Mr D also told the doctor that he and his partner were going through a rocky patch in their relationship. He needed some comforting at this stage. After examining him and discussing what should be done, the GP once again summarized and verbally checked that his understanding matched the patient's understanding about future management. Throughout the consultation, at times, the GP was mentally checking that no serious possibilities were being missed, such as serious illness not considered or suicide risk. The GP brought the consultation to a close by checking with Mr D that his concerns had been covered and by arranging to see him again once some initial investigations had been carried out. Finally, the GP took a few minutes out to have a cup of tea, as this consultation had been quite exhausting. He then felt okay to start another consultation.

This sounds rather an ideal consultation and, in reality, few consultations run so smoothly or cover such ground so successfully, especially on a first meeting. However, it serves to illustrate the stages that Roger Neighbour lists in his model of the consultation from the doctor's perspective.

Below is an exercise that you can use to examine how a consultation addresses the experience of both patient and doctor. It is composed of a number of stages, which means that your tutor will need to organize things quite carefully beforehand.

Practical Exercise

For this exercise, your tutor will need to organize the following:
- ❏ 45 minutes of lightly booked surgery;
- ❏ a space for you to interview patient(s) before and after the consultation(s);
- ❏ time to discuss the process and the consultation(s) with you;
- ❏ receptionists to understand and explain the process to patients and to seek patient consent;
- ❏ one or two patients who would be suitable for the exercise.

This exercise requires you (the student) to:
- ❏ interview a patient briefly before they see the doctor about why they have come for a consultation;
- ❏ accompany the patient into the consultation and observe what happens;
- ❏ talk with the patient afterwards about what happened: find out whether they think their questions were answered and whether they got what they wanted from the consultation;
- ❏ talk about the consultation with the doctor in terms of his or her perception of what happened;
- ❏ discuss your findings with your tutor (who will probably be the consulting doctor as well in this case).

The formal staging of a consultation

We have so far looked at the behaviours that occur and the tasks that patients and doctors hope to address (to a greater or lesser extent) in consultations. Let us now examine the stages of a consultation. By this is meant the route that the consultation takes in order to meet the tasks that are set by patient and doctor. The simplest framework with which to stage consultations is that produced by Byrne and Long in 1976 after they analysed more than 2000 tape recordings of over 100 doctors' consultations. They came up with the following six stages, rarely strictly in this order.

- Phase I: the doctor establishes a relationship with the patient.
- Phase II: the doctor either attempts to discover or actually discovers the reason for the patient's attendance.
- Phase III: the doctor conducts a verbal or physical examination, or both.
- Phase IV: the doctor, or the doctor and the patient (in that order of probability), considers the condition.
- Phase V: the doctor, and occasionally the patient, details further treatment or further investigation.
- Phase VI: the consultation is terminated, usually by the doctor.

Practical Exercise

Try looking at some consultations to see if these stages are in fact dealt with and, if so, in what order. Discuss this first with your tutor. You may also like to discuss whether and to what extent this order is ideal and how and why stages may be missed out or dealt with in a different order in different situations. You may also like to observe and reflect with your tutor how patient-centred or doctor-centred the different stages of the consultation are.

A rather more comprehensive framework that combines both the tasks and the staging of a consultation was produced by Pendleton *et al.* in 1984 and updated in 2003. It details seven aims of the consultation, from the doctor's and patient's viewpoints, which it puts together in a logical, although not necessarily always appropriate,

order. It also talks about the patient's problem. It is worth stressing here that consultations are not just about problems or illnesses. Some are about health rather than illness issues, such as a wanted pregnancy or healthcare for travelling. However, this model is included because it is comprehensive and you might be interested in looking at consultations, in whatever situation, in a more detailed manner.

- *Task 1*: To understand the reasons for the patient's attendance, including:
  1. the patient's problem:
     - the nature and history of the problem
     - its aetiology
     - its effects.
  2. the patient's perspective:
     - their personal and social circumstances
     - their ideas and values about health
     - their ideas about the problem, its causes and its management
     - their concerns about the problem and its implications
     - their expectations for information, involvement and care.
- *Task 2*: Taking into account the patient's perspective, to achieve a shared understanding:
  1. about the problem
  2. about the evidence and options for management.
- *Task 3*: To enable the patient to choose an appropriate action for each problem:
  1. consider options and implications
  2. choose the most appropriate course of action.
- *Task 4*: To enable the patient to manage the problem:
  1. discuss the patient's ability to take appropriate actions
  2. agree doctor's and patient's actions and responsibilities
  3. agree targets, monitoring and follow-up.
- *Task 5*: To consider other problems:
  1. not yet presented
  2. continuing problems
  3. at-risk factors.
- *Task 6*: To use time appropriately:
  1. in the consultation
  2. in the longer term.

■ *Task 7*: To establish or maintain a relationship with the patient that helps to achieve the other tasks.

Practical Exercise

Pick out one of these aims (for example 'how time or resources were used' or 'involving the patient in management decisions') as a focus for a surgery session. Discuss with your tutor the extent to which you both thought this aim had been achieved in a variety of consultations.

Finally, McElvey (2010) has come up with an interesting way to view the consultation, the 'consultation hill'. The five stages of this model are the *preparation*, where the doctor, systems and environment are well prepared and set up for the consultation; the *ascent*, where information is gathered and which is largely patient-led; a *shared summit*, where doctor and patient take a moment to reflect on where they have got to; the *descent*, where management options are discussed and follow-up agreed; and *reflection* on what went well, what could been done differently and what this might mean for future consultations with this patient and with others.

Behaviours that help or hinder a consultation

A number of different ways have been given to assist you in observing consultations in a focused, structured and, it is hoped, helpful way. To complete this chapter on 'the consultation', what you might observe as behaviour that helps or hinders a consultation is briefly summarized and discussed.

Consultations frequently go wrong when the doctor fails to determine the patient's reason for attending, when the doctor fails to grasp the ramifications of the patient's condition, or when the doctor fails to discuss and communicate the options for diagnosis and therapy properly. The patient goes out of the surgery feeling misunderstood and frustrated. The doctor is totally unaware of this, is left with an uneasy feeling that the consultation did not go well, or is left dissatisfied knowing that the consultation was not as effective as it might have been.

Three major skills which will assist a consultation are:

1. listening
2. getting to the real reason for presentation
3. recognizing and understanding cultural differences.

Listening carefully and respectfully to a patient's story, verbal and non-verbal, seems easy, but appears difficult for many of us. Attentive listening will, in the long term, identify and deal with problems more effectively than a hurried interrogation of the patient.

We all know that what the patient presents initially at a consultation is not always the principal problem or issue. For example, somatic problems are often easier to present than psychosocial problems and, in fact, the patient may use a somatic symptom in the initial presentation as a 'ticket of entry'. It has been shown that where a psychosocial issue is initially presented, this is the principal issue in nearly all cases. However, where a somatic problem is initially presented, this is the principal problem in only 53 per cent of cases (Burack and Carpenter, 1983). A more sensitive problem may be presented only indirectly or left until last, even until the patient is at the door. GPs usually become quite adept at picking up these indirect messages. However, sometimes, in fact quite frequently, the real reason or one of the reasons for consultation, if it does emerge, can surprise the doctor, often at the end of a lengthy consultation in the middle of a busy surgery.

Tutor quote

Mr H, a 45-year-old man, opened the consultation by asking for the result of a full blood count ordered by my partner because he had a very prolonged sore throat. The lymphocyte count was just below normal and I spent a long time discussing its significance. I was immensely relieved that he was happy to do nothing and just put up with the nuisance of his sore throat. Then, just as I was about to say 'Is there anything else?' he flattened me with the observation, 'Actually my main reason for coming is that I have a discharge from my penis.' No wonder he wasn't bothered about his lymphopenia!

Practical Exercise

Note the presenting symptoms and the principal problems identified during some consultations. How often do they correlate? Can you detect any indirect presentations? You may detect what your tutor misses.

A common cause of poor communication is cultural misunderstanding. If we consider the term 'culture' in its broadest sense, this includes differences in the doctor's and patient's experience and understanding in terms of such things as age, gender, sexual orientation, physical difference, learning ability, educational background, ethnicity, socio-economic background and prior health experiences and values. Often such behaviours and beliefs, on the part of both the doctor and the patient, are not explicit and we are not consciously aware of them. For other consultations, for example when the patient and doctor do not share the same language, the differences are obvious (see the 'Special communication skills' sections of Chapter 4). It is important that we, as doctors, are aware of difference, valuing diversity and finding pleasure in learning from those of other cultural backgrounds. Valuing diversity also requires a heightened sensitivity to issues of stereotyping and prejudice.

Tutor quote

There is a guy with an Italian second name, nice guy, and he was a student here, ages ago. There was this woman came in, he was sitting in, and she was an elderly Italian woman who I knew pretty well. She was always miserable and I said to the student 'Look, why don't you take her off into the room for half an hour.' So he said 'Yes', and so he did, and later on in the morning I had sort of half forgotten about it and I said absentmindedly, 'Well, did you crack it then?' and he said 'Oh yeah'. 'Well what is the scam?' and he said 'Oh, it is because she is from Venice and her husband is from one of the neighbouring rural villages and therefore this wasn't acceptable in the villagers' eyes, so it was all to do with the sort of class system relating to, you know, the village life in the Venice area.' This was the basis of her disgruntlement with her husband, which had

been lifelong, and that was why she was always disgruntled and it was worse here.

Practical Exercise

Take every opportunity to share with your fellow students and tutors your own beliefs and cultural experiences, especially in the health-related area. As tutors, particularly, we need to provide situations in which such information can be discussed in a respectful atmosphere.

Very early on in your training, you will be encouraged to be with patients and to listen to their stories. As you get more skilled, you will be able to start consulting formally. At this stage, you will be looking at your own consultations in these ways and getting feedback from your tutor to assist this process. You may also be given the opportunity to use video recordings and audiotapes to record your consultations.

Take every opportunity to sit and talk with patients, and discuss with your tutor how to accomplish this in the safest and most appropriate and effective way for both you and the patient. Remember that to be a doctor or to be a patient are just two of the many roles that you have. Doctors are not exempt from being patients at times.

Practical Exercise

A useful way of reflecting on consultations is to write your experiences down and then discuss them with fellow students and tutors. What we have found helpful with our students is to create what we call a log diary of, say, four consultations, each of one side of A4 paper (no more than 500 words). We suggest the following framework:

❑ brief description of presentation, content and process of the consultation (one paragraph),
❑ brief discussion of the outcome of the consultation (one paragraph),
❑ your own response to the consultation (one paragraph),

Practical Exercise continued

❑ what you learnt from the consultation (one paragraph).

In this exercise, the description of your response to the consultation and what you learnt from the consultation are as important as your description of patient presentation and outcome.

The following headings are suggestions for topics you can use to describe your experience of different consultations.

❑ Common self-limiting condition
❑ Long-term condition
❑ Disability
❑ Screening/prevention or health promotion
❑ Life event
❑ Health beliefs
❑ Prescribing
❑ Conflict
❑ Other.

It is also a good exercise to think of a caption that encapsulates your sense of the consultation, for example 'Nothing to fall back on – the physical injury mirrors the emotional difficulty.' We have found it useful to discuss one or more of these case studies in seminar groups, in order to make the task of completing the remaining case studies more enjoyable and rewarding. The resultant log diary can be used for assessment purposes.

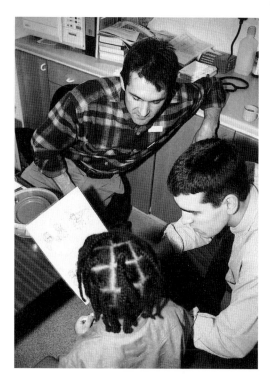

Figure 3.3 Learning from the patient.

Remember that consultations have an emotional element and sometimes they can have quite an effect on you and the patient. Share such experiences with your tutor as they can hold information that can be important in your learning and may need to be followed up with the patient. The Balint Society, founded in 1969, was set up to help GPs towards a better understanding of the emotional content of the doctor–patient relationship (www.balint.co.uk).

The narrative approach to the consultation

The 'stuff' of the consultation is the story, in fact the intersection of stories – those of the patient and the patient's family and community, the doctor and society. Over the last 30 years generally and the last 15 years in the medical world, there has been an increasing interest in the idea of narrative. This 'study of story telling' explores how we construct our stories as individuals and communities, how we tell them to each other, and how stories change over time. The narrative approach challenges ideas that we might have regarding reality and the authoritative voice of Western medicine in defining reality. Could even scientific reality be just a set of stories that a group of people happen to believe for a period of time? The narrative approach invites us as doctors to hold dual respect and an open mind for the worth of both the medical story and the patient's story, the scientific and the patient's explanation of reality and of the meaning of health and illness.

All our talk of the patient's and doctor's tasks and the formal staging of consultations does perhaps give us a sense of order and control – of a process that can be understood and measured

– and knowledge is power. However, is a more open-ended approach to the consultation, with a resultant relinquishing of some of the power that we hold as doctors, more valuable in making sense of health and illness? We, as doctors, may feel safer following the rules of history taking or the staging of a consultation, but what if this differs from what the patient wants to reveal to us? At times, simply witnessing the patient telling their story is all that is required (Figure 3.3). At other times, the stages of the consultation may be reached after many consultations. Even more widely, the story that is told and the actions that follow may belong to a family or a community. The narrative approach broadens our understanding of the consultation.

SUMMARY POINTS

To conclude, the most important messages of this chapter are as follows:
- The consultation is the central activity of a GP.
- It is important to be able to distinguish between the content and process of a consultation.
- The roles that the patient and doctor adopt in the consultation are related to the degree of doctor- or patient-centredness in that consultation.
- The tasks of the doctor and patient in a consultation have different emphases and, for a consultation to be effective, the doctor and patient need to meet as experts.
- Listening, getting to the real reason for presentation and understanding cultural differences are three key areas which contribute to an effective consultation.
- Valuing the stories that we hear helps us all to make sense of the patient's journey.

References

Burack, R.C. and Carpenter, R.R. 1983: The predictive value of the presenting complaint. *Journal of Family Practice* 16(4), 749–54.

Byrne, P.S. and Long, B.E.L. 1976: *Doctors talking to patients*. London: HMSO.

Gask, L. and Usherwood, T. 2002: ABC of psychological medicine. The consultation. *British Medical Journal* 324, 1567–9.

Gregory, S. 2009. *General practice in England: An overview*. London: The King's Fund

Helman, C.G. 1981: Disease versus illness in general practice. *Journal of the Royal College of General Practitioners* 31, 548–52.

McElvey, I. 2010: The consultation hill: a new model to aid teaching consultation skills. *British Journal of General Practice* 60(576), 538–40.

Neighbour, R. 2004: *The inner consultation*, 2nd edn. Newbury: Petroc Press.

Pendleton, D., Schofield, T., Tate, P. and Havelock, P. 2003: *The new consultation*. Oxford: Oxford University Press.

Stewart, M. 2001: Towards a global definition of patient centred care. *British Medical Journal* 322, 444–5.

Further reading

Byrne, P.S. and Long, B.E.L. 1976: *Doctors talking to patients*. London: HMSO.
This is one of the 'classics' in general practice research and is well worth reading if you are interested in the general practice consultation.

Fraser, R.C. 1999: *Clinical method. A general practice approach*, 3rd edn. Oxford: Butterworth Heinemann.
This is a very useful and succinct British text of general practice that has two good chapters on the consultation and the doctor–patient relationship.

Greenhalgh, T. and Hurwitz, B. (ed.) 1998: *Narrative based medicine – dialogue and discourse in clinical practice*. London: BMJ Books.

This challenges our frameworks of the consultation and encourages us to think more deeply about the construction of meaning.

Kai, J. 2003: *Ethnicity, health and primary care*. Oxford: Oxford University Press.

This is a concise and practical introduction to ethnicity and healthcare. The general principles outlined in this book are readily transferable to other healthcare settings and issues of diversity.

Launer, J. 2002: *Narrative-based primary care*. Abingdon: Radcliffe Medical Press.

Both philosophical and practical, this is a good introduction to the narrative approach, challenging our understanding of the consultation.

McWhinney, I.R. 2009: *A textbook of family medicine*, 3rd edn. New York: Oxford University Press.

This is a larger text than that of Fraser. It is based on the North American and British experiences and is more philosophical in nature. It has some wonderful reading on all aspects of general practice, including the consultation.

Morgan, M. 2008: The doctor–patient relationship. In: Scambler, G. (ed.) *Sociology as applied to medicine*, 6th edn. London: Saunders Elsevier.

A good summary of sociological thinking around the doctor–patient relationship.

Pendleton, D., Schofield, T., Tate, P. and Havelock, P. 2003: *The consultation*. Oxford: Oxford University Press.

This is another of the classic general practice texts on the consultation.

Tate, P. 2010: *The doctor's communication handbook*, 6th edn. Abingdon: Radcliffe Medical Press.

This concentrates on how to communicate with patients in whatever setting you meet them. It is easy and fun to read.

Tuckett, D., Boulton, M., Olson, C. and Williams, A. 1985: *Meetings between experts*. London: Tavistock Publications.

This thought-provoking book makes for useful reading for all clinicians and aspiring clinicians. From a study of more than 1000 primary care consultations, questions about the objectives of such meetings are asked and discussed.

SINGLE BEST ANSWER QUESTIONS

3.1 What is the best example of 'process' in the following descriptive excerpts from a consultation?

a) The patient reports hand pain
b) The GP takes a history and examines the patient's hand
c) The patient anxiously waits while the GP hurriedly writes up the notes
d) The GP refers her to the musculoskeletal assessment clinic
e) The GP provides a repeat script for medication for her baby's eczema.

3.2 Patient-centredness is best defined as:

a) The doctor takes into account the patient's desire for taking an active role in the consultation
b) The doctor takes a back seat and lets the patient decide on management
c) The doctor decides what is best for the patient
d) The doctor puts the patient in the centre of their considerations on management
e) The patient is most important in a holistic model of care.

3.3 In a consultation:

a) At the start of the consultation the GP must establish a good relationship with the patient
b) Discovering the reason for the patient's attendance is crucial as a first step
c) A physical examination is an essential part of the GP consultation
d) 'Safety netting' is making sure that the GP is working in a safe environment

SINGLE BEST ANSWER QUESTIONS CONTINUED

e) It is important to reflect on your strong emotional responses in a consultation.

3.4 Ms G. comes to see you and tells you that she has had three colds in the last two months. You examine her and order some blood tests. She returns two weeks later. There is nothing abnormal in her history, examination or investigations that make you think there is a serious physical cause for her recurrent colds. However she is hesitant to leave the consultation. What is the most important thing you should you do in this situation?

a) Reassure her further
b) Reassure her and ask her to return if she has more colds
c) Re-examine her and order more investigations
d) Talk with her about what else is going on in her life
e) Teach her about the natural history and self-care of the common cold.

3.5 The best way of learning about cultural issues presenting in the consultation comes from:

a) Extensive undergraduate medical training
b) Information from books, newspapers and on the internet
c) Listening to patients
d) Sharing information with colleagues
e) Seeking to experience as much cultural difference as possible.

CHAPTER

4

GENERAL PRACTICE SKILLS

- Skills and professional responsibilities
- Acquiring new skills
- How to use this chapter
- Basic professional skills
- Skills used in clinical examination and diagnosis
- Skills used in clinical management and treatment

- Special communication skills
- Summary points
- References
- Further reading
- Appendix: Assessing practical skills in general practice

Skills are essential to general practice. History taking and physical examination are the cornerstones of the consultation and require good communication and examination skills for the satisfactory management of patients. The general practitioner is expected to be competent in a range of skills, the most important of which are explained in this chapter.

LEARNING OBJECTIVES

By the end of this chapter, in relation to each skill listed in the training plan below, you should:
- know what the skill entails;
- understand the basic science of that skill;
- know the clinical indications for the skill;
- know the key steps in performing the skill, having rehearsed the procedure on a model, or volunteer;
- be aware of avoidable pitfalls or hazards of performing the skill;
- know your level of competence by asking your clinical tutor or supervisor to assess you;
- feel competent to practise the skill in a variety of clinical settings;
- know that you treat patients with courtesy and respect when performing a skill.

Skills and professional responsibilities

Examining ears, measuring blood pressure, giving injections, taking blood and syringing ears are all in a day's work for a general practitioner (GP). Some GPs extend their service to patients by acquiring more specialized skills, for example minor surgery, doing electrocardiograms (ECGs) or rectal examination by proctoscopy – procedures for which other patients would be referred to hospital. With busy work schedules in general practice, the management of patients is shared with other members of the primary healthcare team especially practice and community nurses. GP training demands high standards in skills performance as well as responsibility for ensuring competence in staff to whom work is delegated.

Training in clinical skills involves the acquisition of specific technical competencies and an appropriate professional approach, combining both the art and the science of medicine.

Patients should feel reassured and confident in your ability: giving information about the procedure and why it needs to be undertaken, giving your patient an opportunity to ask questions and discuss anxieties and, finally, obtaining your patient's informed consent. The basis of practice is that patients should be actively involved in their care. You have a responsibility to allow them the right to refuse examination and treatment. You also have a professional responsibility to ensure that you are competent in all procedures performed on patients, and that these competencies are maintained and updated throughout your professional career.

Acquiring new skills

When learning a new skill you will work through a set of learning objectives, practise until you feel confident, and then perform the skill in a clinical setting. By revising and applying relevant basic science, you will gain a deeper understanding of the principles and the components of that skill. Working with patients is a real incentive for some preparatory reading!

Begin by practising on a model, then transfer to the consulting room. The adage of 'see one, do one, teach one' has been superseded by 'prepare, practise, perform and perfect'. When you feel ready, ask your tutor to assess your competence. If you fail to achieve a satisfactory standard you should repeat the assessment. However disheartening this may be, minimum standards of competence are important for the safe practice of medicine.

How to use this chapter

The skills described in this chapter are grouped into three sections. The level of undergraduate (UG) or postgraduate training in the Foundation Years 1 and 2 (FY1, FY2) when you would be expected to start performing the skill is indicated in brackets, although timing will vary according to the programme.

Basic professional skills

- How to behave professionally (all years)

- How to maintain patient confidentiality (all years)
- How to obtain informed consent (all years)
- How to examine patients: following a code of practice (all years).

Skills used in clinical examination and diagnosis

- How to take a radial pulse (UG Year 1)
- How to measure blood pressure (UG Year 1)
- How to weigh and measure a patient (UG Years 1, 2)
- How to take a temperature (UG Year 1)
- How to examine an ear (UG Years 3, 4)
- How to use urine and blood dipsticks (UG Years 2, 3)
- How to use a mini-peak flow meter (UG Years 2, 3).

Skills used in clinical management and treatment

- Intradermal, subcutaneous and intramuscular injections (UG Years 3, 4, 5)
- How to syringe an ear (FY1+2)
- How to take a blood sample (venepuncture) (UG Year 3)
- How to write a prescription (UG Year 5, FY1+2).

Special communication skills

- How to write a referral letter (UG Year 5, FY1+2)
- How to sign a Medical Certificate of Cause of Death (death certificate) (UG Year 5 [observe], FY1 + 2)
- How to consult with special age groups (children and elderly people)
  – children (UG Year 4)
  – elderly people (UG Years 3, 4)
- Communicating with patients with limited or no English (all years)
- How to do a home visit (UG Years 1, 2).

Each exercise takes you sequentially through the steps in performing that skill, and is designed as a self-directed learning tool away from your tutor. Try first to observe a competent practitioner demonstrate a specific skill. When you have worked through each exercise, get your tutor to check your technique.

Each exercise has the following format:

1. clinical indications for using the skill,
2. background information on relevant basic science,
3. a list of equipment required,
4. a step-by-step outline of the procedure,
5. points of practice, highlighting commonly encountered problems,
6. a practical exercise or thinking and discussion point to reinforce your learning.

Questions to ask before you start each skills exercise

- *What background knowledge do you need to understand the procedure?* Think of your basic science: the anatomy of the ear, the biochemistry of blood glucose measurement, for example.
- *Have you previous experience?* Are you confident or do you need to improve and if so, how? Whom should you ask for guidance?
- *What are your learning aims and objectives?* How should you do it? What standard of practice is expected for minimum competence? When should you ask to be assessed?
- *What equipment do you need?* Check out what you need before you start. Get the equipment ready.
- *How do you get started?* Arrange for a 'dummy-run', preferably on a model, or staff or student volunteer. When you feel confident, demonstrate your skill to your tutor before transferring to a patient.
- *How do you obtain consent from a patient to let you practise on them?* Your tutor will introduce you to a patient and obtain his or her permission. Common courtesies are an integral part of professional practice. Always introduce yourself and explain what you intend to do before and during the procedure. Offer to help patients who need help positioning themselves on the examination couch. Thank your patients afterwards for their cooperation.

Tutor quote

There are many students who surprise me with their knowledge. It is also good to see when a student is actually caring about patients and I have had lots of students who show little caring touches, like helping an old lady to get dressed or helping somebody with a backache off the couch rather than leaving them until they fall off. This somehow always helps me to spot those doctors I believe to be the caring doctors who won't leave the nurses to go behind them to tidy up the patient.

- *How do you handle difficult questions?* Some patients may confront you with questions that challenge your experience. For example, if you are asked 'Have you done this before? I don't want to be your guinea-pig', you should be honest. Over-confidently telling a patient you have undertaken a procedure numerous times when you are a novice is unacceptable. If you feel uncomfortable, consult your tutor.
- *How can you improve?* After performing a skill, ask your patient and tutor for feedback. If you feel out of your depth, ask for help. Keep calm throughout, even if you are having technical difficulties.

Tutor quote

I remember a student who was anxious about examining patients, to the extent that she was worse than I was when I took my first blood test. She was getting trembly and sweaty and I only realized when I watched her taking a blood pressure that she couldn't really do it. We went through it and in the end we simplified things right down to the point where she just sat with me and checked patients' pulses until she felt calm about holding people's hands and touching people, and that always struck me as being such a small bit of learning in terms of learning but so important as a hurdle to get over.

- *How do you know when you are competent?* Your tutor can help you develop and improve your skills by:
  - arranging equipment, suitable patients, and space to practise,
  - supervising you,
  - advising about correct techniques,
  - monitoring your progress,
  - checking your competence,
  - signing your personal training plan/skills record (see later in this chapter),
  - giving you feedback from the patient.

Tutor quote

Students with confidence ... they can do everything ... no problem ... 'Taking blood ... leave it to me ... I'll take the blood on this patient'. After a few minutes, I pop back to see how the student is getting on and I am horrified to see that there is blood all over the place. They have done the whole thing wrong: they have kept the tourniquet on with the needle out ... blood everywhere ... student not wearing gloves ... a good example of how tutors should make sure to supervise ... somebody should be watching the student.

Basic professional skills

Throughout your medical career it is essential for professional practice that you have good relationships with patients and colleagues:

- always treat patients with politeness and consideration,
- involve patients in decisions about their care,
- show respect for patients and colleagues without prejudice with respect to background, language, culture and lifestyle,
- recognize the rights of patients, particularly with regard to confidentiality and informed consent.

How to maintain patient confidentiality

Throughout your medical career, you will have access to private and sensitive information about patients. Personal details will be shared with you in total confidence on the understanding that information will not be divulged to others except for the purposes of teaching and to other professionals involved in your patient's care. Patients have a right to expect that you will not pass on confidential information without their consent (General Medical Council, 2006, 2009a).

- Confidentiality is central to the trust between patients and doctors.
- Confidential information includes all personal details and data disclosed verbally, in writing or on computer.
- Confidential information used for teaching must be anonymized (i.e. all personal details have been removed from clinical notes, written and oral presentations and project work).
- Confidentiality should be maintained for all time, even after a patient's death.

Practical advice

As most patient files are now electronic, you will need to arrange for password-protected access to patient information. You must not print or photocopy patient electronic records, and never save patient information on USB sticks, or paste into emails.

- Self-written notes on patients for study purposes must be anonymized and secured in a case or folder.
- If you photograph patients for projects, you must obtain their consent, and cover the eyes if used for presentation or publication.
- You must not discuss any patient's personal or clinical details in a public place where confidential information can be overheard.

Remember:

- every patient has a right to confidentiality,
- every student has an obligation to respect that right,
- breaching confidentiality is a disciplinary offence.

How to obtain informed consent

Before you examine, treat or care for competent adult patients, you must obtain their consent. Adults include persons aged 16 years and over. Consent must be given voluntarily and not under pressure from others. Consent may be written, oral or non-verbal. Children who understand what is involved in the proposed procedure can also give consent, ideally with involvement of their parents (General Medical Council, 2007).

- Before you take a history or examine a patient, obtain permission from your tutor or supervisor.
- Introduce yourself to your patient by your full name, stating you are a medical student, your course and place of study. Explain your intentions, whether you wish to take a history, make an examination or carry out a procedure, explaining what is involved and the reason for doing it. Check that your patient understands and ask if they have any questions. Assure your patient of confidentiality and obtain their

consent to proceed. Explain that a patient has the right to decline examination, and that this will not affect their management.

Consent for student undertaking an intimate examination of patient

- If examining an intimate area of the body, for example the breasts, genitalia, vagina or rectum, in addition to obtaining verbal consent, you must always offer the patient a chaperone, preferably your supervisor or other professional. Record in the patient's records your examination and findings and state that consent was given. Sign and date this entry.

Consent for student undertaking a surgical procedure or an invasive examination on a patient

- It may be your medical school policy that students must obtain a patient's written consent before making an invasive examination. If so, ask your patient to sign and date a statement of the procedure to be undertaken, or use an official consent form. This should be counter-signed by your tutor, and scanned into the patient's health record.

How to examine patients: following a code of practice

Patient consultations in general practice tend to be more relaxed than in hospitals. Most GPs and practice nurses do not wear white coats or uniforms. Such informality encourages good rapport between patients and staff and facilitates patient-centred consultations. However, it is important that the patient–doctor relationship is maintained within professional boundaries, and staff need to be aware that over-familiarity with patients may, exceptionally, lead to misinterpretation of the doctor–patient relationship in which allegations of improper behaviour might arise. To avoid this, it is essential that all healthcare staff follow a code of conduct in clinical settings.

Being a student in general practice

- Your identity badge should be prominently displayed at all times. Check the accepted dress code with your GP tutor or trainer before starting your placement.
- You should be a member of a medical defence union. At most medical schools this is compulsory. Once qualified, you cannot be employed without membership of a medical defence union.

Consulting with patients in the surgery

- As a student, always obtain permission from a doctor or nurse before taking a history or examining a patient.
- Privacy is essential. Patient conversations should not be overheard.
- The seating arrangement in the consulting room is important. It is preferable for the patient to be seated to the side of or at an angle to the doctor's chair rather than directly opposite and separated by the desk in a confrontational way (Figure 4.1).
- Using computers: patients prefer to see the screen even if this means slightly turning your back to the patient when inputting data.
- Introduce yourself to the patient by name. Explain your status – medical student or Foundation Year doctor training in the practice. A student should never pose as a doctor.
- Non-verbal behaviour reveals much about you. Maintain eye-to-eye contact throughout the consultation. Looking away momentarily is acceptable, but always refocus on the patient's face, even if not reciprocated. Encourage your patient to respond to questions. Listen attentively, acknowledging you are hearing in an interactive way, such as a nod of the head, smile or murmur of assent. Ensure your body is relaxed, particularly your arms, which are best held open on your lap. Sitting forward, leaning on your desk or folding your arms across your chest suggests aggression and is not conducive to open conversation.
- When your patient is talking, avoid interrupting until there is a natural pause. If patients talk incessantly or ramble, you may need to interrupt and summarize the salient points, to refocus the consultation.
- Keep discussion relevant. Avoid personal or humorous comments or terms of endearment to your patient. It is unprofessional to refer to your own personal circumstances for illustrative purposes, and preferable to phrase a personal experience in the context of a third person.

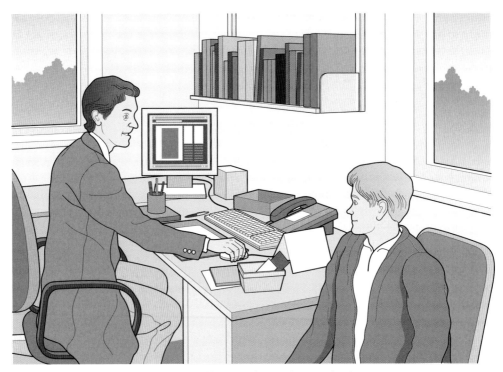

Figure 4.1 Recommended seating in a GP consulting room showing doctor and patient.

■ Avoid writing notes or entering data on the computer while your patient is talking.

Examining patients and professional etiquette

■ Your patient should be allowed privacy to undress and dress. Explain which garments should be removed, where they should be placed. Draw the curtains around the examination couch so you do not observe the patient undressing.
■ Cover the examination couch with clean paper.
■ Ask your patient to let you know when he or she is ready for examination. Minimize patient exposure by providing a cover for exposed body parts when not being examined. You should avoid examining patients underneath their garments.
■ Keep discussion relevant to the examination.
■ If your patient is uncomfortable, distressed or aroused, withdraws consent, makes inappropriate remarks or you feel ill at ease, discontinue

the examination and seek tutor or supervisor advice.
■ After the examination is completed, assist the patient off the couch and ask them to get dressed.
■ Explain your examination findings to your patient, and thank them for their cooperation.
■ Ensure the examination couch has a clean cover for the next patient.

When should you use a chaperone?

Students should never do an intimate examination without a supervising doctor or nurse present who will act as chaperone. Doctors in training such as FY1 should ask their clinical supervisor or other supervising GP to act as chaperone and if unavailable should ask another professional in the practice (e.g. a practice nurse). This includes examination of the genitalia, rectum or female breasts. Established GPs may have difficulty finding a chaperone in practice but a chaperone is essential if the GP is the opposite sex to the patient. One possibility is to offer an examination at a later time when the patient can return with a friend or relative as chaperone, or offer the patient the option of examination by a doctor of the same sex. Surveys have shown that adults of both sexes would prefer a nurse as chaperone and teenagers would prefer a parent. If no chaperone is available, it is preferable to delay the examination rather than be placed at risk.

- Never examine an intimate body area of a patient unnecessarily. This may be misinterpreted.
- If you are a chaperone, observe the examination from the side of the couch. If you have concerns, you should discuss with the examiner and suggest the examination is stopped.

Skills used in clinical examination and diagnosis

How to take a radial pulse

Taking an arterial pulse is one of the most fundamental skills in medical practice and is used in the baseline monitoring of a patient's clinical condition. You will be introduced to this skill in the first year of the undergraduate course. The arterial pulse can be measured at any anatomical site where a main artery runs close to the body surface and is accessible to palpation. These sites include the carotid, brachial, radial, femoral, popliteal, posterior tibial and dorsalis pedis arteries. The pulse most routinely taken is the radial pulse because of its accessibility.

Background knowledge: the physiology of pulse measurement

When the left ventricle of the heart contracts, a column of arterial blood is ejected into the aorta, transmitting a pulse wave into the arterial system. This pulse wave takes between 0.2 and 0.5 seconds to reach the feet, although the speed of the column of blood is about ten times slower. The form of the pulse wave is determined by the quantity of blood ejected into the aorta, the speed of ejection and the elasticity of the arterial wall.

The arterial pulse has four characteristics: rate, rhythm, volume and form. These are most accurately assessed in the main pulses that are closest to the heart (i.e. the carotid, brachial and femoral pulses). The normal adult pulse rate is 60–85 beats per minute. A rapid pulse, or *tachycardia*, is defined as a pulse rate of 100 beats or more per minute, and a slow pulse, or *bradycardia*, is less than 60 beats per minute. The pulse rhythm is the degree of regularity of the pulse. The pulse should be regular, although there may be a noticeable variation with respiration, known as sinus arrhythmia. A pulse is reported as regular or irregular. An irregular pulse is described as *regularly irregular* when the irregularities can be predicted, such as in second degree heart block, or *irregularly irregular*, as in most cases of atrial fibrillation, when there is an erratic pattern. Pulse volume is difficult to assess at the radial pulse. However, a low-volume pulse can be described as 'weak', while a high-volume pulse can be described as 'bounding'. Peripheral pulse characteristics are modified by the properties of the arteries, as in arterial narrowing. Pulse form is a description of the character of the pulse wave (i.e. whether the wave is slow to rise, as in stenosis [narrowing] of the aorta, or falls rapidly, when it is known as a collapsing pulse, as in aortic regurgitation).

Procedure for taking a radial pulse

A radial pulse is measured with your second, third and fourth fingers. Avoid using your thumb as pulsation in the thumb may be confused for the patient's radial pulse and lead to an inaccurate reading. This is less of a problem for stronger pulses such as the femoral and carotid.

1. Ask the patient to rest his or her forearm on a surface with the palm of the hand uppermost. The arm may be supported with your own hand.
2. Feel the patient's radial pulse along the outer border of the wrist using your three middle fingers.
3. The rate is measured with the second hand of a watch by counting the pulse beats in a defined period – usually 15 seconds – and multiplying (in this case by 4) to give the pulse rate per minute. If the patient has an irregular pulse, you should count the rate over one minute for greater accuracy, although measurement by heart auscultation will be more precise.

Practical points

- Use a watch with a second hand for clinical teaching and examinations, otherwise you cannot take an accurate pulse measurement and risk failing a clinical examination.
- Take the radial pulses on both sides of the body (Figure 4.2). It is good practice to compare the two simultaneously, as weakness or delay in one will give a clue about arterial disease.

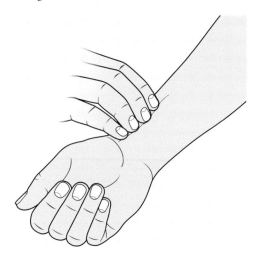

Figure 4.2 Method for palpating the radial pulse. Reprinted from John MacLeod, *Clinical examination: a textbook for students and doctors by teachers of the Edinburgh Medical School*, © 1983 Elsevier Ltd, with permission from Elsevier.

Tutor quote

A tutor was examining third-year students in an OSCE (Objective Structured Clinical Examination). The candidate was fashionably dressed in designer gear. The first question required the student to take the patient's pulse. The student looked at the watch and then at the examiner and exclaimed, 'I can't; my watch has no second hand!' The student scored no marks and failed. Fortunately for the student, the OSCE was an end-of-term formative assessment and not the final qualifying examination. Students cannot undertake full examination of patients in clinical practice without a practically designed watch.

How to measure blood pressure

This is one of the most commonly performed procedures. You may start blood pressure measurement early in the undergraduate course in physiology or in a clinical setting. By the third year, you will be expected to measure blood pressure routinely on patients. Several methods are used, each with advantages and disadvantages, and different levels of accuracy. The most commonly used method is the manual sphygmomanometer based on auscultation. This consists of an inflatable cuff, a measuring unit, either an aneroid gauge or a mercury manometer, and an inflation bulb and valve. Automatic devices use oscillatory methods. Mercury sphygmomanometers are less commonly used now because of the risk of environmental mercury toxicity. Equipment should be regularly serviced every six months.

Common indications for blood pressure measurement include:

- screening at well-person checks,
- assessing fitness for employment or insurance acceptance,
- diagnosing hypertension,
- monitoring treated hypertension.

Because a diagnosis of hypertension has lifelong implications, it is important it is measured accurately. It is recommended practice to measure and report blood pressure after a patient has been resting for 10–15 minutes. If the blood pressure is raised at the start of the consultation, the reading should be repeated after several minutes. A minimum of two measurements should be taken at each visit and 24-hour ambulatory and home readings are now recommended as well. Initially it seems complex in terms of coordination, but becomes straightforward with practice.

Background knowledge: anatomy and physiology of blood pressure measurement

All methods are based on the blood pressure changes that arise from compression of the brachial or radial artery to a pressure above the systolic pressure and from decompression to that below the diastolic pressure (Figures 4.3–4.6). The pressure is applied using an inflatable cuff that encircles the arm and compresses the brachial artery to restrict blood flow. Digital wrist models compress the radial artery.

Systolic blood pressure is indicated by a tapping sound that originates in the artery distal to (away

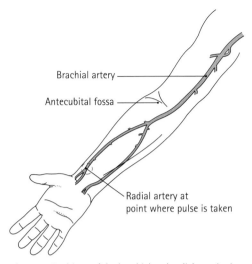

Figure 4.3 Positions of the brachial and radial arteries in relation to surface markings (anterior view).

Cuff pressure more than 120 mmHg

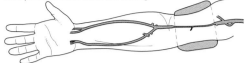

Figure 4.5 The effect of increasing the pressure in the sphygmomanometer above that in the brachial artery. When the cuff pressure exceeds the systolic arterial pressure (120 mmHg), no blood progresses through the arterial segment under the cuff, and no sounds can be detected by a stethoscope bell placed on the arm distal to the cuff.

Cuff pressure less than 80 mmHg

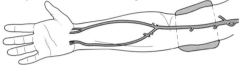

Figure 4.6 The effect of reducing the pressure in the sphygmomanometer below the diastolic artery pressure. When the cuff pressure falls below the diastolic arterial pressure, blood flow is restored to the brachial artery, arterial flow past the region of the cuff is continuous, and no sounds are audible. When the cuff pressure is between 120 and 80 mmHg, spurts of blood traverse the artery segment under the cuff with each heartbeat, and the Korotkoff sounds are heard through the stethoscope.

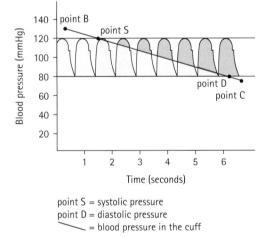

point S = systolic pressure
point D = diastolic pressure
⟍ = blood pressure in the cuff

Figure 4.4 The effect of falling pressure in the sphygmomanometer on the arterial blood pressure. Consider that the arterial blood pressure is being measured in a patient whose blood pressure is 120/80 mmHg. The pressure (represented by the oblique line) in a cuff around the patient's arm is allowed to fall from greater than 120 mmHg (point B) to below 80 mmHg (point C) in about six seconds.

from the centre of the body) the cuff as the cuff pressure falls below the peak arterial pressure. This allows blood to spurt into the compressed artery. *Diastolic blood pressure* is defined as the point at which sounds disappear as the cuff pressure falls below the minimum arterial pressure, allowing blood flow to become continuous.

Oscillatory methods

Oscillatory methods are used in automatic devices. They are based on the principle that blood flowing through an artery between systolic and diastolic pressures causes vibrations in the arterial wall that are transmitted to the air in the cuff. These are detected and transduced into electrical signals to produce a digital readout. Newer models use 'fuzzy logic' to decide how much the device should be inflated to start readings at about 20 mmHg above the patient's systolic pressure. Deflation of the cuff is automatic and occurs at a rate of about 4 mmHg per second. Oscillatory methods may seem slower than the auscultatory methods but are more accurate.

What you will need

- An aneroid or mercury sphygmomanometer.
- An arm cuff with connecting tubing attached to a rubber bulb and to the sphygmomanometer.
- A stethoscope.

About the equipment

- A sphygmomanometer consists of a manometer (either an aneroid model with a pressure gauge or a mercury model with a vertical scale), an inextensible cuff containing an inflatable bladder, rubber tubing, bulb and control valve (Figures 4.7 and 4.8).
- The manometer scale is indicated in millimetres of mercury (mmHg), from 0 to 260 in units of 10 mm and should be read from a distance within 1 metre, with your eye on a level with the meniscus. Recent guidelines recommend that the reading should be to the nearest 2 mmHg.
- Cuffs are of two types: one with a Velcro fastening, and another that is tapered and wraps around the arm, with the end of the cuff tucking under the encircling cuff. Cuffs are available in different sizes to fit small or large adults and children (Figure 4.9). Each consists of a cloth and an enclosed inflatable bladder. The bladder should completely encircle the arm. If it does not, the cuff should be changed for a larger size. The recommended bladder width is 20 per cent greater than the diameter of the limb at the point where the cuff is applied. The cuff is changed by detaching the interconnector and replacing it with an appropriately sized cuff.

Procedure (Figure 4.10)

Your patient should have rested for at least 10 minutes before taking the blood pressure.

1. Explain the procedure and the reason for taking the blood pressure. If this is your patient's first blood pressure measurement, explain that inflating the cuff to a high pressure may feel slightly uncomfortable.

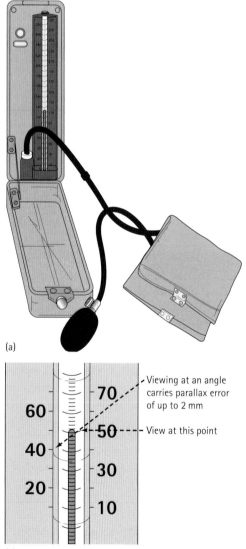

(a)

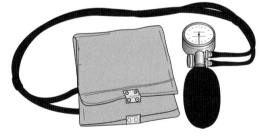

Figure 4.8 An aneroid sphygmomanometer.

(b)

Figure 4.7 (a) A mercury sphygmomanometer. (b) Close-up of a manometer tube to show the scale.

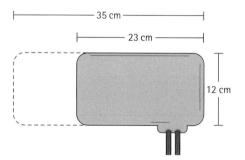

Figure 4.9 Diagram to show the dimensions of a sphygmomanometer cuff suitable for an arm circumference less than 33 cm.

2. Your patient should be seated with his or her arm at heart level. Select the arm closest to a supporting surface for measurement, rest the arm on a surface with the elbow slightly flexed and the palm of the hand uppermost. Ideally, all clothing should be removed from the arm. In reality, with short consultation times in general practice, pulling the sleeve to just below the shoulder without constricting the arm will be adequate. Check that there is sufficient space distal to the encircling cuff for the stethoscope diaphragm in the antecubital fossa without touching the cuff.

3. Wrap the cuff around the arm above the elbow, with the lettering outermost. With an older model, the bladder is placed between the cuff and the skin over the brachial artery, indicated by an arrow on the outside of modern cuffs. It is conventional to position the rubber tubes distal to the cuff, although if positioned proximal to the cuff (towards the centre of the body), it is easier to place the stethoscope diaphragm in the antecubital fossa.

4. The aneroid gauge is free standing and ready to use. With the mercury manometer, open the box with the mercury column vertically placed and facing you, with the middle of the scale, from 180 mm to 60 mm, at eye level. Check that the mercury meniscus reads zero. If not, report this and change your instrument.

5. Locate the radial pulse over the lateral (outermost) aspect of the wrist using your index and middle fingers. To gain an approximate systolic pressure reading, close the valve where the bulb and tubing connect by turning the screw away from you. Inflate the cuff by repeatedly squeezing the rubber bulb. As you inflate, the radial pulse disappears. If you continue to inflate 20–30 mm above this pressure, and deflate, the radial pulse will reappear. This pressure indicates the approximate systolic pressure. Now deflate the cuff.

6. Locate the brachial artery in the antecubital fossa by palpating around the medial (inner) part of the elbow crease (Figure 4.10a and b). Sitting opposite and slightly to the side of the patient, place the stethoscope in your ears and the diaphragm over the brachial artery (Figure 4.10c), steadying it with your thumb or a finger. While listening with your stethoscope, inflate the cuff to a level exceeding the pressure in the artery (Figure 4.10d and e). At this point you will not hear any sounds.

7. Release the pressure in the bulb by turning the control valve slowly, aiming to achieve a fall in the mercury level at a constant rate of 2–3 mm for each heart beat. The column may fall jerkily until you have learnt to control the valve evenly. You will hear faint tapping sounds as the pressure falls. These are known as the Korotkoff sounds, named after the Russian surgeon from St Petersburg who first described them in 1905 (Figure 4.11). Note the reading at the point at which the sounds reappear. This is the *systolic blood pressure* (phase 1).

8. As the cuff pressure falls, you may notice a softening of the sounds (phase 2), which sharpen again as the pressure continues to fall (phase 3), then become more muffled (phase 4) and, finally, disappear (phase 5). The phases are very variable, with sometimes only phases 1 and 5 being discernible. The point of disappearance of sounds (phase 5) is defined as the *diastolic pressure*. There is less inter-observer error with phase 5 recordings.

9. Record both the systolic (phase 1) and the diastolic (phase 5) pressures, writing systolic over diastolic (e.g. 120/80), recording to the nearest 2 mm. For example, readings of 179 systolic over 143 diastolic would be written as 178/142. The blood pressure fluctuates around a mean that is individual for each patient and varies with time and other factors such as the patient's position and degree of relaxation. Fastidiously recording to the nearest 1 mm suggests an accuracy that is misleading.

10. Recheck the readings at least once. If the blood pressure exceeds 140/95 mmHg, repeat in the other arm and again after a further 5–10 minutes. Because the reading may have been taken at the maximum point in the patient's blood pressure range, the pressure should be checked on at least three separate occasions over a period of time of

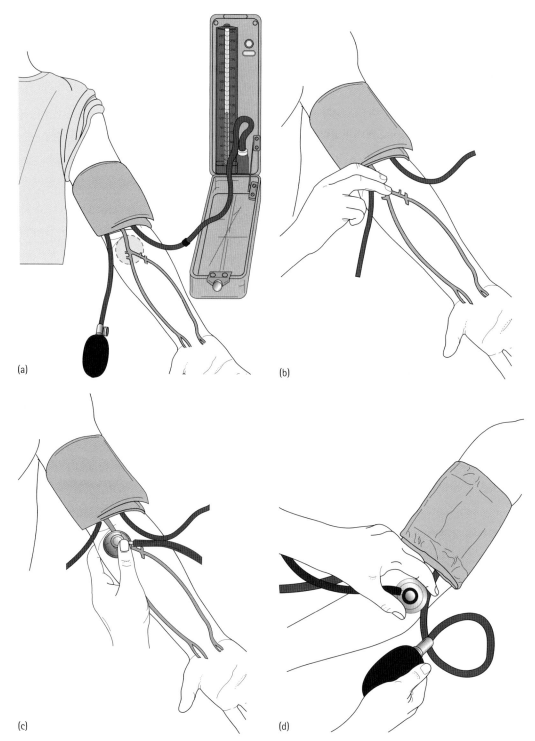

(a)

(b)

(c)

(d)

Figure 4.10 Steps in taking a blood pressure measurement with a mercury sphygmomanometer. (a) Position the equipment and cuff (anterior view). (b) Identify the brachial artery. (c) Place the stethoscope over the brachial artery. (d) Inflate the cuff to a level exceeding the pressure in the artery, as shown in (e).

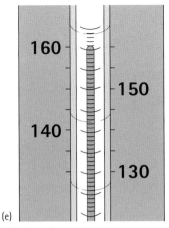

(e)

Figure 4.10 (*continued*)

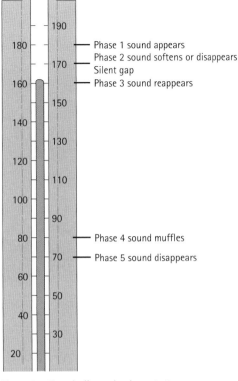

Phase 1 sound appears
Phase 2 sound softens or disappears
Silent gap
Phase 3 sound reappears

Phase 4 sound muffles
Phase 5 sound disappears

Figure 4.11 Korotkoff sounds, phases 1–5.

not less than one month before hypertension is diagnosed; 24-hour ambulatory and home readings are also recommended.

It may be helpful to watch a video or DVD of how to take a blood pressure (British Hypertension Society, 2010) or do some further reading (e.g. Beevers *et al.*, 2007).

Practical points

- Use the correct cuff size for the patient's arm. Too small a cuff gives too high a reading; too large a cuff gives too low a reading.
- The aneroid gauge or mercury meniscus should be read at eye level.
- Inflate the aneroid gauge or mercury column above the systolic by at least 30 mmHg to avoid taking the phase 3 sound as the systolic and under-recording the blood pressure.
- Readings should be taken with the mercury level falling, not rising, recording the systolic pressure first and then the diastolic pressure.
- All bulbs leak slightly, but if the leakage prevents you from halting the mercury column as it falls, the pressure will be underestimated. Report the instrument as faulty and use another.
- If the arm is unsupported, you will obtain a falsely high reading.

Oscillatory blood pressure devices

There are many different models (Figure 4.12). They are battery driven, have automatic inflation and deflation with oscillometric precision measurement, and have display windows for blood pressure and pulse readings. Most have a memory recall facility for up to 14 readings.

Procedure

1. Wrap the cuff around your patient's upper arm, and secure the Velcro fastening.
2. Switch on the start button on the front of the machine and allow the cuff to inflate automatically until it reaches maximum pressure. The pressure will automatically deflate until the blood flows smoothly through the artery in the usual pulses without any vibration in the artery wall.
3. Take the reading from the digital display panel that gives systolic and diastolic readings. The pulse rate may also be displayed.
4. Switch off the machine after completing the measurement to conserve batteries.

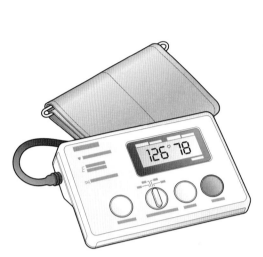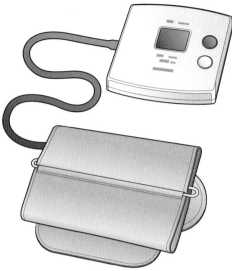

Figure 4.12 Oscillatory sphygmomanometers.

Practical Exercise

❑ Take blood pressure readings on a series of patients and record their Korotkoff phases. What effect will changing the cuff size have? Investigate the difference of cuff size on the readings.

❑ Take the blood pressures of patients of different ages, shapes and sizes. Do you notice any association of blood pressure with (a) age and (b) weight?

❑ Take blood pressure readings on the same patient, varying the position of their arm, for example held horizontally unsupported, horizontally with support, in the overhead and dependent positions. Do you notice any differences?

❑ Take readings with the patient in the following positions: standing, sitting on a chair, lying supine (on the back), sitting on an examination couch with legs horizontal. Are there any differences?

❑ Investigate the effect of exercise and rest on blood pressure. Ask a patient to run up and down stairs several times and measure the pressure immediately after stopping, then every 2–3 minutes for 10 minutes. What happens to the readings, particularly the systolic? Now you can understand why you record pressure after a patient has been sitting still for at least 10 minutes!

❑ Find a patient with an irregular pulse, for example with atrial fibrillation. What effect does this have on serial recordings of blood pressure?

How to weigh and measure a patient

Adult weight and height measurements are used for several reasons, including the long-term monitoring of weight in obesity, recovery from illness when under-nutrition may be a problem, and the assessment of growth in young adults. In general practice, weight measurements are most commonly used for monitoring obesity in adults. Babies and infants are weighed regularly by health visitors to monitor growth and nutrition.

The relationship between weight and height is expressed as an index, the *body mass index (BMI)*.

It is calculated by dividing the patient's weight in kilograms by the square of their height in metres:

$$BMI = \frac{weight\ (kg)}{height\ (m)^2}$$

The BMI is equally applicable to men and women. It is used with a set of charts and nomograms for adults (Figure 4.13); there is a different set for children. Apart from a few muscular individuals who may be wrongly classified as overweight, the BMI is a robust measurement index. Its categories indicate whether weight is in the ideal range of 18.5–24.9 kg/m², underweight (<18.5 kg/m²), overweight (25–29.9 kg/m²) or

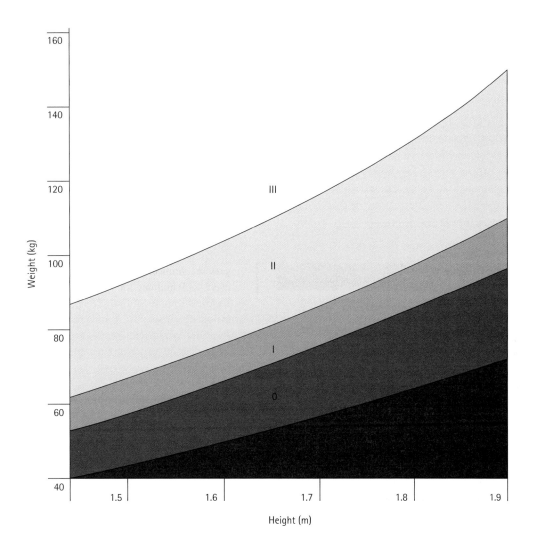

Grade	BMI	Classification
0	19–25	Normal range of weight
1	26–29	Overweight
11	30–39	Obesity
111	40 and over	Severe obesity

Figure 4.13 Use of the body mass index to show grades of obesity.

obese (over 30 kg/m^2). The overweight category is subdivided into: obese class I (30.0–34.9 kg/m^2), obese class II (35–39.9 kg/m^2) and obese class III or morbidly obese (>40 kg/m^2).

Estimates suggest that most adults in England have a BMI above the 'normal' range and that a fifth are obese, with a BMI that exceeds 30 kg/m^2. As obesity is a risk factor for life-threatening medical conditions, patients should be monitored as part of a weight management programme.

Practical points

- A patient's weight should be monitored using the same set of scales to allow comparisons over time. Readings on home or hospital scales should not be compared with surgery or clinic readings because of different sensitivities.
- A patient should be weighed each time wearing similar garments (i.e. with or without coat or shoes).
- Height should be measured with the patient in stockinged feet for greater accuracy, as shoe heels vary.
- Measurements should be read and recorded in the metric system. Despite the official change from avoirdupois to the metric system, patients like to convert to old units.
- Digital systems are preferred because the facility of adjusting the reading to zero between readings leads to greater accuracy. Digital models also allow automatic conversion to the avoirdupois system that is quicker than referring to conversion charts. All machines should be checked annually for accuracy.

How to take a temperature

The normal body temperature extends over a range of values that varies by the site of measurement, by individual and time of day (Table 4.1). A temperature below the normal range is classified as hypothermia (i.e. below 35°C), and above the normal range as pyrexia (i.e. above 37.5°C). Although the body temperature can be estimated crudely by palpation, it is more accurate to use a clinical thermometer.

The following methods are described.

- *Palpation.* Body surface temperature can be measured with the back of the hand to give a crude estimation of local temperature as long as your hand is not cold. This method will detect a local rise in temperature and may offer a clue to underlying pathology that indicates increased blood flow to the area. This occurs with local inflammation, as with skin infections, or increased blood flow in tumours. It will also detect local body cooling in comparison with the opposite side of the body. In a limb this may suggest arterial occlusion.
- *Mercury thermometers* (Figure 4.14a) are commonly used, but, because of concerns about breakage and mercury toxicity, may eventually become obsolete. They have a simple design, with a glass storage bulb for mercury and a connecting column along which expanding mercury flows when the temperature rises. Most have a graduated scale in degrees centigrade, extending from 35 to 42°C. Some have a dual scale in Fahrenheit and centigrade. A special sub-normal reading thermometer that reads from 30 to 35°C or lower is used for diagnosing hypothermia.
- *The digital oral thermometer* (Figure 4.14b) is used for oral temperatures and is quicker to use than the mercury type. It is placed under the tongue, is plastic, waterproof and battery driven. It has a tapered end, a metal sensor at the tip for measuring temperature, a body that displays the temperature in an easy-to-read window, and an on/off button. The temperature range is usually 32–43.9°C. The body temperature is recorded within 10–15 seconds and a beeper sounds when the reading has stabilized.

Table 4.1 Normal temperature ranges by site

Axillary	34.7–37.3°C	94.5–99.1°F
Oral	35.5–37.5°C	95.9–99.5°F
Rectal	36.6–38.0°C	97.4–100.4°F
Ear	35.8–38.0°C	96.4–100.4°F

Because neither mercury nor glass is used in the construction, digital thermometers are safer for use with children. Digital thermometers can also be used to measure body temperature under the arm or rectally (Figure 4.14c).

■ *The ear thermometer* (Figure 4.14d) measures body temperature in the ear and is the recommended method for children, when time and safety are important. It consists of a hand-held body with display window and control buttons for on/off and memory recall, and a cone for insertion into the ear, which is covered by a disposable plastic lens filter. When skin contact is made in the external canal, it will record the temperature within 1 second.

How to take an oral temperature using a mercury or digital thermometer

The thermometer should be sterile (i.e. used after immersion in an antiseptic solution such as chlorhexidine) or used with a protective plastic cover over the thermometer tip and stem.

1. Place the thermometer tip under the patient's tongue, and ask him or her to close the mouth over the thermometer without clamping the teeth onto the glass or sensor tip.
2. Mercury thermometers should be left in place for at least 1 minute to allow the reading to stabilize before removal, and digital thermometers for about 30 seconds or until a beeping sound indicates that the temperature has peaked.
3. Remove the thermometer from the patient's mouth. To read a mercury thermometer, rotate the stem around its longitudinal axis to view the end of the mercury column on the graduated scale. For digital thermometers, take the reading from the display window.

Taking an axillary temperature

When taking an axillary temperature, the thermometer tip is placed in the pit of the axilla and the patient is asked to hold the arm against the chest wall.

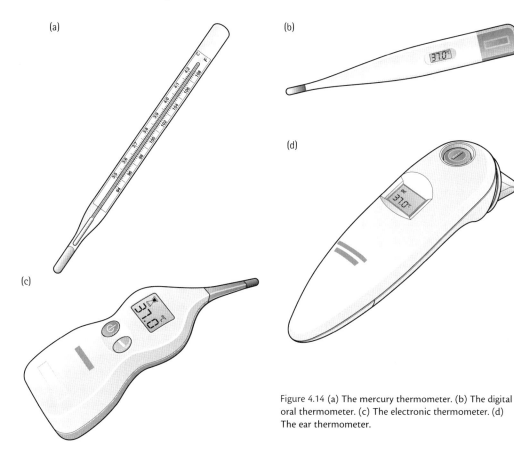

Figure 4.14 (a) The mercury thermometer. (b) The digital oral thermometer. (c) The electronic thermometer. (d) The ear thermometer.

Taking a rectal temperature

A rectal temperature is taken with the patient lying on his or her side. Gently insert the thermometer into the rectum in a backwards direction for a distance of 3–4 cm with the end of the thermometer protruding.

Practical points for all methods of temperature recording

- The thermometer reading must be returned to zero before use (i.e. with mercury thermometers by shaking vigorously until the mercury column has returned to about 35°C and for digital thermometers by clearing the display window using the on/off switch). Failure to do this is a common cause of inaccuracy.
- The time to temperature equilibration varies according to the model. A mercury thermometer should be left in contact with the body for at least 60 seconds before reading; failure to do so causes under-recording of the temperature. The digital and electronic models are much quicker.
- Hot drinks taken immediately before the body temperature is recorded will cause a local rise in body temperature. Check your patient has not recently had a hot drink otherwise you may erroneously diagnose fever. However, it is not unknown for an occasional patient to use this trick to feign illness! Likewise, a cold drink or iced lollipop will cause under-recording of the temperature.

How to take an ear temperature

1. Ensure that a clean probe cover is used with the ear thermometer for hygienic practice.
2. Press the memory button on the handle to turn on the instrument.
3. Straighten your patient's external canal to give the thermometer clear access to the eardrum. For infants, the ear canal is straightened by pulling the pinna downwards and backwards, and for adults, by pulling the pinna upwards and backwards.
4. Fit the probe snugly into the ear canal and press the activation button. This automatically measures the temperature.
5. Release the button when you hear the 'temp beep' and note the reading.

How to examine an ear

Examining an ear includes inspection of both the external ear and the tympanic membrane of the middle ear using an instrument known as an auriscope (otoscope).

Indications for examining the ear

- For diagnosis in patients with ear complaints such as pain (otalgia), itching (pruritus), difficulty hearing, blocked ear, discharge or noises in the ear (tinnitus). The most common ear presentations in general practice are children with earache, ear discharge or pulling at the ear which suggest an underlying problem.
- For diagnosis in infants with non-specific unexplained illness in whom the differential diagnosis includes middle ear infection (otitis media). Parents may have noticed that their child is irritable, cries more than usual, is not feeding, or has an unexplained fever, called pyrexia of unknown origin (PUO).
- To check for wax before ear syringing or hearing aid fitting or review.
- In the assessment of speech disorders to check whether the cause is impaired hearing, for example infants with delayed or poorly developed speech or adults with abnormal speech (dysphasia).
- In routine examination for insurance purposes, pre-employment medical for occupations such as telephonist, or for obtaining a licence to participate in certain sports, such as scuba diving, flying, gliding or parachuting.

Background knowledge

The ear comprises three parts: the outer, the middle and the inner.

The outer or external ear (Figure 4.15) comprises the auricle, which projects from the side of the head, and the external acoustic meatus or canal, which leads to the tympanic membrane of the middle ear. In babies and infants, the auricle and canal are composed of cartilage. As adulthood approaches, only the outer third remains cartilaginous, and the inner two-thirds come to lie in the temporal bone. The canal is lined by skin and in the subcutaneous tissue are hair follicles, sebaceous glands and ceruminous glands that

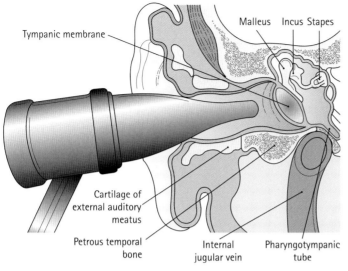

Malleus Incus Stapes

Tympanic membrane

Cartilage of
external auditory
meatus

Petrous temporal
bone

Internal
jugular vein

Pharyngotympanic
tube

Figure 4.15 **The anatomy of
the external and middle ear,
coronal section.**

produce wax. In the adult, the canal is approximately 2.5 cm long and forms an S-shaped curve
that is first directed medially (towards the centre),
forward and slightly upward, and then passes
medially, backwards and upward. Before insertion
of the auriscope, the canal should be straightened
by applying traction to the auricle: in adults, in a
backwards and upwards direction, and in infants,
in a backwards and downwards direction. This
reflects changes in skull shape with growth.

The middle ear (Figures 4.15 and 4.16) consists
of the tympanic cavity in the petrous part of the
tympanic bone and three auditory ossicles: the
malleus, incus and stapes.

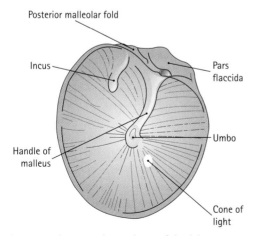

Posterior malleolar fold

Incus

Pars
flaccida

Handle of
malleus

Umbo

Cone of
light

Figure 4.16 **The tympanic membrane of the right ear as
seen through the auriscope.**

What you will see when looking through an auriscope into the ear

You will aim to examine the tympanic membrane.
This separates the outer ear from the ossicles of
the middle ear. Although the membrane is round
and faces downwards and forwards, it appears
oval when inspected through the auriscope due
to a parallax effect. In a normal ear, the tympanic
membrane forms a glistening, semi-opaque sheet
with a cone of light reflected from the lower anteri-
or (towards the front) part. An oblique line passes
in an anterior–posterior (forwards–backwards)
direction. This is the handle of the malleus, which
is attached to the tympanic membrane. Superiorly
(towards the top of the head), the malleus forms
a lax membrane, the pars flaccida. The remaining
membrane is taut and concave where it is pulled
inwards by the handle of the malleus.

What you will need

- An auriscope with charged batteries. Check that
  there is a strong beam of light.
- Set of aural speculae (attachable plastic or metal
  cones of several sizes).

Procedure

Start to gain experience by examining the ears of
symptom-free adults. Children are more easily
upset, tend to fidget, and need a special approach
(see below).

1. Explain the procedure to your patient, demonstrating the auriscope and reassuring that the examination may be uncomfortable but not painful.
2. Inspect the pinna and auricle for skin changes, signs of infection or discharge.
3. Position your patient and yourself. For adults, ask the patient to turn the head to one side or, as the examiner, move to the side of your patient. If you are right handed, it is more comfortable to examine the right ear holding the auriscope in your right hand, leaving your left hand free to pull on the auricle (Figure 4.17). Examine the left ear holding the auriscope in your left hand and pull on the auricle with your right hand. If left handed, try the reverse positions. You may prefer to hold the auriscope in your dominant hand for both sides, but note that when examining the contralateral ear, your arms will cross as you pull the auricle. Hand usage is not a hard or fast rule – do whatever feels comfortable for you.
4. Select a suitably sized speculum (i.e. the largest that can be inserted into the canal without causing pain). A plastic speculum will be comfortably warm, but a metal type may be cold and before use should be warmed in warm water and dried.
5. Turn on the auriscope light. Hold the auriscope between your thumb and index finger, either with the palm of your hand placed vertically or with your palm uppermost. This position difference is a matter of preference. Try both.
6. With your free hand, draw the auricle upwards and backwards to straighten the canal. Insert the speculum gently into the external canal, advancing by a short distance at first. View through the lens in front of the speculum. Use the fourth and fifth fingers to steady the auriscope against the head. What do you see? The skin of the auditory canal should come into view. Sometimes you see deposits of yellow or brown wax. Beyond this you should see a small part of the tympanic membrane. Advance the auriscope along the canal by changing the angle to bring the whole tympanic membrane into view. It will look grey and opaque and you should see a shiny area known as the light reflex. Try to bring this into view by a slight change in direction of either the auriscope or the auricle. The tympanic membrane may appear abnormal – redness usually indicates inflammation; a fluid level or opaque circumscribed area suggests exudates; or a hole in the tympanic membrane suggests a perforation. If you see only wax, the ear canal is probably blocked.

Examining a child's ear (without tears)

An ear examination can be a frightening procedure for a young child. Because children move unpredictably, may be frightened or uncoopera-

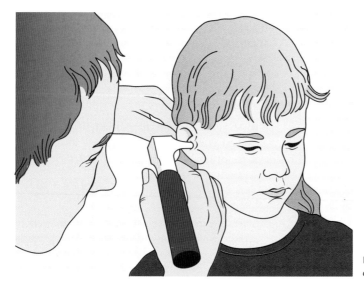

Figure 4.17 An auriscope held in the correct position.

tive, they have to be restrained during the examination. The child's head must be steadied to allow an adequate view of the ear and to minimize the risk of damage to the tympanic membrane by the auriscope. As preparation, explain the procedure to the parent and child.

1. Select a smaller (paediatric) speculum for the auriscope.
2. Befriend your young patient. To avoid a frightening experience, reassure the child about your intentions, perhaps demonstrating your auriscope light on clothing, a teddy, doll or the child's parent. Try turning the encounter into a game.
3. With the parent sitting facing you, ask the parent to sit the child across his or her lap with the child's head and inner arm against the parent's chest, and the parent's arm or hand held firmly across the child's head. The parent's other arm should be placed around the child's chest and outer arm. This is similar to a child's 'cuddling' position (Figure 4.18).
4. You are now ready to examine. Use the same procedure as for the adult, except that to straighten the external meatus, pull the pinna downwards and backwards.

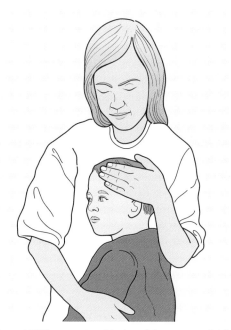

Figure 4.18 The correct positioning of the parent and child for examination of the child's ear.

Practical points

- If the ear is partly or wholly blocked with wax, try removing gently with a cotton bud. If not, the patient should introduce a few drops of oil into the canal daily for about two weeks to allow the wax to soften, before re-examination or ear syringing.
- If you are unable to view the whole tympanic membrane, this may be due to faulty equipment. Although the position of the auriscope in the auditory canal is correct, the main beam of light may not be directed from the end of the speculum because the bulb carrier is bent. Try a different auriscope.
- If a child screams throughout the consultation, what should you do? The kindest approach is to spend time comforting the child or allow a cooling-off period by sending the parent and child back to the waiting room to recover. In reality, you are working to a tight schedule, and regrettably, you may have no alternative but to do a 'go-for-it' examination with the crying child held firmly by an adult. But a warning – avoid ensuing kicks!

Practical Exercise

Examine as many patients as possible. Select a wide range of shapes, sizes and ages. Ask your tutor or other doctors to show you any patients with abnormal ears.

How to use urine and blood dipsticks

Dipstick analysis is an example of 'near-patient' or 'point-of-care' testing performed on urine or blood samples using commercially available disposable reagent strips or kits, and can be done conveniently in a surgery consultation, on a home visit, or on samples left in the surgery. The dipstick method allows results to be used in immediate management decisions. Tests are cheap, simple to use, and save time for both the doctor and the patient compared with sending a patient or sample for hospital testing. However, dipsticks using blood samples are not as accurate as laboratory analysis.

Advances in technology have led to the development of a range of equipment for surgery-based laboratory tests, for example full blood counts and blood chemistry. The equipment requires regular servicing for reliability and calibration to maintain quality control.

Clinical indications for dipstick analysis

Urine

- Screening for urinary proteinuria as found in nephrotic syndrome and nephritis, or for glycosuria as in diabetes (Multistix, Diastix).
- Diagnosis of urinary tract infection, using dipstick urine analysis to detect nitrites, leucocytes and blood (Uristix, Multistix).
- Checking diabetic control through the detection of glycosuria, ketonuria (Multistix, Ketostix, Keto-Diastix).

Blood

- Testing for random or fasting blood sugar (BM-Stix, Glucotide).

How do dipsticks work?

- Test strips are made of disposable plastic with attached reagents that change colour when the substance to be tested is present in the sample. There may be one or several tests combined on each strip.
- In the diagnosis of a lower urinary tract infection, urine bacteria reduce nitrate to nitrite and are detected by the nitrate reductase test. Pus cells in the urine are detected by the leucocyte esterase test.
- In screening for and managing diabetes, the glucose test is based on a double sequential enzyme reaction involving the oxygenation of glucose to gluconic acid and hydrogen peroxide by a catalyst (glucose oxidase). A second enzyme (peroxidase) catalyses the reaction of hydrogen peroxide with a potassium iodide chromogen to produce colours ranging from green to brown.
- Ketone testing is based on the reaction between acetoacetic acid and nitroprusside to produce colours changing from buff pink, indicating a negative result, to maroon, if positive.
- BM-Test 1–44 is based on the glucose reaction described above.

What you will need

- Reagent stick with the associated reagent bottle and colour-coding strip.
- Patient sample container (e.g. for urine).
- A lancet for obtaining a blood sample from the patient.
- A watch or timer that measures in seconds.

Procedure for testing urine

Each test includes simple instructions as outlined.

1. Obtain the urine test sample from your patient. A sample may be passed into any clean receptacle. However, if in addition to dipstick testing a midstream urine specimen is to be sent to the bacteriology laboratory, the sample must be passed into a sterilized bottle and a small volume used separately for the dipstick test.
2. Select the appropriate reagent. Check the expiry date on the unopened bottle; if expired, discard. Sticks should be used within six months of first opening the bottle.
3. Collect a fresh sample as described above.
4. Remove one strip from the reagent bottle and replace the cap on the bottle, noting the time required for the dipstick reading. Hold the plastic end of the strip.
5. If the sample is to be sent for bacteriological culture, the urine should be dripped from the urine container onto the test stick over a sluice or tray, otherwise you will contaminate the urine by dipping the stick into the sample. Note the time with a second hand immediately after testing the sample.
6. After the stated time, read the strip by visually matching the colour on the stick to the colour on the bottle.
7. Record the results in the patient's notes.
8. Dispose of the sample in the lavatory or sluice, not the washbasin used for hand washing – this would compromise hygiene.
9. Wash your hands after completing the test.

Procedure for testing blood

Obtain a blood sample by puncturing a finger or the ear lobe with a lancet, and applying pressure to obtain a drop of blood that is allowed to drip onto the surface of the analysis strip.

Getting the best from BM-test 1–44

Good technique is essential in obtaining accurate results. It is important to follow **all** the instructions below, **carefully**

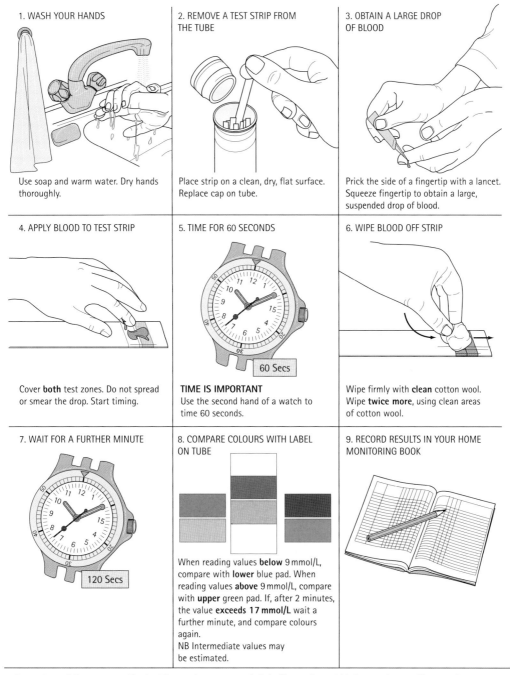

1. WASH YOUR HANDS	2. REMOVE A TEST STRIP FROM THE TUBE	3. OBTAIN A LARGE DROP OF BLOOD
Use soap and warm water. Dry hands thoroughly.	Place strip on a clean, dry, flat surface. Replace cap on tube.	Prick the side of a fingertip with a lancet. Squeeze fingertip to obtain a large, suspended drop of blood.
4. APPLY BLOOD TO TEST STRIP	5. TIME FOR 60 SECONDS	6. WIPE BLOOD OFF STRIP
Cover **both** test zones. Do not spread or smear the drop. Start timing.	**TIME IS IMPORTANT** Use the second hand of a watch to time 60 seconds.	Wipe firmly with **clean** cotton wool. Wipe **twice more**, using clean areas of cotton wool.
7. WAIT FOR A FURTHER MINUTE	8. COMPARE COLOURS WITH LABEL ON TUBE	9. RECORD RESULTS IN YOUR HOME MONITORING BOOK
	When reading values **below** 9 mmol/L, compare with **lower** blue pad. When reading values **above** 9 mmol/L, compare with **upper** green pad. If, after 2 minutes, the value **exceeds 17 mmol/L** wait a further minute, and compare colours again. NB Intermediate values may be estimated.	

Remember... Take your record book with you when you attend clinic. The results could help your doctor achieve good control of your diabetes.

Figure 4.19 Patient instruction sheet on how to use a glucose test strip on blood samples.

Each test kit has instructions written on the side and an enclosed instruction sheet. It is important to follow all instructions carefully to avoid faulty results (Figure 4.19).

Practical points

- Always check the expiry date on the reagent bottle – out-of-date sticks give unreliable readings. When first opening a bottle, write the date on the side and discard after six months.
- Because dipstick tests are not as reliable as laboratory analyses, they should not be used alone for diagnosis. They supplement a high diagnostic index of suspicion from the history and examination.
- Read the strips in good lighting. If the colour falls between two colours, take an in-between estimate.
- False-positive and false-negative readings occur, but are uncommon because the enzymatic methods are chemically specific and quite sensitive. High levels of vitamin C may cause false negatives in the Clinistix and Diastix methods, whereas reducing sugars, such as lactose, fructose and galactose, drugs such as aspirin, tetracycline, cephalosporins and nalidixic acid, and detergents may cause false positives.
- Does colour blindness affect the interpretation of these strips? This may be the case if you have a red/green or mixed colour vision deficiency, and the interpretation of a glucose test strip in this case is unreliable. Blue/yellow defects have little effect on interpretation of the strips. If in doubt, check your colour vision with the Ishihara test. Colour blindness also has implications for self-testing for patients, especially diabetics.

Practical Exercise

- ❏ Sit in the diabetic clinic and test blood and urine samples with available test strips. You will note a wide range of positive readings. For blood sugar, how do the stick readings compare with results from the glucose meter?
- ❏ Sit in a screening or well-person clinic or a general surgery and test samples with dipsticks.

How to use a mini-peak flow meter

Portable mini-peak flow meters are used to diagnose and monitor obstructive airways disease, for example asthma, chronic bronchitis and emphysema. Several models are available, but the most commonly used is the portable mini-Wright peak flow meter. This is a reliable and cheap method of measuring airway obstruction, and is as essential to monitoring of chronic respiratory problems as the sphygmomanometer is to blood pressure. Available on prescription, the meters allow patients to participate in home monitoring. Meters are calibrated in low ranges for use with children.

Background knowledge

Expiratory flow can be measured using the maximum peak expiratory flow rate (PEFR) or the forced expiratory volume in 1 second (FEV_1). The meter measures the maximum flow of exhaled air in a forced expiration to give a PEFR. Changes in chronic bronchitis and asthma increase airways resistance and produce a fall in PEFR. This can be monitored in the surgery with the mini-peak flow meter, although very sensitive changes will only be detected by more sophisticated spirometry. The PEFR and FEV_1 are similar but not identical physiological measures. FEV_1 is measured on a maximally forced expiration using a spirometer and is a more accurate measure of lung function than a peak flow meter. The FEV_1 is disproportionately reduced in patients with airway obstruction. Fixed large airway obstruction is seen most easily in a graph of flow against volume (Figure 4.20). The diagnosis of asthma is made by establishing

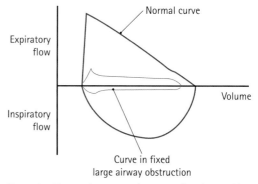

Figure 4.20 Flow–volume curve in a normal patient and in one with fixed large airway obstruction.

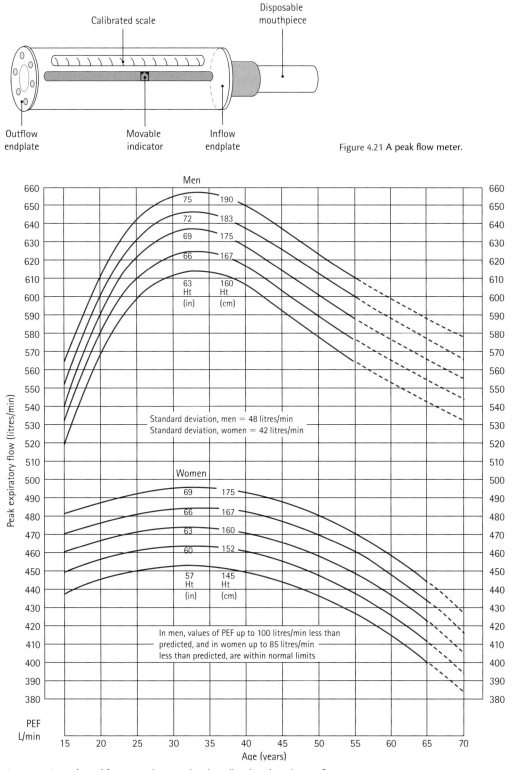

Figure 4.21 A peak flow meter.

Figure 4.22 A graph used for comparing actual and predicted peak expiratory flow rates.

reversibility of airways obstruction in response to a bronchodilator.

What you will need

- Mini-peak flow meter (Figure 4.21).
- A disposable cardboard mouthpiece or plastic mouthpiece that has been disinfected.
- A chart to show normal peak flow readings (Figure 4.22).

Using a peak flow meter involves two steps: demonstrating the use of the meter and teaching your patient how to use the meter (Figure 4.23). The second skill is an extension of the first and is not quite as straightforward as you might think.

Tutor quote

A third-year medical student was asked by his tutor if he knew how to use the peak flow meter. 'Certainly', he replied. 'I've had asthma since I was 7 years of age and often use one.' His demonstration involved three separate steps. 'Stand up, take a deep breath and blow as fast as you can down the tube, like this.' He was then asked to explain to a patient with asthma how to use the meter in preparation for home monitoring. He was surprised that the patient was unable to reproduce his three-stage skill in a way that was reliable. Teaching the same technique and checking the patient's understanding took 11 steps (as described below).

Procedure

1. Explain to your patient the importance of measuring the breathing capacity of the lungs, showing the mini-peak flow meter.

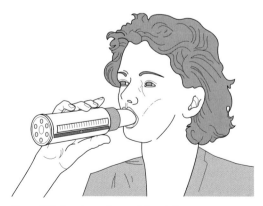

Figure 4.23 A patient using a mini-peak flow meter.

2. Select two separate disposable or sterilized plastic mouthparts and insert one into the meter. This will be your demonstration model. The other will be for your patient.
3. Stand up and demonstrate in slow motion how to use the mini-peak flow meter.
4. With one hand, hold the meter in the horizontal position, ensuring the indicator is free to move. Explain the requirement to take as deep a breath as possible and to hold it. Place your lips over the outside edge of the mouthpiece as if pouting, making a seal between the tube and the lips.
5. Breathe out down the mouthpiece as fast and as forcefully as possible, allowing the indicator to move as far as possible. It is not necessary to continue exhaling until the residual volume is reached, since the peak flow occurs at the start of the process. Repeat this procedure twice more, returning the needle to zero after each attempt, and take the best of three readings as the PEFR.
6. Return the needle to zero.
7. Remove your mouthpiece and replace with the patient's. Hand the meter to the patient.
8. Ask the patient to stand and repeat the demonstration three times, checking technique and returning the indicator to zero after each attempt.
9. Take the maximum recording in litres per minute.
10. Use the peak expiratory flow chart (see Figure 4.22) to plot this value on the ordinate against your patient's age on the abscissa. Determine your patient's predicted PEFR for age and gender on the height curve. Compare the actual with the predicted PEFR and express as a percentage.
11. Enter readings in the patient's record. There is usually a separate asthma file for monitoring long-term treatment.

Practical points

- Hygiene: disposable mouthpieces are preferable, but if plastic models are used, they must be disinfected for each patient.
- Under-recording occurs if air leaks around the mouthpiece. It is therefore important to check that the lips are sealed on the outside of the

tube. Lips may be wrongly positioned inside the mouthpiece.

- Air escapes down the nose, causing under-recording. You can use a nose clip if this is a problem.
- The handgrip impedes the movement of the indicator. Reposition the grip on the meter.
- Poor respiratory effort or low-force blowing causes under-recording. This is more likely in patients who are older or who have a painful chest wall, for example broken or bruised ribs.
- Use of a spitting action down the mouthpiece will move the indicator further than if the flow meter is used correctly. This gives an artificially high reading.

Practical Exercise

Investigate the effects of exercise on PEFR of yourself or a colleague.
- ❑ Take a baseline reading with the mini-peak flow meter.
- ❑ Exercise vigorously for at least 6 minutes, for example by running up and down stairs or in a nearby park. When you feel out of breath, take another reading. Is there any difference? If the post-exercise reading is reduced, is this significant? What criteria would you use for the diagnosis of asthma?

For further reading, see Rees *et al.* (2010).

Skills used in clinical management and treatment

Intradermal, subcutaneous and intramuscular injections

Injections given in general practice are most commonly by the intramuscular or deep subcutaneous route, although occasionally intradermal or intra-articular routes are used. Most vaccines are given by intramuscular or deep subcutaneous injection. Local anaesthetic for minor surgery is given subcutaneously. Injections are sometimes required on emergency home visits to control distressing symptoms, for example a patient with intractable vomiting may be managed with an intramuscular injection of an anti-emetic drug such as prochlorperazine.

Background knowledge

A knowledge of surface landmarks, skin structure and the anatomy of muscles is essential if injections are to be given safely. Be aware of the positions of important structures which, if traumatized with the injecting needle, could be irreparably damaged or result in serious complications such as haemorrhage.

Intramuscular sites

Thigh (Figure 4.24)

Lateral and antero-lateral aspects are formed by the vastus lateralis or rectus femoris muscles, two

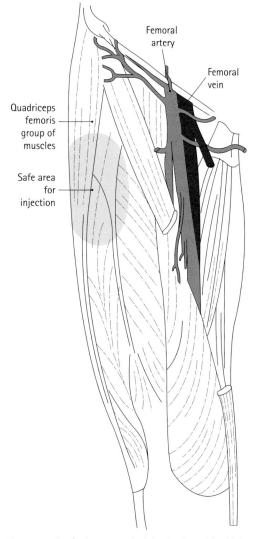

Figure 4.24 Site for intramuscular injection into right thigh (anterior view).

of the four components of the quadriceps femoris muscle (others are the vastus medialis and vastus intermedius), the main extensor muscle of the leg. Inject into the antero-lateral aspect of the thigh into the vastus lateralis or rectus femoris.

■ *Dangers*: avoid the femoral artery and vein (which lie immediately medial to the rectus femoris), and the branch nerve to the vastus medialis.

Buttock (Figure 4.25)

The 'safe' area for injection is the upper, outer quadrant of the buttock. The anatomical contour is formed by the gluteus muscles (maximus, medius, minimus, arising from the posterior gluteal line of the ilium and iliac crest), the natal line and the lateral surface of the greater trochanter. The landmarks are: the iliac crest superiorly, posterior superior iliac spine supero-medially, ischial tuberosity infero-medially and greater trochanter of femur laterally.

■ *Dangers*: sciatic nerve, located inferiorly to two imaginary lines: (i) from posterior superior iliac spine to greater trochanter, (ii) from iliac crest to ischial tuberosity.

Upper arm (Figure 4.26)

The safe area for injection is the deltoid muscle. This forms the contour of the upper arm. The deltoid originates from the anterior aspect of

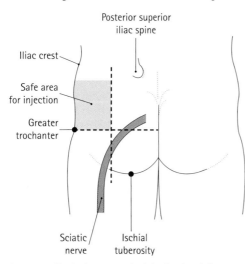

Figure 4.25 Site for intramuscular injection into left buttock (posterior view).

the lateral third of clavicle, the acromion and the spine of scapula and is inserted into the deltoid tuberosity on the lateral side of the shaft of the humerus.

■ *Dangers*: anterior branch of axillary nerve (supplies deltoid muscle), which winds posteriorly around the surgical neck of the humerus, below the capsule of the joint, approximately 6–8 cm below the bony prominence of the acromion.

What you will need

■ Syringe of suitable size: 1 mL, 2.5 mL or 5 mL, depending on the volume to be injected.
■ Needle of suitable size: 21G (green) or 23G (blue) for intramuscular or subcutaneous injections. For intradermal injections, a 25G needle (orange) should be used.
■ Cotton-wool swab.
■ Ampoule of drug to be given.
■ Elastoplast.
■ Sharps box: this is a plastic box, usually yellow, for the safe disposal of needles and syringes.

Choosing the site for an intramuscular injection

Choice of an intramuscular site is a personal decision for the clinician when injecting adults. In infants the antero-lateral aspect of the thigh or the upper arm is recommended. Injection into the fatty tissue of the buttock has been shown to reduce the efficacy of hepatitis B vaccine.

Needle orientation

The needle orientation for intradermal, subcutaneous and intramuscular injections is shown in Figure 4.27.

Procedure for an intramuscular injection

Practise first on models. An old orange or grapefruit is suitable, as the consistency of the peel resembles human skin. Take care to dispose of the fruit after your session to avoid poisoning your colleagues!

1. Before you start, check your equipment. Check the name and dose of the drug on the ampoule. Double-check and, if possible, treble-check with a third-party professional such as a nurse to confirm the drug and

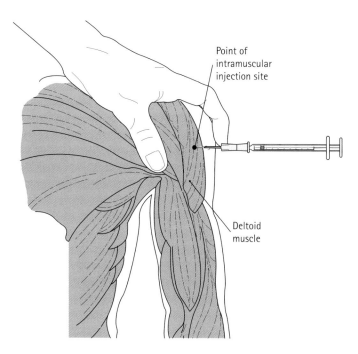

Point of
intramuscular
injection site

Deltoid
muscle

Figure 4.26 Site for intramuscular
injection into the upper arm
(anterior view).

dose. Time spent checking may save much anguish for the patient, relatives and doctor and minimize the risk of litigation.

2. Wash your hands. Use of protective gloves is essential as a precaution against contamination with blood or other body fluids.

3. Draw up the drug into the syringe in the following way. Tap the top of the glass ampoule, or flick your finger against the side, causing the contents to run into the base. Snap the top of the ampoule at the neck. Usually a mark on the neck indicates the point at

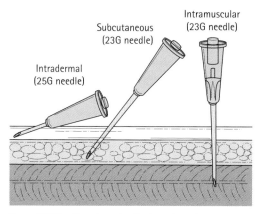

Intramuscular
(23G needle)

Subcutaneous
(23G needle)

Intradermal
(25G needle)

Figure 4.27 Needle orientation for intradermal, subcutaneous and intramuscular injections.

which the glass will fracture most easily. With the needle tip positioned below the surface of the solution, draw up the contents into the syringe by pulling back the plunger. Tilt the ampoule initially to avoid withdrawing air, returning to a vertical position towards the end of the withdrawal process. Upturn the syringe and tap the side to allow air bubbles to coalesce. Advance the plunger to expel air bubbles. The solution should be correctly drawn up and ready for injection.

4. Select the injection site and proceed as follows.

5. Prepare your patient: explain the procedure, stressing that pain will be minimal.

6. Position your patient according to the chosen injection site. For the buttock: lay your patient in the prone position (face down). For the arm: seat your patient with his or her arm relaxed at the side. If you inject in the standing position, it could be traumatic if the patient faints. For the thigh: ask your patient to lie on one side or stand, leaning over a couch with the thigh exposed.

7. Assess the distance between skin and muscle by gently pinching the skin at the point of planned entry and assessing the depth of subcutaneous fat.

8. You are now ready to give the injection. Hold the syringe between the fingers of your dominant hand. Steady the skin at the planned injection site by making it taut.

9. Using a single puncture entry point, advance the needle with the bevel uppermost through the skin at an angle of 90 degrees (Figure 4.28). The needle will pass through the underlying structures of the superficial fascia, deep fascia and into the muscle. Each tissue has a characteristic tension. The depth will depend on the size of the patient and the site. Withdraw the plunger of the syringe to check that blood is not aspirated. If it is, the needle tip may be in a blood vessel, in which case the needle should be withdrawn until no further blood is obtained on withdrawing the plunger.

10. Advance the plunger, emptying the contents into the muscle. Withdraw the needle rapidly. Dispose of the syringe and attached, uncapped needle into the sharps bin. You should not try to re-cap the needle because if you miss, you may have a needlestick injury. If the needle has to be re-capped, for example during a home visit, do so with the cap lying on a surface in the horizontal position, and insert the needle into the cap.

11. Enter details of the injection in the patient's records, to include name of drug, dose, method and site of injection, manufacturer's number from the side of the ampoule and date of expiry.

Procedure for a subcutaneous or intradermal injection

For a subcutaneous injection, follow the above procedure, except that the entry approach of the needle should be at an acute angle of approximately 45 degrees, with the bevel uppermost (see Figure 4.27). The needle is advanced through the epidermis and dermis into the subcutaneous tissue, where the injection is given. For an intradermal injection, the needle approach is an acute angle of about 10 degrees to the skin, with the bevel uppermost (Figure 4.29). When the needle is positioned in the dermis, the solution is injected, and will cause the overlying skin to form a raised area. This disappears as the injected solution is absorbed.

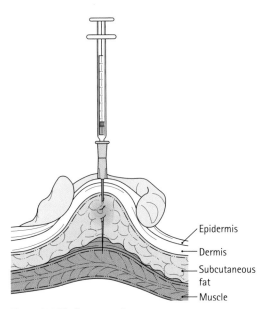

Figure 4.28 The intramuscular route.

- Epidermis
- Dermis
- Subcutaneous fat
- Muscle

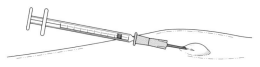

Figure 4.29 The intradermal route.

Practical points

- Contrary to expectation, it is less painful to use a wider bore needle than the finest available. Can you think of an explanation? The pressure exerted through a fine-bore needle is higher than through a larger bore needle in order to deliver the same volume of injectable material. This higher pressure is more painful.

- Should you use an alcohol swab to clean the skin at the injection site? Nowadays, alcohol swabs are considered unnecessary, although you may wish to use a dry cotton-wool swab to apply pressure to the entry point if bleeding occurs.

- How should you remove air trapped in the syringe? Do so by upturning the syringe with the neck uppermost and tapping on the syringe side. Bubbles of air will coalesce, move to the top and escape.

- If you are unable to break the neck of the ampoule, use a small metal blade to etch a scratch at the neck. The glass will usually break at this point.

- If you have a blood spillage, follow the procedure described in the section 'How to take a blood sample'. If you have a needlestick injury, report this to your tutor or trainer and follow the standard workplace procedure.
- After some injections, commonly immunizations, a small hard nodule persists at the injection site for 2–3 weeks. This is harmless and will resolve.
- Could your patient faint?

Student quote

'The first time I gave an injection I was quite nervous, but not, it seemed, as nervous as my patient! First, my tutor made me practise on a grapefruit. Quite simple! Then, the nurse introduced me to Mr W. She ran through the procedure and, as a routine precaution, showed me the resuscitation tray, pointing out the adrenaline syringe to use in the event of anaphylaxis from a severe allergic reaction. She told me this was so rare that she had never seen a case. I reassured my patient that the injection would not hurt, although he did tell me he occasionally felt queasy at the sight of needles. Everything went well until I withdrew the needle. My patient collapsed across the couch. He turned ghostly pale. It occurred to me he might have "dropped dead", although having never witnessed that, I wouldn't have known. My next thought was that he was in anaphylactic shock but the nurse made no move to grab the resuscitation tray. I somehow felt everything would be all right because she was there. She turned my patient on to his back, placed his legs on the couch, and as he opened his eyes she said, 'Just a little faint, Mr W. Take some deep breaths. Can I get you a cup of tea?' What a relief!'

How to syringe an ear

The purpose of syringing an ear is to remove wax or cerumen that is blocking the external auditory meatus, causing pain or hearing impairment. Cerumen is produced by the ceruminous glands of the outer third of the meatus as a waxy protective substance. Wax production is variable and the wax is normally expelled by chewing movements. However, sometimes this process does not occur and the accumulating wax blocks the meatus. It is easier to remove wax that has been softened with oil for 7–14 days prior to syringing. Olive or almond oil is recommended, although some patients prefer an over-the-counter proprietary preparation.

Background knowledge

The anatomy of the ear has been described (see Figure 4.15).

Syringing should be performed with water at or slightly above body temperature (37–38°C). Water warmed or cooled to more than 7°C above or below body temperature will stimulate the labyrinthine system by creating a convection current in the endolymph. This will stimulate the sensorineural epithelium within the ampulla of the horizontal semicircular canal and cause nystagmus (repetitively jerking eye movements), associated with a sensation of imbalance, vertigo and nausea. Patients find these symptoms extremely unpleasant. They are, however, put to good effect when assessing labyrinthine function in a procedure known as the 'caloric test' used in ear, nose and throat departments.

What you will need

- Auriscope and specula.
- Ear syringe with set of nozzles (hand-driven or electric model).
- Collecting dish or receptacle.
- Towel or waterproof cape to place around the patient's neck.
- Water source.
- Water container (reservoir box with electric model; jug with manual model).

About the equipment

Ears can be syringed using an electric pump or a manually operated model. The manual syringe is more cumbersome to use than the electric model and causes soreness and fatigue of the fingers from repeated movements of the plunger. There is also an increased risk of perforating the tympanic membrane. For these reasons, the electric pump is now the preferred method for ear syringing with the manual syringe being increasingly obsolete. However, in the event of equipment or power failure, and in preparation for different styles of practice, both methods are described.

Procedure

1. Take a history of previous ear problems. Has your patient had a chronic ear discharge, a perforated eardrum, or any ear operations, particularly a mastoidectomy for disease within the mastoid cavity? If there is any possibility of a perforated tympanic membrane, do not syringe, because of the risk of introducing infection into the middle ear or damaging the ossicles.
2. Examine your patient's ear to confirm the presence of wax.
3. Explain the procedure to your patient, emphasizing that you should be informed if dizziness occurs.
4. Position your patient on a chair with the ear to be syringed facing you and the head tilted slightly away from you (Figure 4.30). Place a towel or waterproof cape around your patient's neck and shoulders. Decorative earrings should be removed.
5. Ask your patient to hold the receptacle below the ear to be syringed, pushing it against the skin to prevent water dripping down the neck.

Using the electrical ear syringe

1. Plug in the electric pump and turn on the power (Figure 4.31). Fill the reservoir of the syringe pump with tap water at body temperature or slightly higher, 38°C is ideal. Normal saline or sodium bicarbonate can be used instead of water.

2. Select a suitably sized nozzle for your patient and attach it to the syringe handle.
3. Turn on the water supply through the nozzle by switching the control dial on the pump to the 'on' position and adjusting the pressure control dial. Test the flow of water through the nozzle with the stream directed into a sink or receptacle. The flow should be moderately gentle and not too ferocious. Practise controlling the water flow by depressing and releasing the button on the handle of the syringe.
4. Position the spout of the nozzle in the auditory canal with the tip facing upwards and backwards, while simultaneously applying traction

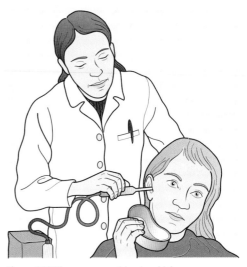

Figure 4.30 The correct position in which to use an ear syringe.

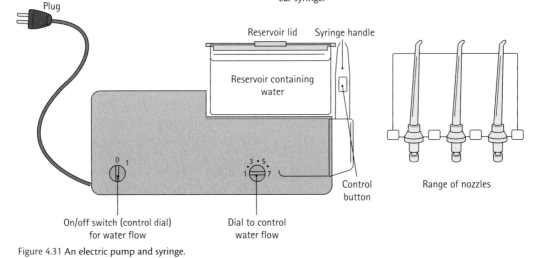

Figure 4.31 An electric pump and syringe.

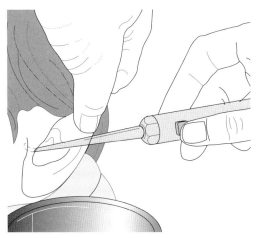

Figure 4.32 The pinna being pulled up and back to straighten the external auditory meatus.

on the auricle in an upwards and backwards direction (Figure 4.32).

5. Direct the flow of water gently towards the roof of the auditory canal. At first, water will be deflected by the wax and run out of the ear into the receptacle, but as wax is displaced, water should flow along the roof of the auditory canal and track around the wax deposit (Figure 4.33).

6. As you continue syringing, flecks of yellow–brown wax will appear in the water. These will become larger, until a single or several larger chunks of wax appear, indicating success removal of all the wax. When you stop syringing, the patient may express delight that hearing has returned. With the auriscope, check whether the meatus is clear. If you can see the tympanic membrane, stop syringing; if not, continue, refilling the reservoir with water as necessary. Examine the ear periodically until the wax has been cleared.

7. Dry the meatus by mopping excess water with gauze or cotton wool. A wet meatal lining predisposes to infection of the external canal and can cause otitis externa (infection of the outer ear canal).

8. Finally, clean the instruments. Wipe the nozzle with gauze or tissue paper, and detach and place in chlorhexidine sterilizing solution. Clean wax out of the auriscope speculum and place in the same solution for 20–30 minutes. Allow to dry thoroughly before re-using to minimize bacterial contamination from the patient's ear.

Using the manual ear syringe

The same principles apply if using the manual ear syringe (Figure 4.34). The models are made of stainless steel and each is supplied with a set of metal nozzles that, unlike the plastic nozzles, are not angled. A jug is used as a water reservoir for filling the syringe; tap water is acceptable.

1. Select a suitably sized metal nozzle and attach to the neck of the syringe.

2. Screw the base with fixed grip rings to the barrel end. By placing your index and middle fingers in the base rings and your thumb in the plunger ring, you will be able to move the plunger relative to the barrel. Check that

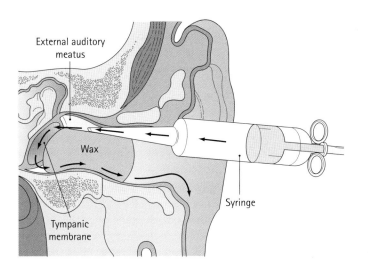

External auditory meatus

Wax

Tympanic membrane

Syringe

Figure 4.33 The direction of water flow in the external canal.

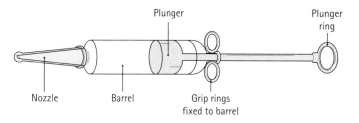

Figure 4.34 A manually operated ear syringe.

the syringe plunger moves freely inside the barrel. Wetting the plunger with tap water or smearing Vaseline on the plunger head will facilitate this movement. Leave in the closed (pushed-in) position.

3. Fill the reservoir jug with tap water at body temperature. Gauging the temperature with your own hand is sufficient, although testing with a thermometer will check accuracy.

4. Position the tip of the nozzle below the surface of the water in the reservoir. Using your dominant hand, place the index finger in the plunger ring. Using your non-dominant hand to grasp the barrel, withdraw the plunger. This will draw up water into the barrel of the syringe. Avoid air entering the barrel. When full, hold the syringe horizontally to minimize leakage.

5. Change your handgrip on the syringe, placing your thumb in the plunger ring and your index and middle fingers in the barrel rings. This frees the non-dominant hand.

6. Advance the nozzle into your patient's external auditory meatus while simultaneously, with your non-dominant hand, applying traction to the auricle in an upwards and backwards direction to straighten the auditory canal.

7. Advance the plunger into the barrel by moving the handle towards the barrel base, approximating the thumb, index and middle fingers. This movement empties the barrel of water. Direct the flow into the auditory meatus towards the roof of the canal.

8. When you have emptied the syringe, withdraw it. Examine the canal with the auriscope to check for persistence of wax.

9. Continue this process of filling the barrel with warm water and syringing the ear until the wax has cleared. This may take as many as 8–12 syringefuls.

10. Dry the canal by mopping with gauze or cotton wool.

11. Clean the syringe with alcohol, particularly the nozzle. Allow it to dry thoroughly before using it on the next patient.

Practical points

- It is essential to use water at body temperature to avoid an attack of caloric-induced vertigo.
- Keep an eye on the water level in the patient-held receptacle. You may be so engrossed in the syringing that you fail to notice that the receptacle has overflowed, with the consequent soaking of you and your patient!
- With the electric model, remember to turn off the water flow in the nozzle when inspecting the ear. If you do not, a jet of water will shoot across the room, targeting anyone in its path, including your tutor or the practice nurse!
- When you have successfully unblocked the ear, your patient may remark about the sudden loudness of noise, especially high-frequency sounds. This abnormal sensitivity to sounds is known as hyperacusis, and will settle after several minutes.

Patients will often warn you when syringing their ears that water is almost certain to shoot out of the opposite ear! This intimation of lack of cerebral content is a joke enjoyed throughout the world. Such hyperbole should not be dismissed without considering the care needed to avoid perforating the tympanic membrane during the syringing process. How could this happen? It is less likely with electric syringes because the angulation of the nozzle tip diverts water away from the tympanic membrane. With the hand syringe, however, unless the stream is directed posteriorly along the roof of the auditory meatus, it is possible for water to impinge on the tympanic membrane with sufficient force that it causes a perforation.

How to take a blood sample (venepuncture)

Venous blood is used for most pathology testing; arterial blood is used for the measurement of blood gases; capillary blood from superficial sites such as the ear lobe for blood sugar; and heel prick samples in neonates for screening of phenylketones. Blood samples are normally taken from the plexus of veins in the antecubital fossa.

The process of taking blood from veins is called venepuncture or phlebotomy and the technician trained to undertake this procedure is a phlebotomist. In the UK, it is now standard practice in hospital and general practice to use a vacuum system (Vacutainer) in which blood flows directly from a vein into a closed tube. This minimizes the risk of contamination from patients' blood.

The use of protective gloves

It is important to take precautions to minimize the risk of contamination of yourself and the immediate environment, such as work surfaces, particularly with hepatitis B and C viruses and human immunodeficiency virus (HIV). When taking blood you should wear protective disposable gloves. Even if you consider a patient to be in a low-risk category for transmissible disease, you can never be sure, as described in the following incident.

Tutor quote

A doctor had a needlestick injury after injecting the shoulder of an 84-year-old patient. She thought this would be of little consequence as the patient was 'low-risk' status. However, the patient had been transfused 8 pints of blood during a hip replacement operation some years ago. As this was immediately prior to the appearance of acquired immunodeficiency syndrome (AIDS), the laboratory had followed her up as a high-risk patient, testing her several times for HIV. Fortunately, all tests were negative and the doctor concerned was hepatitis B immune, having been previously immunized.

'High-risk' patients include those who are:

- known or suspected of being hepatitis B surface antigen (HBsAg)-positive,
- intravenous drug abusers,
- exhibiting high-risk behaviour for HIV,
- on haemodialysis,
- suffering from acute and/or chronic liver disease,
- institutionalized or have Down's syndrome.

All medical students, medical staff and medical personnel who have direct contact with patients or who handle blood products should be immunized against hepatitis B, and should have their hepatitis B immune levels checked one month after completing the primary immunization course. Current guidelines recommend a single booster dose of vaccine every 5 years after the primary course. Medical staff on units where invasive procedures are undertaken (e.g. obstetrics, surgery) may be required to have hepatitis C and HIV testing.

Anatomy

Figure 4.35 shows the superficial veins of the upper limb.

What you will need

- A pair of protective disposable gloves.
- A tourniquet: usually an elasticated strip with fastening buckle, or a length of rubber tubing.
- Vacutainer system: needle 21G (green), needle holder, blood collection tubes.
- Pathology request forms.
- Sealable plastic specimen bag with absorbent pad in case of spillage.
- Soft ball or other object for patient to grip (optional).
- A sharps bin: this is a yellow plastic bin with a white swing-top opening into which are disposed needles or other equipment such as syringes that have been in contact with blood or body secretions. These bins are collected by the Clinical Waste Collections Service in Britain and are incinerated according to the recommendations of the Committee on Substances Hazardous to Health.

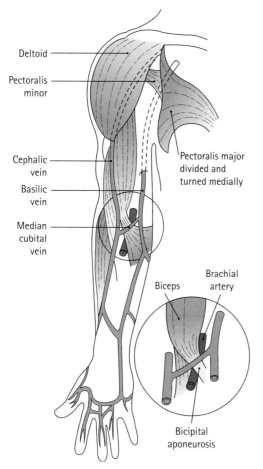

Figure 4.35 The superficial veins of the upper limb (anterior view).

■ For the traditional method: disposable sterile propylene syringe and capped metal needle.

Taking blood with the Vacutainer system

The Vacutainer system is shown in Figure 4.36.

Procedure (Figure 4.37)

1. Explain the procedure to your patient.
2. Select the blood sample bottles for the tests, checking that the labels are blank. The volume of blood required for each test is indicated on the bottle label.
3. Check the request form has been completed.
4. With your patient sitting, select the arm for taking blood, preferably their non-dominant side or the arm closest to a supporting surface. You may support the arm on a small supporting pillow. Apply the tourniquet to the patient's upper arm, about 10 cm above (proximal to) the elbow. The tourniquet should compress the veins but not be so tight distally that the arterial circulation is obstructed. The pulse should be palpable distally. With the arm extended and supported, ask the patient to clench the fist or grip a soft object. This helps to make the veins more prominent. Select a vein for venepuncture in the antecubital fossa. If the veins are compressed for longer than 3 minutes, the results of blood tests may be invalid. If this is the case, release the tourniquet for a few minutes and reapply prior to taking the blood samples.
5. Put on a pair of suitably sized disposable gloves.

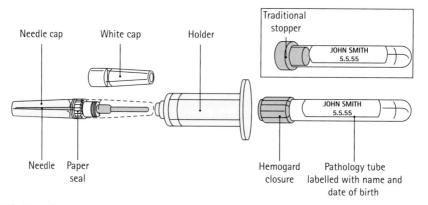

Figure 4.36 The Vacutainer system.

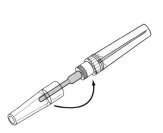

1. Check paper seal is intact as proof of sterility. If seal is broken, **DO NOT USE.** Holding the coloured section of the needle shield in one hand, twist and remove the white section with the other hand **AND DISCARD.**

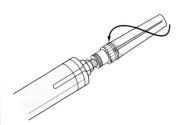

2. Screw needle into holder. Leave coloured shield on needle.

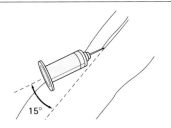

3. Prepare venepuncture site. Remove the coloured section of needle shield. Perform venepuncture in the usual manner with the arm in the downward position.

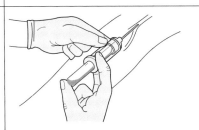

4. Introduce the tube into the holder. Placing your forefinger and middle finger on the flange of the holder and the thumb on the bottom of the tube, push the tube to the end of the holder, puncturing the diaphragm of the stopper. Remove the tourniquet as soon as blood begins to flow into the tube.

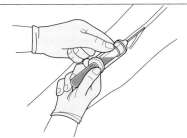

5. When the vacuum is exhausted and blood flow ceases, apply a soft pressure with the thumb against the flange of the holder to disengage stopper from the needle and remove the tube from holder. If more samples are required repeat from step 4.

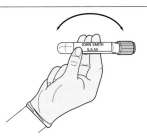

6. While blood is flowing into succeeding tubes, gently invert previously filled tubes containing additives 8 to 10 times to mix additives with blood. Do not shake. Vigorous mixing may cause haemolysis. Remove last tube from the holder before withdrawing needle from vein.

> **Dispose of needles in accordance with local Control of Infection Protocols.**
> **Used needles are dangerous; be safe not sorry.**

Figure 4.37 How to take blood with the Vacutainer system.

6. Select a 21G needle, checking that the paper seal is intact as a sign of sterility. If the seal is broken, discard the needle into the sharps bin. Holding the coloured section of the needle in one hand and the white section in the other hand, twist and remove the white cap and discard.

7. Screw the needle into the holder, leaving the coloured shield on the needle. Remove the cap from the needle. Approach the patient's arm with the needle bevel facing upwards. With the needle and Vacutainer at an angle of approximately 15 degrees from the surface, puncture the skin and advance the needle about 1 cm through the skin and into the vein. You risk perforating the opposite wall of the vein if you advance the needle too far.

8. Introduce the sample tube into the holder. With your forefinger and middle finger astride the base of the holder, place your thumb at the end of the tube and exert steady pressure, pushing the tube towards the end of the holder until you have punctured the stopper at the end of the tube. As soon as blood flows into the tube, remove the tourniquet.

9. Allow the tube to fill to the required level. Apply gentle pressure with your thumb against the base of the holder, and remove the tube and stopper from the needle. When the vacuum is exhausted, the blood flow stops.

10. For further samples, substitute the remaining tubes using the same technique: first tubes without additives, next coagulation tubes, and finally tubes with additives. The latter should be gently inverted about eight to ten times to allow mixing with the blood. Do not shake, as this may cause haemolysis of the blood.

11. When the last tube has been removed from the holder, withdraw the needle from the patient's vein. Apply a steady pressure, or ask the patient to apply pressure over a cotton-wool swab at the puncture site with the elbow extended for 1–2 minutes. Discard the swab into a clinical waste container. If the puncture site is oozing blood, apply a small plaster. Flexing the arm as a method of applying pressure may lead to bruising at the venepuncture site.

12. Dispose of the needle and the needle holder directly into the sharps bin (Figure 4.38) without re-capping. If there is no sharps bin, for example when on a home visit, re-cap the needle by placing the cap on a flat surface and directing the needle into the cap in the same plane. In this situation, an empty soft drinks can makes a good temporary container, and can be disposed of later with clinical waste at the surgery.

13. Label the sample tubes with a ballpoint pen, completing the patient's details. Include full name, date of birth, and other information requested. Ask the patient to confirm these details. Place the samples in a plastic, self-sealing transport bag. These usually have a pouch separate from the sample compartment for request forms and a paper pad to absorb any blood spillage. Blood from a high-risk patient should be labelled 'high-risk', and this should be indicated on the request form.

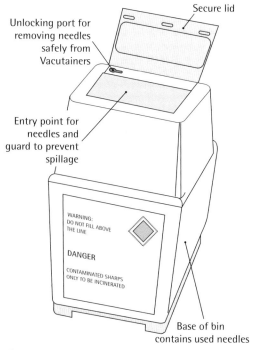

Figure 4.38 A sharps bin for the safe disposal of contaminated needles.

Practical points

- *What if I do not obtain sufficient blood?* An under-filled tube may invalidate the test result. Tubes should always be correctly filled according to volume indicated on the label.

- *How do I know if the needle is in a vein?* As soon as you push the pathology tube onto the holder, if the needle is in the vein, blood will flow immediately. If nothing happens, draw the needle back slightly and if you subsequently enter the vein blood will appear.

- *How do I know whether the vacuum in the sample tube has been lost?* As long as the needle remains under the skin, the vacuum is maintained. If the needle slips outside the skin, the vacuum is lost and you must use a new tube.

- *What should I do if the vein collapses?* Remove the tube, leaving the needle in place in the vein. When the pressure returns in the vein, insert a new tube.

- *What if the veins are too difficult to enter?* This happens with obese patients or patients with sclerosed veins from repeated phlebotomies, intravenous drug use or intravenous treatments such as chemotherapy. After two or three unsuccessful attempts to collect blood, it is advisable to send the patient to the hospital phlebotomy service. Winged blood collection sets with thinner gauge needles and multiple sample adapters for connection to a Vacutainer holder are available in hospitals.

- *What if I puncture the opposite wall of the vein?* A bruise (haematoma) may form at the puncture site. You may have already obtained your sample; if not, it may be possible to continue the phlebotomy. After withdrawal of the needle, the patient should raise the arm above shoulder height, which will cause the veins to collapse and prevent further bleeding into the tissues.

- *What if I spill blood on myself or the immediate environment?* Wash the blood off your exposed areas with soapy water and an alcohol solution (70 per cent) if available. Use sodium hypochlorite solution 10 000 ppm (bleach, Milton) to wipe down contaminated surfaces and leave in contact for 30 minutes. Report any spillage or accidents involving blood or other body fluids to the practice nurse, sister in charge or occupational health officer.

Note. A video recording of phlebotomy will give you a better overview. A copy may be obtainable from your local hospital phlebotomy department.

Taking blood using the traditional needle and syringe

Taking blood with the traditional needle and syringe is done less often nowadays because use of a Vacutainer reduces risk of contamination. It is sometimes necessary to use the traditional method, for example, on a home visit when no Vacutainer is available, or on Elective. The patient is prepared as described above.

1. Protective gloves must be worn.
2. Select a pre-packed, sterile, disposable needle (size 21G) and propylene syringe of sufficient volume for the blood tests (10 or 20 mL). Remove from the packaging.
3. Attach the needle to the syringe. Check the plunger of the syringe can be withdrawn.
4. With the plunger in the closed (pushed-in) position, remove the cap from the needle.
5. Apply a tourniquet as above. Steady the selected vein by applying pressure with your non-dominant hand to the antecubital fossa. With the needle bevel uppermost, puncture the skin over the vein and advance the tip into the vein along its longitudinal axis for about 1 or 2 cm and stop.
6. Steady the syringe against the patient's arm with your non-dominant hand and slowly withdraw the syringe plunger with your dominant hand. Blood should enter the barrel of the syringe. Withdraw the required volume as indicated on the sample tube.
7. Release the tourniquet. Quickly withdraw the needle and attached syringe as an entire unit from the patient's arm. Apply pressure with a cotton-wool swab to the puncture point, with the patient's arm extended as described. Transfer the blood sample into the laboratory sample bottle by inserting the needle through the rubber stopper of the tube. If a Vacutainer tube, the blood will transfer by pressure effect, if not, advance the syringe plunger to transfer blood to the level indicated on the tube label.

Practical points

- If there is insufficient blood for the test, and you need a further sample, it is preferable to re-puncture the patient than disconnect the needle from the syringe in situ and replace with another syringe. Only in extreme circumstances should this be considered, for example in emergencies or when vein availability is poor. This procedure will always result in contamination with blood.
- Surfaces contaminated with blood should be cleaned with sodium hypochlorite.

Special communication skills

How to write a referral letter

Communicating information about patients to health professionals is integral to clinical practice. In general practice, patients with continuing problems may be managed by teams of healthcare professionals based in both primary and secondary care. When a GP involves another professional in patient care – whether for an opinion, transferring clinical responsibility, for investigation, reassurance or management – it is essential to transfer clear information. Conversely, the same applies when a specialist communicates with a GP.

Although informal referrals can be made by telephone or face-to-face contact, for operational reasons and for record-keeping purposes written referrals are accepted practice. In the UK many letters are now transferred electronically via a secure hospital–general practice website to the referring specialist unit using a central electronic appointments system which forwards the referral to the specialist clinic and sends the patient an appointment.

Some hospital and community services prefer referrals using a specialist referral proforma or form with direct entry of patient data onto the proforma. This is easier if the proforma is incorporated into the electronic patient record. Examples include specialist palliative care, psychological therapies and suspected cancer with an option of an urgent referral on a 'two week' fast track system. Most referrals, however, require a personal letter by the GP and so the art of letter writing continues to be an important skill.

Writing clear and concise referral letters needs a great deal of practice. The process involves abstracting information from personal knowledge of the patient and their health record, and presenting this as a logical summary. The letter should have maximum impact in as short a space and time as possible. Time constraints are relevant for both the specialist and the GP. If the letter is too long, the specialist may not have time to read it.

Although everyone has a personal writing style, a few rules should be observed.

- Write in clear, coherent sentences, expressing the problems as accurately and succinctly as possible.
- Use short words and phrases, rather than long words and rambling sentences.
- Use simple language, avoiding colloquialisms. It is acceptable to use the patient's expressions when describing the presentation.
- Avoid medical jargon, for example use 'breathing' not 'pulmonary ventilation'.
- Avoid abbreviations: not everyone understands them.
- Typed letters are required for electronic transfer. Handwritten letters must be legible.

Practical Exercise

Part 1. Think of a patient you have seen with your tutor who needs referral to a specialist. Imagine you are the specialist and have just received the letter. What information would you need from your tutor to allow you to respond appropriately to the request for help? Jot down the information points before continuing with this section. Write a model referral letter for your tutor. Stop here, and attempt to write your letter before reading on. Your outline should have included the following:

- ❏ *Patient details*: name, age, sex, National Health Service (NHS) number, ethnic background, hospital number if you have one recorded for the patient.
- ❏ *Details of GP*: name, address, telephone number and these days perhaps email address.

❏ *Reason for referral*: what help is the GP requesting? What question is being asked of the specialist?

❏ *Degree of urgency for appointment*: state if an urgent appointment is indicated.

❏ *Clinical condition*: important clinical and previous history.

❏ *Findings on physical examination*: include key points and significant positive and negative findings that support your diagnosis or reason for referral.

❏ *Findings on investigation*: results should be included or attached electronically.

❏ *Medication and drug sensitivities.*

❏ *Psychosocial history*: include this if it is likely to help the specialist's management; for example if an elderly patient lives alone, include details of the living arrangements and key carer.

❏ *Explanation given to the patient about the condition and the reason for referral*: this is helpful if the diagnosis may involve breaking bad news, for example if a diagnosis of cancer is likely.

❏ *Expected outcome of the referral.*

❏ *Desirable follow-up*: indicate whether you are expecting the patient to be returned to your care as soon as possible, or prefer the specialist to provide on-going management.

Part 2. Now check your referral letter using the above outline. If you have omitted vital information, amend your letter. Check its suitability and format with your tutor. If your tutor agrees, you could have the letter typed, ready to send to the specialist, remembering that your tutor will need to sign it. When your tutor receives a reply, ask if you may see the letter. Did the specialist interpret the letter correctly? Were all the questions answered? Have you learnt anything from the reply?

Part 3. Recent guidelines for good clinical practice have recommended that patient referral letters from GPs to specialists and replies from specialists to referring GPs should be copied to patients. This has been introduced in some areas.

❏ Can you list at least five benefits to patients of receiving copies of letters?

❏ What factors would a doctor need to take into account in the style and content of the letter?

❏ Are there issues of confidentiality to be addressed in introducing this practice?

How to sign a Medical Certificate of Cause of Death (death certificate)

Background knowledge

When a patient dies, there is a standard procedure for registering the death and for arranging burial. It is a time of personal distress for the deceased's family, and the role of the family doctor is to provide support and guidance to the family. Further information for the family can be accessed on a government website (Directgov, 2010). Before a death can be reported in England and Wales, there must be either a Medical Certificate of Cause of Death, commonly referred to as a death certificate or, if the death was unexpected, a certificate from a coroner after appropriate investigations into the cause of death have been made. A coroner is a lawyer or doctor responsible for investigating deaths.

It is the statutory duty of a registered medical practitioner to complete a death certificate stating to the best of his or her knowledge and belief the cause of death. The certificate is a legal document. If a doctor gives a cause of death that he or she knows to be untrue, charges of perjury (i.e. false declaration) may follow.

If the death was expected and the patient died of natural causes, the procedure is as follows.

1. *Confirmation of death* of the patient by an examining doctor, who may be the patient's medical practitioner or an on-call doctor.

2. Arrangements for *removal of the body* by a funeral director (undertaker) to a funeral parlour. The deceased's family or representative is responsible for deciding on a funeral director.

3. The provision of a *Medical Certificate of Cause of Death* that states the cause of death. This is signed by the attending doctor and is provided free of charge. It must be delivered

to the Registrar of Births and Deaths in the sub-district where the deceased lived. It is the responsibility of the doctor who signs the death certificate to deliver it in person or by post to the local Registrar of Births and Deaths. In most instances however, the doctor arranges for this to be done by an informant of the deceased, usually a relative. A list of eligible persons who can act as informants is given on the reverse of the formal notice of death on the medical certificate.

4. The provision of a formal notice of death entitled *Notice to Informant*. This is attached to the Medical Certificate of Cause of Death as a 'tear-off' section, and is completed by the doctor who signs the death certificate. It is provided free of charge.

5. If cremation is to take place, the provision of a *Cremation Certificate*, signed in two parts by two doctors who practise independently of each other, one of whom will have signed the death certificate (cremation forms 4 and 5). There is a fee for the certificates unless the death is referred to a coroner who provides a certificate for cremation without charge.

If the death was unexpected, or the patient died of unnatural or suspicious causes (see below), the procedure is as follows.

1. *Confirmation of death* by an attending or on-call doctor.

2. Reporting the death to the local *Coroner's Office* by the attending or emergency doctor. If there are suspicious circumstances, the doctor must inform the police. Where there are doubts, the doctor should discuss details with the coroner who has the discretion to decide whether it is permissible to provide a death certificate or to proceed with a post mortem.

3. *Removal of the body* to a mortuary: the Coroner's Office will make arrangements for this.

4. Investigation into the *cause of death* by the coroner, who will provide the necessary certification. An inquest may be necessary to determine the cause of death. Doctors must cooperate fully with any formal inquiry into the treatment of the patient, and not withhold relevant information.

Unnatural or suspicious causes of death must be referred to the coroner and include a death:

- which was violent, unnatural or occurred under suspicious circumstances,
- for which the cause is unknown or uncertain,
- which occurred while the patient was undergoing an operation or before full recovery from an anaesthetic, was related to anaesthesia, or followed a fracture or fall,
- caused by an industrial disease or industrial poisoning,
- which occurred as a result of a medical procedure or treatment, or from a termination of pregnancy,
- which may have been due to lack of medical care or where there were allegations of medical mismanagement,
- where the deceased was not attended by a doctor during the terminal illness or was not seen during the last 14 days of life,
- which occurred as a result of self-neglect or neglect by others,
- which occurred in prison or in police custody.

The Medical Certificate of Cause of Death

This may be the first time as a student or a Foundation Year doctor you are observing the completion of a death certificate in general practice. A book of Medical Certificates of Cause of Death (Form 66) will be kept in the practice and is supplied by the Registrar General through the local Registrar of Births and Deaths. The same form is used in hospitals and the community for all deaths occurring after the first 28 days of life. A different form is used for the deaths of live-born children occurring before 28 days. The Births and Deaths Registration Act of 1953 requires the form to be completed and signed by the medical practitioner who attended the patient during his or her last illness and saw the patient in the last 14 days of life. The certificate has to be accepted by the Registrar of Births and Deaths. If the certificate has not been completed accurately or is unsatisfactory it cannot be accepted.

Procedure

1. Are you eligible to sign the death certificate? If so, you will be registered with the General

Medical Council (GMC) either provisionally as a pre-registration doctor (FY1) or with full registration (FY2). You will have attended the deceased in his or her final illness and have seen the patient in the last 14 days of life. It is not a requirement for you to have seen the body after death. This is necessary only if you sign the cremation certificate.

2. The book of Medical Certificates of Cause of Death (Figure 4.39) is prefaced by a section called Medical Certificate of Death – notes for doctors. This covers your duties as a medical practitioner, completion of personal details about the patient, the circumstances of certification, when to refer to a coroner, the cause of death statement, and any employment-related deaths.

3. You should ask yourself: Do you know the cause of death? Do you feel confident that death was due to natural causes? If 'yes', you may sign the death certificate. Handwrite in ink the following where requested: the full name of the deceased, the date of death as stated to you, the age of the deceased, the place of death and the date when last seen alive by you.

4. If you do not know the cause of death, or did not attend the patient in the last 14 days of life, or you consider that the death was due to violence or unnatural causes, or was a sudden death of unknown cause, you must notify the local Coroner's Office immediately. This includes deaths of patients who sustained a fracture, had an accident or an operation, or had not recovered sufficiently from an anaesthetic. In these circumstances, you should not complete the death certificate.

5. You are next asked to circle an appropriate digit or letter in two lists: confirmation by post-mortem examination and a statement that the deceased person was seen or not seen after death. For information about post mortem, you should indicate one of four options: (1) whether the cause of death takes account of information obtained from post mortem, (2) whether information from post mortem may be available later, (3) a post mortem is not

being held, or (4) you have reported the death to the coroner. Information about whether the deceased was seen after death offers three options: (a) that you as signatory saw the body, (b) that another medical practitioner saw the body, or (c) that the body was not seen after death by a medical practitioner. If you have reported the death to the coroner for further action, you should initial Statement A on the reverse of the form.

6. The next section asks for details of the cause of death. It is completed in two parts: Part I covers the condition(s) leading to the cause of death, and Part II asks for information on other significant conditions contributing to the death but not related to the disease. Part I may confuse even the most experienced doctor. The form asks for the 'underlying cause of death' to be completed in I(c) and the disease or condition directly leading to death in I(a). You are asked to indicate at I(b) any other condition, if any, leading to I(a). The 'underlying cause of death' is the disease or injury that initiated the series of morbid events that led to the death. In I(a) you are asked for the disease, injury or complication causing death and not the mode of death, as in asphyxia. If two conditions have contributed to the death, both causes should be written on the certificate. An example is 'I(a) Chronic bronchitis, coronary atheroma'. If you are awaiting further information for confirmation of cause of death, such as a histology report, you should initial Statement B on the reverse of the form.

7. On the right-hand side and opposite the section 'Cause of Death', you will notice a box in which you are asked to state the approximate interval between the onset of each condition listed and death. For example:

I(a) Myocardial infarction   5 days
I(b) Coronary atheroma   5 years
I(c) Influenza   2 weeks
II Chronic bronchitis   18 years

8. Below the section 'Cause of Death' is a box in which you are asked whether you believe the death may have been due to or contributed to by the employment followed at some

COUNTERFOIL

For use of Medical Practitioner, who should complete in all cases.

Name of deceased ....

Date of death ....

Place of death ....

Age ....

Place of death ....

Last seen alive by me } ....

Post-mortem† *   1   2   3   4
Coroner

Whether seen after death*   a   b   c

Cause of death:—

I   (a) ....

     (b) ....

     (c) ....

II ....

Employment? [ ] *Please tick where applicable*

B. Further information offered?

Signature ....

Date ....

Ring appropriate digit(s) and letter.

Register to enter No. of Death Entry [ ]

BIRTHS AND DEATHS REGISTRATION ACT 1953

(Form prescribed by the Registration of Births, Deaths and Marriages (Amendment) Regulations 1985)

MEDICAL CERTIFICATE OF CAUSE OF DEATH

For use only by a Registered Medical Practitioner WHO HAS BEEN IN ATTENDANCE during the deceased's last illness, and to be delivered by him forthwith to the Registrar of Births and Deaths.

Name of deceased ....

Date of death as stated to me .... day of .... 19 ..... Age as stated to me ....

Place of death ....

Last seen alive by me .... day of .... 19 .....

1   The certified cause of death takes account of information obtained from post-mortem.

2   Information from post-mortem may be available later.

3   Post-mortem not being held.

4   I have reported this death to the Coroner for further action.

Please ring appropriate digit(s) and letter

a   Seen after death by me.

b   Seen after death by another medical practitioner but not by me.

c   Not seen after death by a medical practitioner.

[See overleaf]

CAUSE OF DEATH

The condition thought to be the *Underlying Cause of Death* should appear in the lowest completed line of Part I.

These particulars not to be entered in death register

Approximate interval between onset and death

I(a) Disease or condition directly leading to death† ....

(b) Other disease or condition, if any, leading to I(a) ....

(c) Other disease or condition, if any, leading to I(b) ....

II Other significant conditions CONTRIBUTING TO THE DEATH but not related to the disease or condition causing it. ....

The death might have been due to or contributed to by the employment followed at some time by the deceased. Please tick where applicable [ ]

†*This does not mean the mode of dying, such as heart failure, asphyxia, asthenia, etc: it means the disease, injury, or complication which caused death.*

I hereby certify that I was in medical attendance during the above named deceased's last illness, and that the particulars and cause of death above written are true to the best of my knowledge and belief.

Signature ....

Qualifications as registered by General Medical Council } ....

Residence .... Date ....

For deaths in hospital: Please give the name of the consultant responsible for the above-named as a patient. ....

(Form prescribed by the Registration of Births, Deaths and Marriages Regulations 1968)

NOTICE TO INFORMANT

I hereby give notice that I have this day signed a medical certificate of cause of death of

....

Signature ....

Date ....

This notice is to be delivered by the informant to the registrar of births and deaths for the sub-district in which the death occurred.

The certifying medical practitioner must give this notice to the person who is qualified and liable to act as informant for the registration of death (see list overleaf).

DUTIES OF INFORMANT

Failure to deliver this notice to the registrar renders the informant liable to prosecution. The death cannot be registered until the medical certificate has reached the registrar.

When the death is registered the informant must be prepared to give to the registrar the following particulars relating to the deceased:

1. The date and place of death.

2. The full name and surname (and the maiden surname if the deceased was a woman who had married).

3. The date and place of birth.

4. The occupation (and if the deceased was a married woman or a widow the name and occupation of her husband).

5. The usual address.

6. Whether the deceased was in receipt of a pension or allowance from public funds.

7. If the deceased was married, the date of birth of the surviving widow or widower.

THE DECEASED'S MEDICAL CARD SHOULD BE DELIVERED TO THE REGISTRAR

A

I have reported this death to the Coroner for further action. ....

Initials of certifying medical practitioner. ....

The Coroner needs to consider all cases where:

The death might have been due to or contributed to by a violent or unnatural cause (including an accident);

or   the cause of death cannot be identified;

or   the death might have been due to or contributed to by drugs, medicine, abortion or poison;

B

I may be in a position later to give, on application by the Registrar General, additional information as to the cause of death for the purpose of more precise statistical classification. ....

Initials of certifying medical practitioner. ....

or   there is reason to believe that the death occurred during an operation or under or prior to complete recovery from an anaesthetic or arising subsequently out of an incident during an operation or an anaesthetic;

or   the death might have been due to or contributed to by the employment followed at some time by the deceased.

LIST OF SOME OF THE CATEGORIES OF DEATH WHICH MAY BE OF INDUSTRIAL ORIGIN

MALIGNANT DISEASES	Causes include:	INFECTIOUS DISEASES	Causes include:
(a) Skin	– radiation and sunlight – pitch or tar – mineral oils	(a) Anthrax	– imported bone, bonemeal, hide or fur
(b) Nasal	– wood or leather work – nickel	(b) Brucellosis	– farming or veterinary
(c) Lung	– asbestos – nickel – radiation	(c) Tuberculosis	– contact at work
		(d) Leptospirosis	– farming, sewer or under-ground workers
(d) Pleura	– asbestos	(e) Tetanus	– farming or gardening
(e) Urinary Tract	– benzidine – dyestuff – chemicals in rubbers	(f) Rabies	– animal handling
(f) Liver	– PVC manufacture	(g) Viral hepatitis	– contact at work
(g) Bone	– radiation	BRONCHIAL ASTHMA AND PNEUMONITIS	
(h) Lymphatics and haematopoietic	– radiation – benzene	(a) Occupational asthma	– sensitising agent at work
POISONING		(b) Allergic Alveolitis	– farming
(a) Metals	e.g. arsenics, cadmium, lead	PNEUMOCONIOSIS	– mining and quarrying – potteries – asbestos
(b) Chemicals	e.g. chlorine, benzene		
(c) Solvents	e.g. trichlorethylene		

NOTE:—The Practitioner, on signing the certificate, should complete, sign and date the Notice to the Informant, which should be detached and handed to the Informant. The Practitioner should then, without delay, deliver the certificate itself to the Registrar of Births and Deaths for the sub-district for the sub-district in which the death occurred. Envelopes for enclosing the certificates are supplied by the Registrar.

PERSONS QUALIFIED AND LIABLE TO ACT AS INFORMANTS

The following persons are designated by the Births and Deaths Registration Act 1953 as qualified to give information concerning a death:—

DEATHS IN HOUSES AND PUBLIC INSTITUTIONS

(1) A relative of the deceased, present at the death.

(2) A relative of the deceased, in attendance during the last illness.

(3) A relative of the deceased, residing or being in the sub-district where the death occurred.

(4) A person present at the death.

(5) The occupier* if he knew of the happening of the death.

(6) Any inmate if he knew of the happening of the death.

(7) The person causing the disposal of the body.

DEATHS NOT IN HOUSES OR DEAD BODIES FOUND

(1) Any relative of the deceased having knowledge of any of the particulars required to be registered.

(2) Any person present at the death.

(3) Any person who found the body.

(4) Any person in charge of the body.

(5) The person causing the disposal of the body.

**"Occupier" in relation to a public institution includes the governor, keeper, master, matron, superintendent, or other chief resident officer.

Figure 4.39 Medical Certificate of Cause of Death.

time by the deceased. It does not ask you to provide details, only to tick the box and report to the coroner. Details of the categories of death that may be of industrial origin are given on the reverse of the death certificate and in fuller detail at the back of the certificate book. However, you should have medical confirmation that this is the case because the coroner will ask you to submit a medical report. In the event of a suspected industrial disease, there will probably be an inquest.

9. Sign and date the form, certifying that you were in attendance during the deceased's last illness and that the details on the form are true to the best of your knowledge and belief. You are asked to give your qualifications as registered by the GMC, and to state your residence: this means the general practice address, not your home address.

10. Complete the counterfoil adjacent to the Medical Certificate of Cause of Death that asks for a copy of the details on the medical certificate.

11. Finally, you should check whether the back of the certificate form needs to be completed: Box A that you have reported the death to the coroner; Box B that you may be in a position later to provide the Registrar General with additional information as to the cause of death for statistical purposes.

Practical points

■ A symptom or a mode of dying, such as heart failure, is not acceptable as a cause of death. The underlying disease must be stated.

■ When recording a tumour, you should state the histology and whether benign or malignant.

■ Avoid the word 'accident', as in 'cerebrovascular accident', as this alarms relatives and implies violence. Instead you are advised to use 'stroke'.

■ Avoid ambiguous statements such as the cause of death was 'old age'. The registrar has a list of accepted causes of death and if your stated cause of death is not included on the list, the registrar is required to notify the coroner. This may cause distress to the relatives and it would have been more considerate to discuss the wording with the Coroner's Office first.

Communicating with relatives

It is good practice to see or telephone the deceased's next of kin to explain the details on the death certificate and to enquire about who will be the informant. This contact provides an opportunity for relatives to ask questions about the cause of death and for you to clarify concerns. You should check that the informant knows what to do with the death certificate and the Notice to Informant. It is also an opportunity to enquire about the relatives' health and to offer support. Finally, thanking or commending the family if they have provided care will assist the bereavement process and will be appreciated.

How to consult with special age groups (children and elderly people)

Consulting with patients at the extremes of age requires an adaptation of your approach with adults. Though separated by an age span of several decades, there are similarities in history taking when consulting with infants and elderly people who depend on others for part or all of their care. With both groups, communication involves a third party – babies with their parents or guardian, elderly dependent people with a relative or other key person with caring responsibilities. The sharing of information takes place as a trio of doctor, patient and informant. Even if your patient cannot talk, you can establish rapport non-verbally through eye contact, by touching, miming or writing if the patient can read. Use information gleaned from observing your patient, interaction with the carer and the home environment to supplement your history. The malodours of an incontinent patient, young or old, are distinctive. A healthy baby with normal muscle tone handles differently from the acutely ill, floppy child. Nurses in close contact with immobile elderly patients describe how they intuitively 'feel' their patient's condition; for example patients with a stroke and disabling loss of speech (aphasia/dysphasia) may offer greater than normal resistance to being positioned if suffering pain.

Consulting with infants and elderly people requires special skills, which you will develop with experience.

Consulting with children

General approach

- Every child has the right to be treated as an individual with particular needs and potentialities.
- Every child has the right to have his or her wishes taken into account, and the right to speak and be listened to.
- It is the duty of professionals to take account of age, sex, health, personality, race, culture and life experiences when planning services for children (Children Act, United Kingdom 1989).

These principles underpin the approach to managing children. Whatever a child's age, each consultation is a partnership between the child, the child's parent(s) or guardian(s) and the doctor.

Children's personalities, behaviour and ability to communicate vary widely and are dependent on their stage of development, cultural background, education and understanding. In addition, children and their parents may have unpredictable responses to illness. Parents often seem unduly upset and communicate a great deal of anxiety when their children are ill, to a degree which may appear disproportionate to the child's state of health. With the intense early bonding between parents and babies, it is emotionally disturbing to observe a previously responsive child deteriorate and, furthermore, frustrating when a child is unable to describe symptoms. Parents have an innate fear of losing a child – a fear that may be fuelled by sensationalist reporting in the media, particularly during epidemics. In addition, parents may be exhausted through disturbed sleep in caring for their child, leaving them emotionally vulnerable. These factors need to be considered when consulting with parents and children. Each consultation should be handled sensitively and with an individual approach tailored to the needs of each situation.

Children and babies are particularly changeable. They may appear ill one moment and bouncing with energy the next. They may be fractious in the consulting room and difficult to talk to, or be so excited when visiting the surgery that they show a dramatic improvement. Parents will often say that the child 'just wasn't like that when I left home. He's proving me a liar!' Remember, however, that parents are the experts in their child's health, and are the most qualified to give an accurate description of their child, even if not confirmed in the surgery. Communicating with children calls for patience and flexibility. Praising good behaviour throughout the consultation encourages cooperation.

As children grow older, communication patterns with parents and people in authority change in a complex way that reflects their move towards independence. While some teenagers appear to be forthcoming in the consultation, others may display a grudging resentment, play a manipulative 'game' with their parents or doctor, or be overwhelmed by anxiety and embarrassment, especially if asked about personal matters or required to undress. All this is a normal part of growing up and needs to be allowed for in the consultation by offering an explanation for the reasons for your questions or examination. The age at which teenagers prefer to consult alone varies according to the nature of the presenting symptom, the degree of maturity and the relationship with their parents and doctor. Over the age of 16, teenagers have legal responsibility for their personal medical care. Despite this, many prefer to be accompanied in the consultation. To respect confidentiality, teenagers should be given the opportunity to talk alone when accompanied. Older children are quick to identify adults as patronizing through what might be misinterpreted glances of disapproval or comments. For this reason, it is advisable to avoid personal comments or passing judgement.

Practical tips

- Greet your young patient by name in a friendly way, introduce yourself and explain where he or she should sit.
- Observe the child's behaviour and interaction with his or her parents and with yourself as you bring the family into the consulting room. This will provide useful information before you begin the consultation. Is the child shy, avoiding eye-to-eye contact, hiding behind or clinging to the parent, or is the child friendly, confident and chatty from the start? Nowadays, children are drilled into not talking to strangers so that, if this is your first contact, the child will probably appear unfriendly while at the same time recognizing your tutor as familiar.

To understand how to respond to such a typical child, it will help to consider the impact of entering your consulting room.

Thinking and Discussion Point

- Spare a thought for the child. Imagine yourself as a small person in a grown-up world. Think of how the doctor and the consulting room would appear to you, looming at your small feet as you walk in through the door, holding the hand of a towering adult. Literature affords many illustrations of disproportionate sizing – *Alice in Wonderland*, *Gulliver's Travels* and *Mrs Pepperpot*!

- Show restraint. Children need time to adjust to 'strange' people seated in what appears to be a vast room dominated by intriguing instruments and computers. At first, avoid overwhelming the child with personal comments or by being over-friendly, as this approach may be rejected and the child may burst into tears rather than reciprocate. While initially greeting the child by eye contact and name it may be preferable to initially focus attention on the parents and allow the child time to absorb the surroundings. Once you have passed the test of acceptability, your small patient may begin to relate, and you can then shift the consultation from a two-way to a three-way exchange.

- Physical contact. It is sometimes tempting to pick up babies, but they may sense unfamiliarity and not settle. Parents may also object if you treat their baby as a cuddly toy. Unless they ask you to help by holding their baby, or you wish to examine the baby, it is advisable to leave the infant undisturbed in the parent's arms. Likewise, with older children it is best to avoid physical contact unless they spontaneously climb onto your lap. Exceptionally, parents may misinterpret contact as manhandling of their child rather than an expression of your goodwill.

- Diversions. Toys help divert attention and encourage a child to settle into the consultation. Children usually prefer to discover toys alone rather than having them thrust into their hands. A nearby box or surface with a small number of toys appropriate for a range of ages may tempt. When examining a child, diversionary games such as 'peek-a-boo', demonstrating examination on a doll or teddy or, if none is available, on a parent will reassure and encourage cooperation. Sometimes the whole consultation has to be turned into one big game in order to obtain the necessary information and enlist cooperation, but this is often hard work and time consuming.

History taking and examination of a child

Having settled the family group into the consulting room, you can proceed with history taking. The use of open questions helps to identify the parent's expectation from the visit early on in the contact. The age when a child is sufficiently mature to give a reliable history varies, but may be around 7–10 years, although the child may not share the parents' concern about his or her medical condition. With a younger child, questions should be directed towards the parent, while allowing the child to contribute spontaneously. It is wise to cross-check the child's information with the adult and, conversely, to check the adult's information with the child.

It is acceptable to examine children in an opportunistic way rather than follow a systems procedure, particularly when time is limited. You may be able to examine more thoroughly if the child is cooperatively sitting or lying on the parent's knee than if distressed lying on an examination couch. If you need to examine the ears or chest, do so first, because once a child starts to cry these procedures will be difficult. Procedures that may be uncomfortable, for example inspecting the mouth or taking blood, should be left to the end of the examination.

A common difficulty is knowing how to express to a child the parents' concern without making the child feel ashamed or guilty. It is best to address the problem and the parents' anxiety directly, while involving the child in the decision-making process. For example with a 7-year-old child who is bed-wetting (nocturnal enuresis): 'Charlie, mum is worried about you wetting the bed at night. Many children do this at your age. They can't help it. One day you will grow out of it; it will stop and everything will be all right. Because it's a lot of work for mum to wash the sheets, shall we see if we can find someone to help you get dry?'

Practical Exercise

During your time in general practice, try to gain experience in taking histories from the following groups:

❑ a parent/parents and baby aged under 12 months,
❑ a parent/parents and toddler aged 1–3 years,
❑ a parent/parents and primary school child aged 3–11 years,
❑ a parent/parents and pubertal child aged 12–15 years,
❑ an adolescent consulting alone.

Compare the contributions made by the child towards the consultation at each age.

Thinking and Discussion Point

Taking histories from this age group allows you to assess your attitude towards older people. Do you regard them with:

☐ Affection as you would your grandparents or an aunt or uncle?
☐ Respect or fear because of their great age, wisdom and dignity?
☐ Curiosity as a source of history pre-dating your own existence?
☐ Frustration because speech and hearing loss prevent effective communication?
☐ Contempt because they have no role in life, may be unkempt, incontinent or grumpy?
☐ Disdain because they appear old-fashioned, speaking and dressing differently from you?

If 'ageism' is defined as prejudice or discrimination against people of a certain age, consider how the outcome of a consultation with an older patient may be influenced by the negative views of the interviewer.

Consulting with older patients

Most older people take care of themselves, plan their own lives and make their own decisions. However, a small proportion suffer from serious conditions such as strokes or Alzheimer's disease, which have such a devastating effect on their life that they need help to cope with everyday needs. For some, communication is made difficult by deafness, speech disorders or memory impairment.

At times you may experience some negative feelings when communicating with older people. Negative feelings must be addressed, even in the most adverse circumstances, for example when visiting a neglected person in distressingly dirty conditions. It helps to understand why people live in this state. What are the medical circumstances? What were this person's previous personality and lifestyle? How can their quality of life be improved despite having an irreversible medical condition? Whatever the patient's state, courtesy is essential. Older patients dislike being patronized, but they may be too courteous to tell you.

The question of whether to address an older patient by first name or surname with title sometimes arises. Although you may feel rapport would be established more quickly by using first names, most older people believe the use of surnames is a mark of respect. If in doubt, the use of names should be discussed with your patient. What is important is that both you and your patient feel at ease.

Observation provides clues about communication difficulties. Spotting a hearing aid may prompt you to adjust your voice, but if you do this check that the patient can hear before proceeding with the interview. A patient with a hemiplegia may have visual loss on one side (hemianopia), and you may need to change position if your patient is to see you.

A keen eye during home visits may supplement your history taking and provide valuable information about a patient's social circumstances. Is the house clean or cluttered? How do the relatives and patient interact? Are there signs that the patient is not coping with everyday activities?

Communicating with patients with limited or no English

The UK population is increasingly cosmopolitan and multi-racial. Patients with limited or no English are more likely to present in metropolitan and tourist areas. Patients with language difficulties represent a range of circumstances: people working on secondment from overseas, migrant workers from abroad seeking short-term employment, refugees or asylum seekers, holiday visitors, relatives visiting families in the UK, and indigent families whose first language is not English and whose English is limited. All groups are entitled to registration with a GP. Holiday visitors register temporarily with the NHS if their country of origin has reciprocal arrangements with the UK, or privately if this is not the case. Refugees are entitled to the full range of NHS healthcare services free of charge and are encouraged to have permanent registration with a GP.

Communicating with patients with limited English is difficult, and can lead to misunderstanding and frustration for healthcare professionals and patients. In addition, patients may not understand the UK healthcare system, and may originate from a country where expectations and experience of medical care differ from those in the UK, for example, direct access to specialist rather than GP care.

It is important for healthcare professionals who consult with patients with limited or no English to understand the cultural differences and the patient's expectations. Tolerance of cultural and racial diversity is essential for making effective contact. This is particularly so for refugees and asylum seekers, who may have difficulty accessing healthcare and communicating needs. Refugees represent diverse populations including those applying for refugee status, allowed temporary admission to the country while immigration status is considered, or with the right to stay indefinitely. Refugees are a vulnerable group because many have health problems that are complicated by personal and psychological distress arising from torture, separation from their families, loss of status, poverty and the 'cultural bereavement' of leaving their country of origin.

If receptionists identify patients with language difficulties on first contact, special arrangements can be made. They can book to see a doctor who speaks the same language, if available; it can be arranged for an accompanying friend or relative to act as interpreter; or they can be offered a professional interpreter in person or from a telephone interpreting service. In addition, patients may belong to an ethnic group that states a preference to consult with a doctor of the same gender. Muslim and Hindu women prefer a woman doctor when consulting with gynaecological problems, and this request should be respected.

For reasons of confidentiality, patients should be offered the choice of a professional, a relative or a friend as interpreter. However, use of a close family member as an interpreter raises confidentiality issues and may not be in the patient's or relative's best interests. The use of children may pose particular problems, as patients may need to discuss sensitive topics of a sexual or personal nature or, in the case of refugees, discussion may be around brutality or torture in their persecuting country and may be upsetting.

How are interpreting and translating services used?

Although the terms 'language interpretation' and 'translation' are often used interchangeably, by definition *interpretation* refers to the spoken language and *translation* to the written language. In the UK, professional interpreters are pre-booked for the patient's appointment time using a telephone interpretation service (such as Language Line Services) which has available at short notice professionally trained interpreters in up to 170 languages. These interpreters are proficient in their language and have a general knowledge and familiarity with the culture of that language. The service is remunerated on a pro-rata hourly rate by the NHS. In addition most GPs in the UK also have access to a translation service and a web-based sign and language support (SignTranslate, 2010). This service offers registered practices access to British Sign Language interpreters who can communicate with deaf patients if the practice has webcam facilities.

If no interpreter is available, or the patient is seen without forewarning of language difficulties, communication may need to be non-verbal, using facial expression, miming or drawing. Although this may establish rapport with the patient and address basic needs, it is an unsatisfactory and unreliable way to conduct a consultation.

Consulting through an interpreter is difficult, time consuming and stressful for the doctor within the constraints of short consulting times in general practice. The logistics of arranging an appointment with doctor, patient and telephone interpreter simultaneously are not easy. It is recommended that appointment times be extended up to 30 minutes for patients with language problems because of the increased time needed.

Your approach

Before the consultation begins, check the arrangements for accessing an interpreter. Has a receptionist pre-booked a telephone interpreter, or should the GP to contact a language interpretation service prior to the consultation? Once telephone contact has been made the interpreter will introduce him- or herself by first name and state their interpreter's reference number. Start by introducing yourself and checking the interpreter's language. Give the interpreter a brief summary of the patient's age, nationality and gender from the registration details, and any clues you have about the clinical problems.

You are now ready to start the consultation with your non-English-speaking patient and an interpreter using a three-way communication system. Welcoming the patient by shaking hands and indicating where he or she should sit will help break down barriers. If a personal interpreter accompanies the patient, indicate where they should sit. It is preferable to seat the patient closest to yourself with a full view of your face so that lip reading and facial expression can enhance communication. The interpreter should sit next to the patient, facing you. Check that your patient consents to the use of an interpreter. If a telephone interpreter is used, the consultation will involve passing the telephone from the patient to you, or using the telephone speaker, and allowing time to talk to and listen to the interpreter. Allow the patient an opportunity to talk about presenting problems. Interpreters are familiar with the structure of the

consultation and will initiate the process. A good start is to acknowledge the patient's problems.

Supplementing verbal exchange by observing body language will provide clues about symptoms such as pain, distress, anxiety, depression or the anatomical location of symptoms. Keep communication to a minimum and give instructions clearly via the interpreter when you have made a diagnosis and need to explain your management. At this stage you should check the patient's understanding of the UK health service and, if necessary, explain how the system works, particularly in relation to general practice. It is helpful to write down your name, diagnosis and instructions in English, including drawings and diagrams, and follow-up arrangements. The patient or family then has the option of getting a translation later. If you give the patient a prescription, you should explain the location of the pharmacy. Information leaflets in the patient's language are helpful, but if unavailable, a leaflet in English allows later translation. Before you say goodbye and thank your interpreter, offer your patient a last chance to ask questions.

How to do a home visit

As a student, you may visit patients at home for a variety of reasons. You may make a pre-arranged visit alone or paired with a student colleague to gain experience in routine history taking from a housebound patient, to follow up a patient recently discharged from hospital, to undertake a project, to accompany your tutor or other member of the primary healthcare team to assess a chronically ill patient or to gain emergency 'on-call' experience.

Visiting a patient at home is a very special experience. Indeed, it is a privilege enjoyed by few. Although some members of the primary healthcare team (for example community nurses, midwives and health visitors) visit defined patient groups, what makes general practice unique is the access doctors have to the homes of registered patients. Patients are a microcosm of society, representing all backgrounds and ages. Doctors have the advantage of being invited and usually welcomed into the home. Many students feel nervous about home visiting, partly because of feelings of insecurity, lack of self-confidence about social and communication skills and, with pre-arranged visits, a feeling of imposing on patients. However, most patients enjoy talking to students, there being mutual benefits.

This topic is further discussed in Chapter 10 on treating people at home.

Thinking and Discussion Point

Can you think of other occupations that have access to homes? Under what circumstances would visits be made?

Every home reflects individual and family values. Visiting a cross-section of society you may be surprised at the wide range of lifestyles and living conditions. Some visits will fascinate, as they offer insight into cultures different from your own, but in other homes you may react adversely, particularly where a patient's personal cleanliness is compromised due to incontinence or cognitive impairment. Whatever your impression, you need to handle the situation sensitively, remembering that you are a guest and that you are there to help a patient made vulnerable by illness or disability. Whoever and whenever you visit, you need to be prepared for all eventualities.

Common questions from students about home visiting

- How safe will I be? Because you are in an unprotected environment when visiting, you should be aware of personal safety, especially when travelling. Observe the same ground rules as you would when socializing in the community generally. Avoid risks such as walking alone in alleyways, being confrontational with strangers or appearing lost. Obtain clear directions before you set out. Look confident without appearing arrogant. Always inform someone of where you are going and when you expect to return. Take the surgery telephone number with you in case you need help, and your mobile phone.
- Should I carry identification? Patients, especially older people, are naturally suspicious of strangers who knock at their door. They have a right to expect confirmation that you are the student sent by your tutor. You must wear an identity badge with photograph. In addition, a letter of introduction from the surgery is reassuring. Patients appreciate a quick telephone call before you set out. When the patient opens the door, greet the patient by name and announce who you are, where you are from and why you are visiting. Check whether there is a relative in the house and, if so, that he or she is aware of your visit before starting your interview. If you are visiting a patient living in sheltered housing, a residential or nursing home, always introduce yourself on arrival to the warden or manager as a security measure.
- What shall I wear? This should be discussed with your tutor beforehand as dress codes may differ from practice to practice. Patients expect you to be clean, tidy and professional. They may feel threatened if you wear outrageous fashions. For safety reasons, avoid appearing too conspicuous in the area you are visiting: not too smart in a depressed area, not too scruffy in a smart part of town.
- How shall I respond if a patient is abusive or I feel threatened? Occasionally the interview may go wrong. Your patient may misunderstand or misinterpret your conversation through no fault of your own. If you sense that you are no longer welcome or that the relationship with your patient or a relative feels uncomfortable or threatening, leave the house as soon as is courteously possible. There is a tendency to underestimate feelings of resentment so it is better to leave rather than attempt to repair the situation. If possible, sit between the patient and the entry door of the room so that, in the event of a patient becoming physically aggressive, you can make a speedy exit.
- What happens if the conversation runs dry? Many students worry about this more when taking a history in a patient's home than in hospital or the surgery. This is probably because the patient has greater control in the home situation. The use of open questions and summarizing techniques will maintain conversation. Pauses in the conversation are quite natural and may be helpful. They may seem embarrassingly long but they are usually much shorter than you imagine.

- Should I examine the patient? It is recommended that you do not examine a patient at home unsupervised by your tutor. There is no insurance cover for this in the event of an accident, for example if the patient falls or makes a false allegation.
- What shall I do if the patient becomes acutely ill during the visit? Patients who become acutely ill may agree to continue with a student visit so as not to disappoint but it is appropriate to stop the interview and offer help. You may need to call a relative in the house. If you are unsure, call the surgery for advice.

Checklist for home visits

- The patient's name, address and telephone number.

- The carer's name, address and telephone number, if appropriate.
- The practice telephone number and your mobile.
- A map of the area visited with directions for finding the patient's address.
- Personal identification and a letter of introduction.
- A print-off of the patient's electronic record – usually medical summary and medications. If the practice maintains hard copy records take these with you.

After a pre-arranged visit, it is courteous to write and thank the patient.

SUMMARY POINTS

To conclude, the most important messages of this chapter are as follows:

- The patient is at the centre of your learning and must be treated with courtesy and respect.
- General practice requires an understanding of the basic science underlying any skill.
- Be aware of the clinical indications for using a skill.
- To learn a skill, you need close supervision and expert knowledge.
- It is important to rehearse and repeatedly practise any skill.

References

Beevers, G., Lip, G.Y. and O'Brien, E. 2007: *ABC of hypertension*, 5th edn. London: BMJ Books, Wiley-Blackwell.

British Hypertension Society 2010: Blood pressure measurement DVD. www.bhsoc.org (accessed 12 September 2010).

Department of Health 2010: *The UK Foundation Programme reference guide*. www.foundationprogramme.nhs.uk (accessed 12 September 2010).

Directgov 2010: *What to do after a death*. www.direct.gov.uk/en/Governementcitizensandrights/Death?WhatToDoAfterADeath (accessed 12 September 2010).

General Medical Council 2006: *Good medical practice*. London: GMC. www.gmc-uk.org (accessed 12 September 2010).

General Medical Council 2007: *0–18 years: Guidance for all doctors*. London: GMC. www.gmc-uk.org/static/documents/content/0-18_0510.pdf (accessed 9 April 2011).

General Medical Council 2009a: *Confidentiality*. London: GMC. www.gmc-uk.org/static/documents/content/Confidentiality_0910.pdf (accessed May 2011).

General Medical Council 2009b: *Seeking patients' consent*. London: GMC. www.gmc-uk.org/static/documents/content/Consent_0510.pdf (accessed 3 June 2011)

General Medical Council 2009c: *Tomorrow's Doctors*. www.gmc-uk.org/TomorrowsDoctors_2009.pdf_27494211.pdf (accessed 9 April 2011).

Language Line Services 2010: www.languageline.com/page/industry_healthcare (accessed 23 September 2010).

MacLeod, J. 1983: *Clinical examination: a textbook for students and doctors by teachers of the Edinburgh Medical School.* Edinburgh: Elsevier.

Rees, J., Kanabar, D. and Pattani, S. 2010: *ABC of asthma*, 6th edn. London: BMJ Books, Wiley-Blackwell.

SignTranslate 2010: *Online sign language interpreting.* www.signtranslate.com (accessed 23 September 2010).

Further reading

Foundation Programme 2010: *Training and assessment.* www.foundationprogramme.nhs.uk/pages/home/training-and-assessment (accessed 12 September 2010).

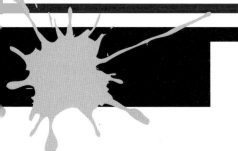

APPENDIX

Assessing practical skills in general practice

Undergraduate level

Medical schools implement their own methods of assessment for the core clinical skills and procedures that medical students are expected to have acquired on graduation. Some will be acquired predominantly in hospital and others in general practice. Small group or individual teaching in general practice makes this setting ideal for the learning and assessment of skills. Most schools have student logbooks which list core skills and procedures. Skills required in the undergraduate programme are listed in *Tomorrow's Doctors* (General Medical Council, 2009c)

Evaluation of skills competencies may be through 'in-course' assessment, as in the sign-ups in a logbook, or 'end-of-course' assessment, as in an Objective Structured Clinical Examination (OSCE). You are required to demonstrate minimum competence in the skill being assessed and that you have achieved a standard required for safe clinical practice with patients.

What constitutes minimum competence? Assessment of a skill is undertaken against standards of performance that are shared by the community of practitioners of that skill. This process is known as criterion referencing and involves an observer checking your performance against a set of listed criteria or descriptors. You may find it helpful to cross-check your skills against these OSCE questions.

Measurement of pulse and blood pressure

Instructions to candidate. Examine this patient's pulse and blood pressure using the equipment provided and report your findings to the examiner.
Marking schedule: criteria for the measurement of blood pressure and pulse.

Adequate/Inadequate/Not performed

- Introduces him/herself to patient.
- Establishes rapport with patient.
- Explains procedures and ensures consent.
- Ensures patient has rested for 10 minutes where appropriate.
- Positions patient and equipment appropriately.
- Applies cuff correctly.
- Locates brachial pulse.
- Puts stethoscope in antecubital fossa.
- Blows up cuff to appropriate level.
- Measures systolic and diastolic readings in mmHg.
- Removes cuff.
- Reports reading and interprets correctly.
- Encourages patient's questions and deals with them appropriately.
- Acknowledges patient's concern.
- Uses appropriate language.
- Documents blood pressure.

Peak flow measurement and instructions to patient on use of an inhaler

Instructions to candidate. Assess this patient's peak expiratory flow rate using the equipment provided and instruct him in the use of an inhaler.
Marking schedule: criteria for assessing measurement of peak flow and instructing patient on use of inhaler.

Adequate/Inadequate/Not performed

- Introduces him/herself to patient.
- Establishes rapport with patient.
- Explains importance of technique and ensures understanding.
- Checks patient's understanding of asthma.
- Prepares meter appropriately.
- Asks patient to take deep breath and seal lips around mouthpiece.
- Asks patient to blow as fast as possible into meter.
- Reads meter correctly.

- Checks peak flow against standard chart or patient's personal record.
- Indicates whether peak flow reading is as a result of a satisfactory technique and comments on its value.
- Suggests reasons for inhaler to be used.
- Shows patient how to shake inhaler.
- Asks patient to breathe out fully before using.
- Shows patient how to coordinate inhaler action while breathing in.
- Instructs patient to hold breath for 10 seconds after inhalation.
- Explains how to repeat after 1 minute.
- Indicates how often to use inhaler.
- Uses appropriate language.
- Checks patient has understood procedure.
- Encourages patient's questions and deals with them appropriately.
- Acknowledges patient's concerns.

Urine analysis

Instructions to candidate. Test this urine sample and report your findings to the examiner.
Marking schedule: criteria for assessing urine analysis.

                Adequate/Inadequate/Not performed
- Puts gloves on.
- Ensures urine sample is fresh.
- Checks container for correct stick and expiry date.
- Opens container and takes single stick out, closing bottle.
- Dipsticks urine for 1 second and taps off excess urine.
- After dipping, holds strip horizontal until test is complete.
- Reads stick after appropriate time.
- Records the result.
- Disposes of stick and gloves.
- Washes hands.
- Interprets results appropriately.
- Acknowledges need to send urine to laboratory or otherwise.

Measurement of blood glucose

Instructions to candidate. Measure the blood glucose and report your findings to the examiner.

Marking schedule: criteria for assessing measurement of blood glucose.

                Adequate/Inadequate/Not performed
- Introduces him/herself to patient.
- Establishes rapport with patient.
- Explains procedure and ensures consent.
- Ensures patient is sitting or lying down.
- Assembles equipment.
- Inserts strip and calibrates machine as appropriate.
- Chooses an appropriate place for test and ensures site is warm and well perfused.
- Washes hands and puts on gloves.
- Takes lancet and inserts sharply into skin, drawing blood.
- Obtains a hanging drop of blood without undue squeezing of puncture site.
- Drops blood onto test strip.
- Waits until the machine records a reading.
- Disposes of sharp safely.
- Checks haemostasis.
- Disposes of strip and gloves.
- Reads appropriately and records.
- Appropriate interpretation of value.

Ear examination

Instructions to candidate. Examine this patient's ear including the use of the auriscope.

Marking schedule: for assessing ear examination.

                Adequate/Inadequate/Not performed
- Introduces him/herself to patient.
- Establishes rapport with patient.
- Explains examination to patient and ensures consent.
- Enquires about hearing loss, characteristics and impact on life.
- Enquires about associated features, tinnitus and vertigo.
- Enquires about possible causes.
- Tests hearing with speech.
- Tests with tuning fork.
- Holds auriscope and patient's ear correctly.
- Identifies normal anatomy.
- Appropriate use of questions, open, closed and clarifying.
- Acknowledges patient's concerns.
- Encourages questions from patient and deals with them appropriately.
- Appropriate summary and analysis of findings.

Postgraduate level

In the first two years after graduation, UK graduates follow the Foundation Programme curriculum in Foundation Years 1 and 2 (FY1 and FY2). The curriculum is available online and covers the syllabus, core competences and approaches to assessment. Each doctor has an electronic portfolio in which his or her clinical supervisor records the level of competence in assessed skills using descriptors (Department of Health, 2010).

Procedures that FY1 doctors should be competent and confident to do and teach to undergraduates are listed. Those appropriate to general practice are indicated by *.

- Venepuncture* and intravenous cannulation
- Local anaesthetics*
- Arterial puncture in an adult
- Blood cultures from peripheral and central sites
- Subcutaneous*, intradermal*, intramuscular * and intravenous injections
- Intravenous medications
- Intravenous infusions, including the prescriptions of fluids, blood and blood products
- ECG*
- Spirometry and peak flow*
- Urethral catheterization
- Airway care, including simple adjuncts
- Nasogastric tube insertion.

FY2 doctors should maintain competence in the above procedures and extend skills to include the following within their subspecialty rotations.

- Aspiration of pleural fluid or air
- Skin suturing*
- Lumbar puncture
- Insertion of a central venous pressure line
- Aspiration of a joint effusion.

CHAPTER

5

DIAGNOSIS AND ACUTE MANAGEMENT IN GENERAL PRACTICE

- The patient walks into the room ... what next?
- What is a diagnosis?
- Why make a diagnosis?
- Levels of diagnosis
- What about diagnoses in general practice?
- How are diagnoses made in general practice?
- What are your objectives in planning your patients' care?

- Management in general practice
- Management by the whole primary care team
- Evidence-based medicine in general practice
- Guidelines and protocols
- Summary points
- References
- Further reading
- Single best answer questions

Although there are many facets of general practice, sound diagnostic reasoning and effective and informed decision making are cornerstones of good medical care. This chapter shows how your clinical skills are the starting point for developing your management plan with the patient. It explores the ways in which investigations, referral and therapy contribute to the process of management. Understanding ways of using research evidence and linking this to good clinical judgement will inform your decision making and help you to provide high-quality care for each of your patients.

LEARNING OBJECTIVES

By the end of this chapter, you will be able to:
- understand the nature of diagnosis;
- use elementary clinical skills to diagnose many of your patients' problems;
- learn the nature of investigations and how to ensure you use them effectively;
- plan a programme of management for your patients;
- understand the place of referral in patient management;
- understand the role of evidence-based medicine and guidelines in supporting patient care in general practice.

The patient walks into the room ... what next?

In general practice, the reason that the patient has walked into your consulting room is that he or she has taken the decision to consult a doctor. This is very different from hospitals, where a patient can only be seen by referral from another doctor (with the exception of accident and emergency/casualty and certain other self-referral clinics). In general practice, the patient makes the decision to see the doctor and the reasons vary widely, as discussed in Chapter 7 on common illnesses in general practice. In this chapter, we consider the processes of making diagnoses and managing patients with acute problems. The principles of patient diagnosis and management are common to many clinical situations; here we focus on those that are of special significance or different in the primary care setting.

Reasons for seeing the doctor can include:

- a new medical problem or issue;
- an acute episode in a chronic problem;
- follow-up of a previous acute consultation;
- concern about a symptom (perhaps after reading something in a magazine or on the internet);
- discussion about a visit to another doctor (usually a specialist);
- discussion of investigation results;
- to obtain repeat medication;
- for a medical examination (e.g. for life insurance or taxi driver medical);
- to complete a form or letter.

Practical Exercise

Make a record of each consecutive patient you see during a surgery. What was the main reason for consulting? Do you consider this a valid reason for coming to the doctor? Compare with your tutor each of your perceptions of the reason for consultation and whether it was an appropriate use of your GP's time. Later, you will use this list again to consider which of these consultations might have been better undertaken by other members of the primary healthcare team.

What is a diagnosis?

'I stood at the end of the bed and said, "This is Obstreosis of the Ductal Tract! It's a tertiary case and Coreopsis has set in". They were all amazed of course but it was a barn door case.'

(after James Thurber, 1965)

It is not unusual to hear this sort of claim, usually from a registrar trying to impress someone. Sooner or later, they find they are talking to their beer and starting to believe their own stories.

Perhaps surprisingly, it is unusual to make an absolute diagnosis. Most diagnoses are actually a balance of probabilities, based on evidence drawn from a number of sources. This is part of the evanescent entity called *clinical judgement*. When patients are better, the fact that they were treated with medication appropriate to the working diagnosis lends confirmation to the diagnosis. If the patient has either recovered or died, there is less pressure to make a definitive diagnosis. If the patient fails to improve, the problem is explored further and further explanations are proposed until a diagnosis is made or events render it unnecessary.

Why make a diagnosis?

While it is academically satisfying to make a precise diagnosis, the overriding reason for our work as doctors is that of helping our patients. In this light, a firm diagnosis is helpful but not the sole or even necessarily the most important consideration. For instance, we are taught to differentiate between direct and indirect inguinal hernias; in practice, clinical differentiation is of little practical importance, as it does not alter the management. Or consider the problem of an elderly smoker with an acute exacerbation of chronic obstructive pulmonary disease (COPD). He is treated with antibiotics, bronchodilators and steroids, and recovers. Was this an exacerbation of bronchitis or bronchopneumonia? Since the presentation and management are more or less identical, the precise diagnosis is arguably immaterial here. If the diagnosis lies between acute bronchitis (often with a lot of bronchospasm) and asthma, it is of much more significance, as longer term management will be different. In other situations, it may be important to act before making a diagnosis. For instance, temporal arteritis presents with a severe headache, but the symptoms are not pathognomonic. Definitive histological diagnosis by temporal artery biopsy will take at least a few days. Treatment is by high doses of steroids with potentially serious side effects, but the risk of delaying is of sudden and irreversible blindness. Treatment is therefore commenced on clinical suspicion.

In each of these cases, the safe management of the patient is the critical issue, as part of which making a formal diagnosis has varying levels of priority.

Levels of diagnosis

We can think of diagnoses as being made at various levels, as in Table 5.1. As a student, you should be able to get progressively to higher levels as your learning proceeds, but for all doctors there are situations in which they are only able to make an elementary diagnosis, and in those situations it is more important to have a strategy for handling that situation based on a sensible working hypothesis, rather than being 'stuck' on making a diagnosis.

You should only make the inferences that the diagnostic information you have collected allows you to make. If you assume that you have to make a firm diagnosis when the information is simply not strong enough, you will help neither the patient nor yourself. Rather, you need to use the information that you have obtained as a summary of your thinking so far. Unless you are clear on what you do and do not understand about your patients' problems at each point, you will be unable to ask the right questions to take you to the next stage.

What about diagnoses in general practice?

Because of the nature of general practice, diagnoses are more frequently of the 'working hypothesis' kind. This is sometimes crudely interpreted as hospital doctors making 'proper' diagnoses and general practitioners (GPs) failing to do so. However, the nature of general practice is such that diagnoses will rarely be as clear when a patient first presents to the surgery as they will be when the patient goes to a hospital clinic. There are a number of reasons for this.

- The patient usually presents at an earlier stage of the illness at the surgery than at the hospital when symptoms and signs are less developed.
- The patient is less clear in his or her mind at presentation as to the nature of the problem. As this is discussed with the patient's primary care physician, the nature of the problem is clarified.
- The GP is considering the whole patient, the psychological, the social and the physical; specialists, by their very nature, focus on one aspect of the patient's problems.

Table 5.1 Levels of diagnosis

Diagnostic level	Features	Examples
Pathological diagnosis	Pathological material has been examined which is pathognomonic of the condition	Dermatophyte infection from culture of affected skin
		Crohn's disease from surgical specimen of diseased bowel
Clinical diagnosis	Symptoms and signs of condition are so suggestive that treatment can be confidently undertaken	Acute asthma attack
Differential diagnosis	Several possibilities exist which are listed in order of likelihood	An acute abdomen: – peritonitis – acute pancreatitis – perforated peptic ulcer A chronic running nose: – allergic rhinitis – vasomotor rhinitis – chronic sinusitis
Problem list	The various problems cannot be made to fit into a diagnosis or diagnoses by the doctor or student	An unhappy child: – headache – tummy ache – just changed schools – awake at night with cough

Tutor quote

Somebody came in with a cough who was a grand-mother of 54. I asked if she smoked and, yes, she did. She smoked excessively, and she said she had to smoke because of the stress. I made some enquiries about the stress and she said she was stressed out because her son drank excessive amounts of alcohol and he was beating his wife. They had two children, a baby of 4 months and one of 7 years. The outcome of the consultation was that she needed a place of safety for those two children. So the consultation went from the presentation of a productive cough to, within 10 minutes, the need to alert the social workers and get a Place of Safety Order for the children.

Alarm point: It is always helpful to have a firm diagnosis but your most important goal is the safe management of the patient in which a diagnosis may not be the highest priority.

How are diagnoses made in general practice?

Doctors in any situation have three essential tools to help them understand their patients' problems:

- they listen to the patient's story and views of their illness: the history;
- they physically examine the patient: the examination;
- they perform various kinds of tests: the investigations.

Different disciplines use these approaches in varying amounts. Some doctors, such as haematologists, rely heavily on investigations to make diagnoses (how else can you work out the cause of an anaemia?); others, such as surgeons, place considerable reliance on the examination (how else do you diagnose a lump in the groin?); but the most important basic information, even in these disciplines, is obtained from the history, and every clinician relies on this as the major diagnostic tool. It has been estimated that 80 per cent of all diagnoses are based on the history, 15 per cent on the examination and 5 per cent on investigations.

The history in general practice

> ### Practical Exercise
>
> Listen to your tutor take a history from some patients. To which part of the history does your tutor give greatest weight?
> - ❑ The presenting complaint?
> - ❑ The systems review?
> - ❑ The past history?
> - ❑ The family history?
> - ❑ The therapeutic history?
> - ❑ The social history?
> - ❑ The patients' knowledge and beliefs about their conditions and their attitudes to them?

Often, a GP does not need to take past, family or therapeutic histories, as these are well known to them. This is one of the features of the continuing care relationship found in general practice. In well-organized GP records, these details are recorded on a summary page of the computer record.

You will also notice that your GP tutor assesses patients very quickly, often asking relatively few questions along the way, but building up a surprisingly thorough view of the patients' problems. This is a function of the expertise that GPs (and other experienced doctors) develop over time. This approach to gathering information is sometimes called the 'focused history'. Although it develops with experience, you should understand the principles on which it is based to develop your own clinical skills. General practice is a good place to practise this, however do not simply go for speed: the most important thing is to have the breadth and depth of understanding of the patient's problem that allows you to commence management: speed will come with time.

When you first learn to clerk patients as a student you learn a long list of questions which you go through in more or less the same way with every patient. This is fine as a beginner with limited medical understanding, but it is time consuming, often does not give you adequate detail of the key areas and it does not need a doctor to simply work through a list. In a focused history you focus your questions on areas relevant to the patient's problems. You are thus making a judgement about what to ask and what to leave out. The advantage is that you build up a much fuller and more relevant picture: the problem is that in making a judgement about what to include and what to leave out you may make the wrong judgement. As your experience and medical knowledge develop that becomes less of a problem, but in the mean time it is worth practising a focused history approach to develop your diagnostic acumen.

Taking a focused history

You will often hear the request 'take a focused history', particularly in exam settings. What that means and how you do it are not often discussed. Below is an approach to taking a focused history.

The 'LiCkERM' model of history taking stands for:

- Listen
- Clarify
- Explore
- Review
- Manage.

Listen

Start with an open question. In general practice it is worth keeping it very broad as you never know quite what is going to present: 'How can I help?' or 'What can I do for you today?' are good. Resist the temptation to start asking questions, rather encourage the patient to keep talking about their problem from their perspective. Try to obey the 'golden minute' rule of letting the patient do all the talking for the first minute of the interview. If the patient has come to a stop, phrases like 'go on …' or 'tell me more …' will encourage them to speak. Reflection can be useful: if a patient has come to a stop, repeat their last few words back to them to get them going again: 'you were saying it's worse in the mornings'.

In emotionally charged situations the patient may need time to collect their thoughts and cope with the emotions of it all. Do not be afraid of that silence: it is doing a lot of your work for you.

Tutor quote

I hate the old 'what seems to be the trouble?' starter question. It all seems to imply that you (the simple-

ton patient) are telling me your problems in your own pathetically ill-informed way, but it takes me (the physician of genius) to understand what the real problem is and to put it into proper medical terms.

Tutor quote

So what I am thinking about is a student who was just unable to get out of the way of asking leading questions, technical questions. So, after a battle, we agreed that he would say nothing, that he would introduce himself and say hello to the patient and that he would say nothing, and he was completely flabbergasted by what happened then. He was shocked by how much patients told him. We then had this sort of game using just gestures to encourage people to say things. He also had a list of phrases that he could use, like 'Tell me more about that' and 'Is there anything else you want to tell me?'. And so we went through this list of questions and we agreed it and he really thought this was cracked and he went along with it because I used my authority to force him. But he was just completely flabbergasted by this and shocked. It was very exciting for me, too, as it seemed to me that the questions that were left out of the clinical examination are 'Tell me all about it', 'Is there anything else you want to tell me?', 'What did it feel like?', 'What did it look like?' and so on. And the second part of the agreement that I made with this particular student was that before he could ask any technical questions he had to summarize back to the patient what the patient said, and so he would summarize by saying, 'Now, if I have heard you right, what has happened to you is this and I would like to ask you some questions, but before I do is there anything else you want to tell me?' So that was a revelation for both of us really.

Clarify

Analyse what each symptom means. Patients often use medical terms but may not be using them to mean the same as you. If you ask 'What do you mean by "blood pressure"?', for example, you may find that the patient is talking about their headaches or flushes. This not only ensures you are talking the same language as your patient, it begins to explore each symptom in detail. I certainly found this useful on one particular occasion when a patient's alleged diarrhoea turned out to be constipation!

There are plenty of mnemonics to remind you how to analyse a symptom: I like WWQQAAB – where, when, quality, quantity, aggravating and relieving factors, associated manifestations and beliefs.

Asking the patient about their beliefs or ideas, concerns and expectations about the condition is essential in any setting, but especially so in primary care. Yet many students feel uncomfortable doing so. It is discussed further below.

Clarify the time frame. 'When were you last completely well?' gets you to the starting point. 'What happened then?' Be clear about the duration of episodes and the time between them. Were they completely free between episodes or merely less bad?

Explore

Depending on the symptoms you have elicited, ask for 'RED FLAG' symptoms – symptoms that if positive would have a sinister implication. For instance, with back pain ask (amongst other things) about weight loss and night sweats, which suggest tuberculosis or malignancy as a cause.

Past medical history is vital, but not as a list of random diseases. 'Have you had anything serious?', 'Have you seen a specialist or been admitted to hospital?' are much more revealing. Use a similar approach to family history.

Treatment history is important for three reasons. (1) Drugs cause many problems and may be the cause of your patient's symptoms. (2) As a foundation doctor you will be writing up admission drug charts based on the information you have gleaned. Studies have shown errors of up to 50 per cent doing this. Care taken at this stage can save your patient a great deal of potential danger and suffering. Do your best to find out the name of the drug, the frequency of taking it and the strength of tablets. Fortunately in general practice you will normally have this on record, but there will be frequent occasions when a new drug has been started by another doctor who has not yet told you about it. (3) Finally, the treatment history is a double check on the past medical history: the amlodipine for overlooked hypertension, the

mesalazine suggesting that irritable bowel was in fact inflammatory bowel disease.

Social history: As a minimum find out how this problem affects and is affected by the patient's home and work situation and how it affects other family members.

Exploring beliefs: Many students feel uncomfortable or question the relevance of exploring ideas, concerns and expectations, yet it is often crucial to managing the problem. Patients who come to you with a headache are often little bothered by the headache itself but worried about what it means – often either brain tumours or meningitis. Telling the patient 'Don't worry, it's nothing serious' may be true, but is unlikely to reassure the patient who thinks you have just overlooked their brain tumour. Patients are often reluctant to say what is really bothering them, maybe out of fear, maybe in case they look silly. At the same time you cannot assume you know what it is. Reassuring the patient that it is not a brain tumour when they were worried about blood pressure and strokes is not likely to help the situation (see the case study below).

It is often useful to ask 'What are you worried this might be?' or 'In your darker moments, what are you most worried this is?'. Many doctors make the mistake of assuming they know why the patient is there; they may come up with brilliant diagnoses, but if they have not dealt with the patient's concerns, the job is only half done.

Alarm point: Time spent unpicking the patient's story is never wasted. Eighty per cent of your diagnostic information is there: examination and investigations cannot take the place of a careful history.

Case Study 5.1

A 73-year-old woman was admitted to hospital about once a month for investigations of sudden acute chest pain. It did not sound cardiac and the electrocardiogram and cardiac enzymes were always normal. Her husband had died of a heart attack some years previously as a result of which she was reassured by everyone that 'your heart's fine' and sent back to her flat. If reassurance was all it took, she had overdosed on it. But back she came again month after month. One day, the houseman sat down with her and naively asked,

'What do you think the problem is?' After a prolonged silence, she said, 'It's cancer, doctor'. 'Why do you say that?' 'My brother had lung cancer'. The houseman (wising up): 'Did he have pain with it?' 'Terrible pain'. 'Was it like yours?' 'It was exactly the same!' Everyone was absolutely right that there was no organic pathology, but wrong in assuming that it was her heart and the memory of her husband's death that had precipitated her symptoms.

Case Study 5.2

The husband had diabetes and developed a phimosis. He had the usual circumcision and all appeared fine. One day his wife appeared and asked 'So how long will it take to grow back doctor?' I wonder how many people would have guessed that was her big worry.

Thinking and Discussion Point

Why does telling a patient there is 'nothing wrong' often not result in the reassurance that the doctor was intending?

Review

Having gathered all this information, you now need to fit it all together into a coherent story. Having got it together in your own head the best thing is to play it back to the patient. Not only will vocalizing it reveal gaps to you as you tell it, but it will allow the patient to 'edit' their story, adding missing parts and clarifying others. It has a second benefit in that the patient will be reassured to know you understand what they have been experiencing.

You know you've finished your history when you have the information you need to move on to think about how you are going to manage the patient.

Systems review? 'The greatest argument against the systems review is that experienced clinicians do not use it' said a former Royal College of Physicians president (Hoffbrand, 1989). Routinely asking a shopping list of questions is often of little benefit. You will not often hear experienced clinicians make use of it, but you should not write

it off, particularly at your early stage of learning medicine and diagnostic method.

Cognitive psychologists have proposed that we can use a dual model of clinical reasoning. For an experienced clinician working with a straightforward problem, the clinical reasoning becomes almost intuitive, which is why you will hear experienced clinicians moving from presenting problem to diagnosis and management with very few questions or intervening steps. If you are inexperienced, however, or if you are dealing with an unusual presentation (which may be a common condition not presenting straightforwardly or a rarer condition with which you are unfamiliar), then you can resort to the slower hypothetico-deductive approach, where you explore slowly and widely before drawing conclusions. As a beginner you will spend much more time in this mode, but as you gain experience you will find you ask fewer questions but gain better answers and move more to the intuitive approach.

However experienced you are you will always need to return to the hypothetico-deductive approach from time to time when rare conditions or unusual presentations crop up (Sinclair and Croskerry, 2010).

Manage

You will note I tend to think of examination as part of the investigation of the patient rather than as part of the clerking. If so, bear with me – you may yet come to sympathize with this aberration.

The whole purpose of your exploration of the patient's story is to get you to the point where you have enough information to make decisions about how you are going to proceed. So the question is not 'What's the diagnosis?' or 'What blood tests shall I do?' but more generally 'How do I take things forward from here?'.

There are two options: (1) You have a clear enough view of what is going on to propose a management plan. (2) You need to gather more information from a physical examination or from investigations.

The examination in general practice

'He never examined me' is a frequent complaint of patients who found a consultation unsatisfactory. There is little time for each consultation in general practice; although the average has gradually moved upwards from 6 minutes in the 1970s to 11.7 minutes (The Information Centre, 2006/7), it is still a short period of time in which to accomplish a great deal. GPs respond by honing their clinical technique to include only those things that are of significant diagnostic value. As we saw above, the examination only contributes 15 per cent to the diagnosis, as opposed to 80 per cent from the history.

Practical Exercise

As your tutor talks to successive patients, decide what examination (if any) you would make. Compare this with what your tutor does and discuss the differences with him or her. You should not assume that the tutor's decision is necessarily the only one. Often, a number of approaches could be made, and understanding the differing merits and objectives of each is useful.

❑ Discuss with your tutor how useful it is to: take the blood pressure of a patient complaining of headache; listen to the chest of a child with a cough; palpate the abdomen of a young man with acute diarrhoea.

❑ Why else might you want to examine the patient apart from to make a diagnosis?

❑ What is the value of carrying out a 'full physical' as a screening exercise?

You should think of an examination in the same way as an investigation: how will carrying out this examination improve my understanding of the patient's problems? Does the patient need the examination for reassurance? The focused examination is therefore much like the focused history: you make a judgement about what is likely to be worthwhile and focus your attention there.

Investigations in general practice

Investigations can be used in two main ways: for diagnosis and for management. For instance, a single random blood sugar test is useful for the diagnosis of diabetes. It will detect the bulk of cases (although a blood sugar taken 2 hours after eating is better still). However, in the management

Thinking and Discussion Point

'General practitioners under-investigate and hospital doctors over-investigate.' Discuss the truth (or otherwise) of this assertion with your tutor and with a hospital doctor. How will you ensure you investigate appropriately?

of diabetes, the blood sugar changes so quickly that a single test is of little value, especially since the result may not be available for some days. In managing diabetes, a rapid assessment of blood sugar is required and must be repeated frequently if it is to inform management. Indicator strips used for the self-measurement of blood sugar are much more useful, even though they are considerably less accurate. Where precision is required for diagnosis, an immediate result is more important for management.

Interpreting results: normal or abnormal

Few investigations give an absolute result or are pathognomonic. For the most part, they will help you build up your evidence for a diagnosis, but only when interpreted in the light of the whole of the patient's story. For instance, an electrocardiogram (ECG) is a useful test in suspected myocardial infarction, but it does not always show characteristic changes in a confirmed myocardial infarction, and it sometimes shows changes when no infarction has taken place. This under-diagnosis or over-diagnosis by the test are known respectively as the *sensitivity* and *specificity* of the test. While one does not need to know the exact values, it is important to have an approximate idea of the limitations of any test. An awareness of sensitivity and specificity is helpful in judging these limitations. (There are definitions of sensitivity and specificity in the glossary section of this book.)

Often, sensitivity and specificity are inversely related. For instance, the erythrocyte sedimentation rate (ESR) is a sensitive test but a very poorly specific one. It is usually elevated to high levels in a condition such as polymyalgia rheumatica (it is sensitive), but is frequently elevated for a host of unrelated reasons (poorly specific). A

Paul–Bunnell test is very specific: when positive, it is highly indicative of glandular fever, but many people with established glandular fever have a negative test (it is insensitive). Other assays (such as assays of thyroid-stimulating hormone) are both specific and sensitive and, as such, approach the ideal. Any test you order should be done in the light of your knowledge of its limitations of specificity and sensitivity.

When presented with an individual who has a positive result in a screening test, what may be of more interest to a clinician are the positive and negative predictive values (see the glossary for definitions).

Who's for screening?

With increasing access to private healthcare, there has been a considerable increase in the vogue for 'screening' tests. With modern laboratory technology, a large number of tests can be done quickly and relatively inexpensively on a single sample of blood. American medicine (see any relevant soap opera) gets through acres of such tests. As well as American medics, there are UK foundation doctors ordering every test under the sun in case the consultant should ask for it. There are problems with this approach. Every test has a probability of producing a false-positive result. The more tests carried out, the more false-positive results you will obtain. You then have to deal with these, sometimes by ordering more elaborate, expensive or invasive tests. To minimize spurious results, only carry out a test when there is a clear clinical indication. An example of the failure of screening tests comes from the early days of human immunodeficiency virus (HIV) infection. With the disease then relatively rare and tests relatively unsophisticated, there was considerable political pressure from some quarters to screen people for HIV *en masse*. The number of undiagnosed true positive cases in the community was below the rate of false positives for the test. At the same time, there were significant numbers of false negatives, both because of the technical limitations of the test and because it was unable to detect early infections. Thus the test caused distress to people who would turn out to be uninfected, while failing in its aim as a screening test.

Effects of tests on awareness of health

Another reason to avoid unnecessary tests is that they can increase anxiety and concern about health. Stoate (1989) showed that screening for blood pressure increased anxiety about health, as reflected in an increased frequency of consultations in those screened. In the case of blood pressure, such screening arguably justifies the health anxiety caused; for many tests done 'just to see', it certainly does not.

Deciding whether to request a test

As a student or doctor, the most important question you can ask about any investigation is, 'Will it change my management?' If the answer is 'yes', you then need to ask, 'Could I get the same information cheaper, quicker or less invasively another way?' If the answer is 'yes', you should think again.

Who is the investigation for: patient or doctor?

We have stated that investigations have the two prime functions of diagnosis and management. In addition, you may have seen investigations used to 'reassure the patient'. It is important to consider whether or not the patient will be reassured by your action. In the same way as doctors sometimes assume, rather than ask, what their patients' real worries are, they equally may assume that a patient will be reassured by a negative test (such as a cranial X-ray to reassure the patient that there is no brain tumour). The same message applies: find out what the issues are that actually concern the patient and deal with those. As a *British Medical Journal* editorial put it, 'Unless their true fears are addressed, diagnostic tests may leave them more anxious than before' (Fitzpatrick, 1996).

The range of investigations available in general practice

An increasing range of investigations is available to GPs. These may be carried out in the following ways:

- By the patients themselves: for example blood sugar monitoring using indicator strips, peak expiratory flow rate monitoring via mini peak flow meters (both available on prescription).
- In the doctor's surgery: for example indicator strips for urine testing for a wide variety

of substances, immunological detection kits for pregnancy testing, ECGs and audiograms; there are mini auto-analysers available allowing 'near patient testing' for basic biochemical and haematological indices such as cholesterol, haemoglobin and creatinine.

- In a clinical laboratory (usually based at a hospital, but sometimes contracted out to an independent laboratory): some complex or unusual assays, such as certain endocrine or genetic tests, are only carried out at specialist centres. The availabilities of laboratory-based tests to GPs vary from laboratory to laboratory.
- In specialist departments: most kinds of X-rays are available directly to the GP; other sophisticated tests, such as endoscopy and echocardiography, are examples of an increasing range of tests often available directly to GPs without consultant referral. The exact availability varies from area to area, depending on factors ranging from the availability of the investigation locally to the prejudices of the person in charge of the investigating unit. The reasons why certain tests are not available may be highly idiosyncratic. The hospital may believe that to allow GPs to use certain tests would be to waste money (this assumes the GPs are using them excessively or inappropriately). It may be 'protectionism', as a specialty tries to protect its interests from others treating those conditions. In the better-regulated establishments, a dialogue will be established between the laboratory or department offering the test, and the GPs and others who wish to use it to ensure it is correctly used and appropriately available.

Do 'good' doctors use more or fewer investigations?

There can be a kind of machismo in ordering every investigation under the sun or, conversely, refusing to have anything at all to do with them. There is a certain feeling, prevalent among foundation doctors starting their first job, that more is always better. If you are used to using an investigation, you can get blasé and use it more frequently than justified by the clinical situation. Huge numbers of routine urea and electrolyte samples taken during inpatient stays have little clinical value. Conversely, examinations may be under-used by

those who are not aware of the potential they offer. Thus, you cannot judge a doctor by the quantity of investigations he or she uses, but by the quality of use. So aim to know the potential and the drawbacks of each investigation and, armed with that knowledge, investigate appropriately.

Thinking and Discussion Point

Should investigations replace clinical examination? How accurately can you assess a heart murmur or an ovarian cyst in a clinical examination? Should we be considering the sensitivity and specificity of our clinical examination along with investigations?

Alarm point: Never order an investigation without a clear idea what you expect it to tell you. Always consider how limitations of specificity and sensitivity will affect your interpretation of the result.

What are your objectives in planning your patients' care?

Two first-year medical students gave the following opinions after a visit to a hospice.

Student quotes

It was depressing, all those people dying and nothing the doctors could do.

It seemed incredibly peaceful; although people knew they were dying, they seemed really peaceful and content.

The two views above show completely different opinions on what was going on. Too often, our views of what constitutes management are from one direction only. Let us look at the different goals that a doctor might be trying to achieve in managing a patient.

- *To cure the patient's disease.* This is the most usual view of the doctor's role. Television soaps, society in general, patients, relatives and sometimes the doctors themselves believe this is their role. Sometimes it is: if you have bacterial meningitis, you want the doctor to move fast and eradicate the organisms before they do you permanent harm.

- *To prevent disease.* If one can prevent a disease developing, it is far better than curing it once it is there. This is a prime role for the GP, who has access to a population in both sickness and health, as described in the chapter on health promotion. There is an opportunity to intervene with screening, education and lifestyle advice before disease starts. Cervical screening, education about safe sex and advice on smoking have all had an important impact on the lives of individuals. However, this role is unglamorous. There is a much less tangible reward for the GP preventing coronary artery disease than for the surgeon with a large team and high-tech facilities.

- *To slow the progressions of a chronic disease and to prevent complications.* It may be impossible with existing medical knowledge to prevent or cure a disease (see Chapter 9 on dealing with chronic illness). In an ageing population, chronic disease puts an increasing burden on the health service. Slowing the progression of such disease and preventing its complications are key treatment aims. Diabetes is a good example. Insulin-dependent diabetes can neither be prevented nor cured at present, but the important aims of management remain to prevent the serious complications of blindness and renal disease and fatal ones of stroke and myocardial infarction.

- *To alleviate symptoms.* Some illnesses are brief and self-limiting; they do no long-term harm, but are unpleasant while they are there. An example is sore throat. Approximately 65 per cent of cases are viral (Ross *et al.*, 1971) and no antiviral treatment is available. Thirty-five per cent are bacterial, but studies of antibiotics show that they only reduce the duration of symptoms by 1 day. Thus curative treatments are either non-existent or limited in their efficacy. Prevention is not a practical possibility. To enable patients to function as well as possible while they have the infection is the objective. Thus treatment is with analgesics, antipyretics and anti-inflammatories, most conveniently provided by aspirin, which has all three effects (although this is not used

in children under 16 years of age because of the association with Reye's syndrome). Paracetamol is a safe alternative, being an analgesic and antipyretic, and despite the absence of anti-inflammatory properties, it is probably of comparable efficacy. Locally acting agents such as soothing or local anaesthetic throat pastilles or sprays may be helpful. Alleviating symptoms has an equally important role to play in major illnesses. The management of pain resulting from a terminal illness or surgery is of tremendous importance to the patient. The doctor may have other priorities, especially if a patient is having difficult or dangerous postoperative problems. Historically, doctors have not always managed pain very well, sometimes disregarding it in favour of what they consider to be more pressing issues or being poorly informed about its management. An important goal of the hospice movement has been to develop ways of alleviating symptoms for which there is no ultimate cure.

- *To educate and inform.* The doctor has an important role in educating patients and thus helping them to manage their illness. In the example of the sore throat and other minor illnesses, patients need to be helped to learn to manage their illness, but this is equally important in major illnesses. Diabetes management relies crucially on the patient's understanding of his or her illness and its management. The aim is for the patient to understand how to manage the illness from day to day by the use of an appropriate diet and exercise, by monitoring blood sugar values and by manipulating the insulin regime. To do so, the patient needs to understand something of the nature of the illness, but much more about the practicalities of what to do and when. In many conditions, patients are encouraged to take a more active role in their own management, and there is a vocal lobby from patient groups demanding such changes. While this may appear laudable, it is not always clear how effective it is. For instance, numerous studies attempting to educate patients about asthma have shown little effect in preventing hospital admissions or symptoms.

Thus, in managing any patient, there are a variety of objectives that may be pursued, and often more than one. Being clear about which objective you are pursuing will help to ensure that each aspect of the patient's problem is appropriately dealt with.

Alarm point: Planning patient care has a range of objectives of which 'curing' the disease may not be the most important and indeed may not be possible.

Management in general practice

Assessing the patient

The first step in managing your patient is your assessment of the patient's situation. Taking the history, making the examination and arranging diagnostic investigations are the major part of this process, as discussed above. Your further assessment will depend upon the objectives you have established for your patient's management.

If, for example, your objective is patient education, you will need to assess what the patient understands about his or her condition. You will have some knowledge of this from the history, especially your exploration of the patient's ideas, concerns and expectations about the condition. But you may need to go into more detail at this stage, and begin a dialogue with the patient comparing your understanding of the condition to the patient's.

If your objective is the alleviation of symptoms, you will need to have measures of their severity against which the effects of your therapeutic manipulations can be compared. For instance, for the patient with intermittent claudication, you need measures of exercise tolerance (such as how many stairs can be climbed before the pain starts). Attempt to quantify your patient's symptoms in terms that have a meaning for both you and your patient. (For a patient living in a bungalow, the above may be unhelpful, and the number of stops on the way to the shop may be better.) This allows you and your patient to have a way of comparing progress. Laboratory investigations may define this more precisely, such as Doppler imaging and angiography in the case of the patient with intermittent claudication, but they should augment

clinical understanding rather than attempt to replace it.

Case Study 5.3

A 19-year-old man, Mr G, complains of breathlessness and a night-time cough. You have assessed the patient by taking a history that has revealed an episodic pattern of breathlessness, worse early in the morning and when playing football. It is worse in the spring when the pollen count is high and much worse when he visits his aunt and her cats. On examination, there are no physical signs in the chest, but he has a peak flow of only 300 L/min. He believes he has asthma, but is alarmed by the reports he has read in the paper of the rise in asthma deaths. You lend him a peak flow meter, which later shows consistently lower morning than evening values, and arrange skin tests, which confirm his allergies to cats, pollen and to house dust mite.

Planning treatment

Having assessed your patient's condition, you are now in a position to initiate treatment. Consideration of any treatment's effectiveness is vital. Much treatment offered to patients is of no proven efficacy. Later in this chapter we consider how evidence-based medicine and clinical guidelines ensure your patient receives treatment that is likely to be of benefit.

What are the risks and benefits of treatment?

What are the possible adverse consequences of the treatment you are proposing? Will your treatment be worse than the disease it is intending to cure? If the treatment is important but side effects inevitable, how will you ensure your patient is compliant with that treatment? You and your patient need to take a view of the risks and benefits of the treatment you are considering. For a rapidly fatal disease such as meningitis, the antibiotic chloramphenicol with its associated risk of aplastic anaemia may be a justifiable risk. (Chloramphenicol is now virtually never used in the UK. However, in the developing world it remains an affordable and effective antibiotic choice.)

So far, we have assumed your patient requires drug treatments, but other treatments are possible and often desirable. A change in lifestyle may be of considerably greater importance for the insom-niac patient than the prescription of any drugs. Relaxation techniques, such as yoga, can produce significant and sustained falls in blood pressure that may be more acceptable to the hypertensive patient than a lifetime of tablets. A spectrum of treatments from the orthodox, such as surgery and physiotherapy, through osteopathy and chi-ropractic to acupuncture and homeopathy are all offered with more or less scientific justification. (These options are discussed further in Chapter 6 on prescribing.)

Your job as a doctor is to help patients find a treatment that:

- they find acceptable,
- has good evidence for its efficacy, and
- has acceptable adverse risks.

Negotiating with the patient

If your plan for the management of the patient is to go ahead, the patient is the person most respon-sible for implementing it. Following through your management plan requires not just telling your patient about it, nor even listening to their concerns, but is an active process of negotiating with the patient around the various options that are available and the benefits and shortcomings of each.

Tutor quote

I was running a seminar with some students. We were talking about compliance and the word 'bar-gaining' came in. Some students went for it; some students said that they would bargain. One student said that we should be ashamed of our view. He said, 'We should say "This is what you need, these are the tablets, this is the dose you take", and the patient will take it if you tell them'. So the discus-sion went on, and I said, 'But aren't patients differ-ent? Different patients make decisions in a different way'. What he said then was, 'If you give all patients exactly the same information then their decisions will be identical'. Now we were coming to the crunch, so I said, 'What do you mean? If you took a 40-year-old man who has recently lost his wife because she took penicillin and died of anaphylactic shock and somebody who had recently had a child who recovered from pneumonia because of penicillin

and if you gave them the same information, would they make the same decision?' and he said, 'Yes, if you give them the statistics, they will still make the same decision'. So he was still not prepared to accept that patients make decisions differently. So then he said that he believed that they would make the same decision as him. So one of the other students then said, 'You want your patients to be like you?' and that is what stopped him – 'Do I want the patients to be like me? Does everybody have to be like me for me to accept them?' I could see that there was this expression change. I said to him that, as a doctor, you respect the patient, that they are different, they have autonomy, they make their own decisions; respect them and if you find that their decision is going to be different from yours, that means you have to bargain. I think he definitely learnt that people make different decisions, they come from dif-ferent places and information is not everything, and even if they do make a different decision, so what?

Evidence for the failure of doctors to take this part of management seriously is found in statistics that reveal that up to 20 per cent of prescriptions given by GPs are never taken to the chemist, and of those that are, a significant percentage of patients do not take some or any of the medica-tion as prescribed (Fry, 1993).

Typically, a negotiation about treatment with a patient means the doctor will present his or her assessment of the problem and proposed solution to it. The doctor may present alternatives and dis-cuss with the patient the risks and benefits of each option, and will check the patient's understanding and views about the preferred form of treatment. Then the patient and doctor between them will come to an agreement about the treatment to be undertaken.

Alarm point: Your brilliant diagnosis and treat-ment plan will only work if the patient buys into it: negotiating concordance is a vital part of effec-tive medicine.

Case study 5.3 (continued)

Tests confirm that Mr G has moderately severe asthma and a number of allergies. You propose a regular steroid inhaler and beta-2 agonist as required. Mr G is unhappy with this; he has read about the side effects of steroids and anyway prefers to avoid drugs and favours homeopathy. You discuss with Mr G the lack of scientific evidence that homeopathy can be of benefit in this situation, but agree with him that he is perfectly at liberty to try this, if he should so choose.

You discuss the possibility of preventing his asthma by avoiding contact with allergens and conclude that, apart from avoiding his aunt's cats and reducing house dust mites at home, the effects of doing this are likely to be fairly limited. You discuss Mr G's fears of medication with him, and particularly corticosteroids when used in low doses in inhaled form. You eventually agree that Mr G will use a beta-2 agonist inhaler, will try to avoid contact with specific allergens and will continue to monitor his peak flow. He will also discuss things with his homeopath.

Monitoring progress

Having negotiated treatment and initiated it with the patient, the doctor needs to monitor its effectiveness. This may range from the very simple to much more highly organized schemes of testing and monitoring. At the simple end of the spectrum, the doctor who sees a child with an apparently uncomplicated upper respiratory chest infection will discuss with the mother the appropriate, usually non-prescription, remedies and will invite her to call the doctor or return to surgery if the child is not showing improvement within a certain time. The doctor may warn the mother of things to look out for which suggest something more serious is going on.

Even in this very simple example, the doctor has:

- made a plan,
- shared it with a patient,
- set up criteria by which its success or failure will be judged,
- considered arrangements for following up the patient.

In more complex situations, these same principles are followed, but in ways appropriate to the situation. For example, when a newly diagnosed diabetic is started on insulin, the doctor needs to know that the patient is able to measure and inject the dose of insulin. The patient needs to monitor his or her blood sugar using finger-prick samples. A specialist diabetes nurse can visit the patient at home to check how he or she is coping with these tasks. The patient needs an appropriate diet and is given brief advice on this in the surgery and an appointment is made with the dietician for more detailed advice. The doctor knows the appointment will not be for a number of weeks, which gives the patient time to learn about all the other aspects of treatment. There are now education programmes specifically for patients to learn about their diabetes. Unlike the previous example where it was left to the mother to return if things were not going well, here it is important that a definite meeting is arranged to review progress quite soon. The patient may have things that are important to discuss, the insulin dose will almost certainly need modifying, and the doctor or practice nurse will want to find out how the patient is getting on with the different aspects of treatment.

In these early days, there will be a number of meetings at frequent intervals. As the diabetes comes under control and the patient becomes more confident, so these intervals will be extended, and day-to-day responsibility for care may be taken over by the specialist nurse. When everything is stable, a different pattern of visits will be initiated at intervals of perhaps a year. The patient will be seen and checked for evidence of visual or renal impairment, the feet will be checked for vascular or neuropathic changes, and the patient and the doctor or nurse will discuss diet and medication. This pattern can be maintained for as long as the patient is well, but if the patient becomes acutely ill, the plan will change to allow effective monitoring and treatment of the condition.

Alarm point: Even in simple situations have a clear plan of management and agree it with the patient, have a fallback and consider the need for follow-up.

Management by the whole primary care team

This section focuses on the role of the doctor; we have already mentioned the role of specialist nurses and the dietician in the patient's management.

It is important to be aware that management is an issue for the care team as a whole and not just the doctor. Only by working together as a whole are the patient's best interests served. The relationship between the doctor and the primary healthcare team is discussed in Chapter 2 on general practice and its place in primary care.

Case Study 5.3 (continued)

Mr G gets considerable benefit from his beta-2 agonist inhaler, but has frequent worsening attacks of asthma that result in two brief admissions. Partly as a result of the fright this gives him and partly through his good relationship with the practice nurse who runs the asthma clinic, he accepts the need for inhaled steroid therapy. Regular reviews in surgery are arranged by the nurse, but in addition the practice manager ensures that the receptionists are aware of the patient's need to be seen urgently whenever he requests it. Mr G avoids further admissions, but he continues to call out the doctors fairly frequently at night and makes considerable use of the practice nebulizer.

Thinking and Discussion Point

Is this the best we can do? What further steps would you wish to take to improve Mr G's treatment? Discuss these with your tutor.

Making referrals

Reasons for referring

The GP has two main options in dealing with the problem that the patient brings: doing so in-house or seeking assistance from other resources. It is impossible to give cut and dried rules about which is the 'correct' solution, as there are often a number of ways to deal with a problem, all of them equally valid and any of which may be chosen for a variety of reasons in different situations. Such reasons may emanate from the GP, the patient or the local situation.

- Different GPs' training, experience and personality will give them different approaches to the same problem.

- A patient may find one solution much more acceptable than another theoretically equally good one.
- Local facilities vary widely, and a service that may be well provided for in one area may be poor or non-existent in another.

Thus, a GP with experience of counselling or child psychiatry may be perfectly happy to tackle a complex psychological problem without outside help, but may refer to a specialist a child with something relatively straightforward about which the GP is uncertain for some reason. Allergy problems may be dealt with swiftly and efficiently by a special clinic in one area; in another there may be a virtual absence of such help, throwing the GP back on his or her own resources. A mother may be incapable of accepting reassurance about her child's condition until a specialist appointment is arranged in one situation, while another, similar situation is resolved by a brief chat with the doctor.

Few referrals good; more referrals bad?

There is no straightforward relationship between the apparent abilities or training of a doctor and the number of referrals he or she makes. The assumption that better trained doctors refer less was challenged when it was found that GPs with specialist ear, nose and throat (ENT) training referred more ENT problems than those without. This may have been because of the need for specialist diagnostic equipment and operative surgery. We can hypothesize that GPs trained in specialties not requiring this sort of resource, such as dermatology, might refer less. Part of the explanation for different referral patterns amongst doctors lies in the ability of individuals to deal with uncertainty. The doctor who is comfortable living with a degree of uncertainty over diagnosis will refer less; the doctor who cannot cope with uncertainty will refer more. For the patient, neither approach is without consequences. In the former case, it may mean not getting referred when it would have been advisable, and in the latter it may mean being referred unnecessarily. Secondary care depends upon primary care restricting the numbers presenting, so the GP is obliged to make a decision about what requires referral and what does not.

The referral letter

A practical exercise in how to write a referral letter can be found in Chapter 4. However, in terms of what to say rather than how to say it, there are a number of points.

- Avoid long letters; few people read them. Choose only information that will be useful to the doctor receiving the letter.
- Be clear about why you are making the referral – what you hope to gain from it. There may be a number of factors:
  - you may need a service undertaken, such as an operation or an endoscopy;
  - you may require a second opinion to confirm an unclear diagnosis: you may feel happy about the diagnosis, but the patient may not, so the second opinion is for the patient's benefit;
  - you may be asking the specialist to take over the management of the patient problem, or one aspect of it – this may be appropriate for the patient who is moving from a chronic phase to an acute phase in an illness, such as someone with previously stable angina which has now become unstable and requires operative intervention.

It is important that the consultant should be aware of your reasons for the referral and what you expect to get back from him or her. The letter itself needs to be a coherent précis of the patient's condition, with relevant past, social and therapeutic histories. It is written to give the person to whom you are referring a clear view of the patient's problems rather than to show how clever you are. At the conclusion of this summary you will give your diagnosis, differential diagnosis or problem list.

Writing a referral letter is a useful exercise for a student, as it challenges you to produce a concise and accurate summary and think through the management of your patient, as well as helping you master the skill of writing the referral letter itself.

Alarm point: be clear what you want from a referral. Make your request concise and relevant.

Reviewing patients after a referral

For the GP, the relationship with the patient is an ongoing one, so he or she will see the patient again after the referral has been made and will have to put into action any new plans that have been decided upon. In well-ordered circles, the specialist will write back to the GP with an opinion about the patient's problems and answering the questions the GP has raised. Things do not always work out like that, and the letter may not deal with the things that the referring doctor considered to be important and may not answer the questions that were raised. Occasionally, the GP may not have the courtesy of a reply at all.

When a reply has been received, it is a good time to review the patient and consider the various changes in his or her management. This is an important exercise to:

- check that the patient has understood what the consultant has proposed;
- ensure that new information has been added to the patient record, such as details of changes to medication;
- make sure that the management plan for the patient has been updated to take account of the changes.

The doctor must also consider how the management will be shared if the patient is to continue being seen by the specialist as well as by the GP. This is a critical area of communication and is frequently handled poorly. Mistakes and misunderstandings easily arise in areas such as changes of drugs and changes in dosage.

Thinking and Discussion Point

How often do you communicate by letter with anyone? Is sending bits of paper through the post the best way to link a patient's treatment across primary and secondary care?

Evidence-based medicine in general practice

Since the last edition of this book the use of evidence-based decision making has grown

Thinking and Discussion Point

Think about the last time you considered how to treat a particular patient. On what did you base your decision? Your own experience? The teaching of your GP tutor or hospital consultant? But on what did these 'oracles' base their teaching?

rapidly. This has in turn been accelerated by the 'pay for performance' Quality Outcomes Framework which pays doctors who reach targets in collecting data and managing patients. These targets have been largely based on evidence-based criteria for the management of common conditions, for instance, for regularly measuring the practice population's blood pressure and for treating those in whom – according to the guidelines – it is too high.

Evidence-based medicine is a process that explicitly uses research evidence to guide medical decision making. This is not to say that clinical judgement is obsolete; evidence-based medicine should integrate best research evidence with clinical expertise and take into account individual patient circumstances and values.

The practice of evidence-based medicine can be divided into five steps (Sackett *et al.*, 2000).

- *Step 1*. Having identified a need for information (e.g. about diagnosis, causation, prognosis, therapy or prevention), frame it into an answerable question.
- *Step 2*. Search for the best evidence with which to answer that question.
- *Step 3*. Critically appraise that evidence for its validity (closeness to the truth), impact (size of the effect) and applicability (usefulness in your clinical practice).
- *Step 4*. Integrate the results of the critical appraisal with your clinical judgement and with your patient's unique circumstances and values.
- *Step 5*. Evaluate your effectiveness/efficiency in steps 1–4 and seek ways to improve next time.

While these steps seem clear enough, working them through in a real clinical situation may not be straightforward. For example, in general practice, the clinical question may not be easily identified; patients frequently have multiple, ill-defined problems involving complex psychosocial factors, and a definitive diagnosis may not be made. Many minor illnesses seen in general practice are poorly researched. Data from hospital studies may not be applicable in the general practice setting. Available trials may have set exclusion criteria which make them of uncertain relevance for your population. For instance, trials frequently exclude elderly people (maybe because of the greater likelihood of comorbidities), who may be the very group about whom you need evidence to manage effectively.

Moreover, GPs have to cover the whole spectrum of illness and, unlike specialists, have limited time to focus on a particular area. GPs tend to rely on guidelines and protocols developed by others (such as academic departments of general practice) to allow them to use best evidence to care for their patients.

It would be wrong to assume that GPs are poor users of evidence-based practice medicine: as long ago as 1996 Gill *et al.* showed that most interventions in a training general practice are based on evidence from clinical trials.

Practical Exercise

1. Choose a clinical problem and frame an answerable question. This should focus on a common problem based on a patient you have seen in general practice. Possible examples might be: 'Should antibiotics be given for sore throats?' and 'Should patients in atrial fibrillation be anticoagulated?'
2. Search the literature. If you do not know how to do literature searches, now would be a good time to learn; the library at your medical school will probably offer training.
3. Critically appraise the literature. When you have collected a sheaf of references, you will need to evaluate the validity, impact and applicability of their results.
4. Integrate the evidence with your clinical expertise and your individual patient's unique circumstances and values.
5. Discuss your findings with your GP tutor. Does the existing patient management plan

Practical Exercise continued

fit with that suggested by your research? If not, should it be altered? What factors other than the research evidence affect that particular patient and how should treatment be individualized?

Alarm point: While guidelines and protocols derived from evidence-based studies are an invaluable aid to good management, patients' needs are individual and therapy should be tailored to meet individual situations.

Guidelines and protocols

GPs rely extensively on these 'pre-digested' summations of available evidence. They are intended to be 'extensive, critical and well balanced information on the benefits and limitations of various diagnostic and therapeutic interventions' (WHO-ISH Mild Hypertension Committee, 1993). As part of the guideline it should be clear what 'level of evidence' was used by its developers. The pyramid diagram (Figure 5.1) is a helpful illustration of this, the pyramid shape indicating that while at the bottom there is no shortage of low-grade evidence and opinion, the availability of the meta-analyses at the top of the pyramid are in much shorter supply.

Sources of guidelines include expert panels from the Royal Colleges, professional associations and medical audit advisory groups. Groups have come together with the specific purpose of developing

guidelines for clinical practices such as SIGN – the Scottish Intercollegiate Guidelines Network. The government's establishment of the National Institute for Health and Clinical Excellence (NICE) in 1999 (www.nice.org.uk/) has produced a large number of guidelines, particularly targeted at the needs of the NHS and many of direct relevance to general practice.

One effect of having different groups producing guidelines is that the guidance can vary. For instance, the Joint British Societies' Guidelines on Prevention of Cardiovascular Disease in Clinical Practice (British Cardiac Society *et al.*, 2005) are more stringent than those produced by NICE, which takes a more pragmatic approach to setting a minimum acceptable standard of care.

Despite the 'evidence-based' tag there are inevitably assumptions and prejudices that influence the final recommendations. These will not be obvious if you rely solely on the 'cookbook' summary. For instance NICE's dyspepsia guideline recommends using a proton pump inhibitor (PPI) for 'uninvestigated dyspepsia' (NICE, 2004). The full guideline explains that uninvestigated dyspepsia responds to a PPI in 55 per cent of cases. However, PPIs are a major cause of expenditure for the NHS (£425 million in England in 2006). The guideline also notes that 37 per cent respond to much cheaper antacid remedies. There would be a strong financial case for recommending antacids as first line treatment in this situation, based on precisely the same evidence.

In using guidelines you should consider:

- the quality of the evidence from which they were developed;
- the academic rigor of the development process;
- the assumptions that the developers will have made (which they should have discussed in the guideline, but of which they may have been unaware);
- whether they apply to your patient or local population.

Many general practices have developed protocols or set ways of dealing with particular conditions, such as asthma and diabetes, often based on a local implementation of existing guidelines. The advantage of such protocols is that they help ensure uniformity and quality in patient care,

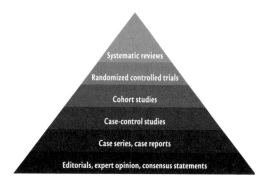

Figure 5.1 The Pyramid Diagram.

especially where many different health professionals are involved.

For further information on guidelines and protocols, see Chapter 9 on chronic illness and Chapter 13 on quality assurance.

Practical Exercise

1. Choose a topic based on a patient you have seen in general practice.
2. Find out whether any guidelines exist on this topic and whether copies are available in the practice.
3. Does the practice have a protocol for dealing with patients with this condition?
4. How was this protocol developed?
5. Interview a selection of the GPs and nurses in the practice to see whether they use these guidelines/protocols and their views of them (and of guidelines/protocols in general).

SUMMARY POINTS

To conclude, the most important messages of this chapter are as follows:

- Patients choose whether to see their doctor: the reasons vary greatly and are not necessarily medical.
- Diagnoses exist at various levels: a firm diagnosis may be impossible to reach initially, and the early management of your patient may involve clarifying the diagnosis by various means; a firm diagnosis is not always required for good management.
- Most diagnoses are made through the careful use of basic clinical skills: taking a history, making an examination and performing investigations are the starting point and basis of all patient management.
- Investigations contribute to your patients' care when they are relevant, sensitive and specific: batteries of random investigations provide little additional information and may mislead.
- Good patient management is your overall goal: it is not intrinsically difficult; the diagnostic information you have gathered is integrated into a detailed picture of your patient's problem; having developed this, you are able to develop a management plan that allows you to inform, reassure, treat and, where necessary, refer your patient.
- Making a referral is an important communication between primary and secondary care: this chapter has considered the decision to refer and the objectives of a referral.
- Decisions on patient care should be based on a combination of clinical judgement and research evidence and should take into account individual patients' unique circumstances and values.
- Evidence-based medicine provides strategies to ensure the best of contemporary medical research is available to each patient.
- Guidelines condense best evidence into useable formulations. Their limitations should be appreciated, but they have huge potential to improve patient care.

References

British Cardiac Society, British Hypertension Society, Diabetes UK, HEART UK, Primary Care Cardiovascular Society, The Stroke Association 2005: Joint British Societies' guidelines on prevention of cardiovascular disease in clinical practice. *Heart* 91, v1–v52.

Fitzpatrick, R. 1996: Telling patients there is nothing wrong. *British Medical Journal* 313, 311–12.

Fry, J. 1993: *General practice: the facts.* Abingdon: Radcliffe Medical Press.

Gill, P., Dowell, A., Neal, R., Smith, N., Heywood, P. and Wilson, A. 1996: Evidence based general practice: a retrospective study of interventions in one training practice. *British Medical Journal* 312, 819–21.

Hoffbrand, B.I. 1989: Away with the systems review, a plea for parsimony. *British Medical Journal* 298, 817–19.

NICE (National Institute for Health and Clinical Excellence) 2004: Management of dyspepsia in adults in primary care. www.nice.org.uk/nicemedia/live/10950/29460/29460.pdf (accessed 3 June 2011).

Ross, P.W., Christy, S.M. and Knox, J.D. 1971: Sore throat in children: its causation and incidence. *British Medical Journal* 2(762), 624–6.

Royal College of Radiologists 2003: *Making the best use of a department of clinical radiology: guidelines for doctors,* 5th edn. London: Royal College of Radiologists.

Sackett, D., Straus, S., Richardson, W., Rosenberg, W. and Haynes, R. 2000: *Evidence based medicine: how to practice and teach EBM,* 2nd edn. Edinburgh: Churchill Livingstone.

Sinclair, D. and Croskerry, P. 2010: Patient safety and diagnostic error: tips for your next shift. *Canadian Family Physician* 56(1), 28–30.

Stoate, H.G. 1989: Can health screening damage your health? *Journal of the Royal College of General Practitioners* 39(322), 193–5.

The Information Centre (2006/7) UK General Practice Workload Survey. www.ic.nhs.uk/webfiles/publications/gp/GP%20Workload%20Report.pdf (accessed May 2011).

Thurber, J. 1965: The secret life of Walter Mitty. In *The Thurber carnival.* London: Penguin Books.

WHO-ISH Mild Hypertension Committee 1993: *Guidelines for the treatment of mild hypertension. Memorandum from a WHO-ISH meeting.* Geneva: World Health Organization.

Further reading

Diagnosis

Epstein, O., Perkin, G.D., Cookson, J. and de Bono, D. 2003: *Clinical examination.* Edinburgh and New York: Mosby.

Gray, D. and Toghill, P. (eds) 2000: *Introduction to the symptoms and signs of clinical medicine.* London: Arnold.

Evidence-based medicine

ACP Journal Club: American College of Physicians and BMJ Publishing Group.

  A regularly updated electronic database that provides access to all issues of the ACP Journal Club and back issues of the *Evidence-Based Medicine Journal.* These summarize individual studies and systematic reviews from a large range of medical journals. Studies are selected according to explicit criteria for scientific merit and clinical relevance. Your library may subscribe; see www.acponline.org for more information.

Clinical evidence 2003: London: BMJ Publishing Group. www.clinicalevidence.bmj.com

  A compendium of evidence based on systematic reviews of the literature.

Cochrane Library. Oxford: www.thecochranelibrary.com/

  A compendium of evidence based on systematic reviews of the literature.

Greenhalgh T. 2006: *How to read a paper: the basics of evidence-based medicine.* Oxford: Wiley-Blackwell.

A superbly helpful introduction to evidence-based medicine.

Sackett, D., Straus, S., Richardson, W., Rosenberg, W. and Haynes, R. 2000: *Evidence based medicine: how to practice and teach EBM*, 2nd edn. Edinburgh: Churchill Livingstone.

An excellent introduction to evidence-based medicine, it uses a case-based format focusing on general medicine, but the accompanying CD-ROM contains cases relevant to general practice. The book has a regularly updated website at http://www.cebm.utoronto.ca/

Guidelines and protocols

There are many useful websites providing clinical guidelines. The three below will be a good starting point:

Health Information Resources, www.library.nhs.uk/default.aspx

National Institute for Health and Clinical Excellence (NICE), www.nice.org.uk/

Scottish Intercollegiate Guidelines Network (SIGN), www.sign.ac.uk/

Acknowledgements

Thank you to Dr Joanna Collerton who was co-author in previous editions.

SINGLE BEST ANSWER QUESTIONS

5.1 Ms Jilly L, aged 23, attends the surgery with intermittent epigastric pain for six weeks. She is overweight (although she thinks that she has lost a little weight since the pain started) and smokes 10 cigarettes a day. On examination she has mild epigastric tenderness. The best intervention at this stage is:

a) A course of proton pump inhibitor (PPI, e.g. omeprazole)
b) Advise her to stop smoking
c) Advise her to lose weight
d) Arrange an outpatient upper GI endoscopy
e) Arrange helicobacter testing.

5.2 Mrs Joyce L, aged 63 (Jilly's mother), attends the surgery with intermittent epigastric pain for six weeks. She is overweight (although she thinks that she has lost a little weight since the pain started) and smokes 10 cigarettes a day. On examination she has mild epigastric tenderness. The best intervention at this stage is:

a) A course of PPIs (e.g. omeprazole)
b) Advise her to stop smoking
c) Advise her to lose weight
d) Arrange an outpatient upper GI endoscopy
e) Arrange helicobacter testing.

5.3 Mr Michael L, aged 27 (Joyce's son), comes to you complaining of 'chronic stomach ache' for six weeks. He describes pains in his upper abdomen which come and go with no very clear pattern and no relieving or exacerbating factors. He admits that he is both smoking and drinking alcohol more recently. He has not lost weight and on examination there is nothing to find. The best intervention at this point is to:

a) Prescribe a trial of PPIs
b) Explore the patient's beliefs
c) Reassure the patient that there is nothing serious likely to be wrong
d) Reassure the patient that the risk of malignancy is minimal
e) Advise on dietary modification for probable irritable bowel syndrome.

5.4 Mr Michael L (the same one) accepts that he has irritable bowel syndrome of which the stress and anxiety caused by his mother's illness is partly to blame. He has found little benefit from dietary modifications and the anti-spasmodics you prescribed don't help much either. A work colleague has been seeing a 'nutriopathic physician' who he says is absolutely brilliant. He asks for your advice about what to do:

SINGLE BEST ANSWER QUESTIONS CONTINUED

a) It's worth pursuing, if only for the placebo effect

b) Explore the claims made for the therapy before advising the patient

c) Warn the patient to steer clear of alternative remedies

d) Encourage the patient to attend to relieve the burden on the surgery and local NHS

e) Give strong endorsement of the therapy which will increase any placebo effect and the likelihood of success.

5.5 Mr ML, aged 72 (Michael's and Jilly's father), has mild COPD and presents with a purulent cough, breathlessness and fever. He has no drug allergies. He has a dull percussion note, bronchial breath sounds and whispering pectoriloquy at his L lung base.

a) Give a prescription for amoxicillin and clarithromycin in line with best practice guidelines

b) Prescribe doxycycline as he is more likely to comply with a single drug regime

c) Elicit the patient's ideas and concerns about treatment and prescribe accordingly

d) Stress the importance of taking antibiotics according to the instructions and to avoid alcohol

e) Discuss the effective options and come to an agreement about which he is happy to take.

CHAPTER

6

PRESCRIBING IN GENERAL PRACTICE

- Introduction
- The scale of medication use in the UK
- Guidelines for good prescribing
- Prescribing for special groups
- Generic prescribing
- Prescribing support in primary care
- Writing a prescription
- Repeat prescribing
- Abuse of drugs and controlled drugs
- The doctor's bag
- Dispensing practices

- Prescribing by nurses in practice
- The role of the community pharmacist
- Over-the-counter medication
- Communicating about medications between primary and secondary care
- Prescribing costs and monitoring
- Summary points
- References
- Further reading
- Single best answer questions

The scale of medication use in the UK is enormous. While it has brought huge benefits, the problems caused by side effects, drug interactions and drug errors are a major cause of illness for patients and a significant burden to the health service. This chapter outlines these problems and discusses a number of strategies to ensure you develop good prescribing habits.

LEARNING OBJECTIVES

By the end of this chapter you will be able to:
- understand the scale of medication usage in the UK;
- develop good prescribing habits;
- find sources of help with prescribing in primary care;
- write a prescription;
- understand how computers in primary care are used to aid acute and repeat prescribing;
- understand the importance of communications about medication between primary and secondary care;
- understand the legal and practical approaches to prevent the problems of drug abuse;
- understand self-prescribing and over-the-counter medication and the role of the community pharmacist and other healthcare professionals in prescribing.

Introduction

Miss Molly had a dolly, who was sick, sick, sick,
So she called for the doctor to come quick, quick, quick.
The doctor came with his bag and his hat,
And he knocked on the door with a rat a tat tat.

He looked at the dolly and he shook his head,
He said, Miss Molly, put her straight to bed,
He wrote on the paper for a pill, pill, pill,
I'll be back in the morning with my bill, bill, bill.

An old skipping song, its origins clouded with time, reveals an iconic view of the general practitioner (GP). While hospital doctors may be associated with the stethoscope, GPs are identified by their bag, their bill and their prescription pad. Of these, the bill has gone, the bag is fading, but the prescription pad remains a pervasive symbol. This is not necessarily a positive image: 'The moment I sat down he started writing out a prescription' is a well-aired complaint.

Prescribing new and repeat medications to patients is a major part of general practice, but it is important to understand that drugs are not the only approach to patient therapy. This chapter discusses the range of therapies available to the GP and the range of issues involved in prescribing medication effectively.

The scale of medication use in the UK

The scale of medication usage is vast. Two-thirds of the population are taking some kind of medication at any time, whether prescribed, purchased over the counter from a chemist or from alternative therapists (Fry, 1993):

- At any one time, 66 per cent of the population is taking some form of medicine; half of this medicine is prescribed and half purchased 'over the counter' (Kohn and White, 1976).
- A prescription is issued in 66 per cent of general practice consultations and a similar volume is generated using the repeat prescription system.
- The average person receives eight prescription items per year.
- The most widely prescribed drugs are cardiovascular, dermatological and anti-asthma preparations, and antibiotics. The most widely purchased 'over-the-counter' (OTC) drugs are analgesics, vitamins and cough medicines.
- Drug costs consume 10 per cent of the total National Health Service (NHS) budget, of which 18 per cent is spent in hospitals and 82 per cent in general practice.
- Up to 20 per cent of patients do not take their prescription to be dispensed.

The total budget for pharmaceutical supplies to the NHS in England was £11 billion (2007–8) (DoH website http://www.dh.gov.uk/en/Healthcare/Medicinespharmacyandindustry/Pharmaceuticalpriceregulationscheme/DH_4071841). It is estimated that it costs the NHS in England £300 million a year for medicines that are wasted, dispensed but never taken (York Health Economics Consortium, 2010), and this is in a system which the authors conclude is reasonably well managed.

In summary, the scale of prescribing is large and the costs are high. Drugs are beneficial in many conditions, but can also have side effects. How can you ensure that you prescribe effectively and safely?

Guidelines for good prescribing

Good prescribing is not a particularly difficult task. It relates more to attitude: fastidiousness in considering a series of questions each time a drug is prescribed and a desire to do the best for each individual patient. While as a student the list of drugs you need to learn about seems endless, in practice most doctors use only a limited number of drugs, which they therefore get to know well. This list is often based on a local formulary (see below). Advice on good prescribing is available from many sources including the *British National Formulary* (BNF.org).

Every time you reach for your prescription pad consider the following:

- Is a drug necessary?
- Is a drug the right choice?
- Is the drug effective?
- Is the drug safe?
- Is therapy economical?
- Do you and your patient agree on your management plan?
- Does your patient understand how and when to take the medication?
- Is there a long-term plan?

Alarm point: always ask yourself whenever you consider prescribing: Is a drug necessary, is it the right solution, is it effective, is it safe, and is it part of an agreed plan?

Is a drug necessary?

Have you made a diagnosis?

In the chapter on diagnosis and management (Chapter 5) we considered how management decisions can be made with and without a diagnosis. Ideally, in choosing therapy you will have a diagnosis, but life is not always ideal.

Treatment may be initiated:

- on a firm diagnosis,
- on a provisional diagnosis,
- to relieve undiagnosed symptoms, or
- as a trial of therapy (helping confirm the diagnosis if it works).

The less certain you are of what you are treating, the less chance you have of successful treatment. At the same time, the risk of adverse effects from your chosen medication is not diminished.

Symptomatic treatment

There are many situations in which it is entirely appropriate to treat the patient's symptoms. For instance, pain usually requires symptomatic treatment in addition to any treatment of the underlying cause. So in an acute myocardial infarction, opiate analgesics for pain are as essential to treatment as drugs to limit infarct size. Occasionally symptomatic treatment is of particular importance when there is little that can be done for the underlying disease. The relief of pain and breathlessness in lung cancer offers a major contribution to the patient's quality of life. For many self-limiting conditions seen in general practice, symptomatic treatment, often as self-treatment, is all that is appropriate (see below).

Remember that the same considerations of necessity, effectiveness, safety, economy and patient review apply to symptomatic treatments as to other therapeutic interventions.

Self-limiting conditions

Many of the patients seen by GPs present with self-limiting conditions. These are minor conditions that will resolve by themselves without necessarily requiring the GP's intervention.

It is the GP's role:

- to educate patients about the nature of their condition and how to recognize it themselves next time;

- to empower patients to deal with the problem by themselves and without recourse to medical services.

In doing so, the GP is not only helping the patient, but also aiming to manage demand for consultations. If patients deal with the problem by themselves next time, it contributes to reducing the burden on the surgery and other healthcare services.

Upper respiratory tract infections (URTIs) in adults and children are very common examples: the doctor's aim should be to help patients recognize the symptoms and treat themselves. The doctor will need to become involved if the illness becomes protracted or severe or unexpected complications arise, and will need to discuss with the patient the boundaries for safe self-management.

While a condition may be self-limiting, it may not be common (so there is little point in teaching patients to recognize it themselves); the symptoms may be disturbing and merit treatment in their own right. Moreover, appropriate medication may only be available on prescription. For example, acute vestibuloneuronitis presents with dramatic vertigo, sometimes leading to falls and injury. Although it rarely lasts more than a few days, accurate diagnosis, symptomatic treatment (with vestibular sedatives) and appropriate advice from the GP (e.g. avoiding driving) are usually required, despite it being a self-limiting condition.

The increasing number of former prescription drugs now available over the counter has increased the range of minor conditions patients can treat themselves. For instance, topical antifungal treatments are available over the counter.

Is a drug the right solution?

We are fortunate in the UK to practise in an age in which numerous highly effective medications are available and in a country where they can be afforded. Doctors have a particular expertise in using drugs and it is therefore not surprising that they turn to them frequently. However, drug treatment is often not the only option, and often not the option of first choice. Although this chapter is principally about prescribing drugs, the section below reviews some of the non-drug approaches that the GP and his or her patient may turn to.

Options for non-drug therapies in practice

Physical therapies

- *Physiotherapy*. Physiotherapists are practitioners in their own right. A physiotherapist will not merely carry out a request for treatment, but will make his or her own assessment of the patient's condition and treat accordingly. Generally, physiotherapists are based at hospital or in community clinics. Some are practice based by local arrangement.
- *Osteopathy* and *chiropractic* are sometimes available through the NHS by local arrangement. The GP is often asked to advise on their usefulness or otherwise. The limited evidence base for their efficacy rightly limits their availability on the NHS.
- *Alternative physical therapies*, such as Alexander technique or reflexology, may sometimes be available by local arrangement within the NHS. Using public money to pay for unproven therapies is controversial. The role of alternative therapies is discussed below.
- *Exercise* is now seen as having a critical role in health, from maintaining bone mass in postmenopausal women to gaining cardiovascular fitness and treating depression. GPs may be able to 'prescribe' exercise through local links with a fitness centre or similar.

Psychological therapies

- *Counselling* is frequently available as a service within a practice. Counselling services are also widely available in the community as local government-run services, or run by voluntary groups such as the church, and private counsellors. There is a wide variation in the qualifications of counsellors, and the GP has a role advising on reputable sources of help.
- *Specialist counselling*, for alcohol, smoking, drugs, etc. often operates as an extension of local psychiatric services or as part of the community provision of the local health service. Patients may self-refer or require GP referral. The GP has an important role in knowing about the availability of such services and directing patients to them.
- *Psychotherapy* is widely available privately, from many different theoretical foundations, from Freudian psychoanalysis to behavioural approaches, and shading at the edges into alternative therapies and religious-type organizations. Of the more orthodox therapies, the theoretical approach seems to have less bearing on outcome than the individual qualities of the practitioner. Mainstream psychotherapy is usually available within the NHS, although cost constraints may allow only a limited number of sessions for a patient and delay in getting a first appointment.
- *Support and counselling from the GP*. The GP him/herself is a source of emotional and psychological support for patients. Many consultations with a partly or wholly psychological basis are dealt with by the GP in everyday consultations. Some GPs undergo additional training in counselling and psychotherapy and offer this as a service to their patients. Psychological issues in general practice are discussed in Chapter 8.

Self-help

Many patients attempt, often successfully, to sort themselves out through their own efforts. The GP may act as a source of support and encouragement, may help the patient find self-help groups, and advise on the course of actions they propose. The internet is now a major source of advice for patients. Advice ranges from the excellent, to drug company advertisements, to the ravings of the probably insane! To the patient, it may not be clear which sort they have discovered. For example:

> 'Toddlers are to be inoculated against six diseases at once in a bid to boost vaccination rates. Recently uncovered evidence suggests as many as 400 children have died from a vaccine and 21,000 experienced an adverse reaction in the UK alone.' (vactruth.com)

Alternative therapies

A huge variety of alternative or complementary therapies are available to patients. It is important for the GP to be aware of the claims each makes and the evidence to support them. Because of the nature of complementary practices, many have little formal scientific evaluation. The dictum 'first do no harm' is of prime importance. Harm can be caused either by the effects of a therapy (it is worth remembering that orthodox therapies have much greater potential for harm than most complementary therapies) or by using an ineffective remedy and refusing an effective one. (Some homeopaths warn their clients not to take conventional therapies while taking homeopathic remedies.) Tragic and unnecessary deaths have resulted from an insistence on a particular type of therapy. Many therapies that started life as 'alternative' have moved, as prejudices have changed and evidence emerged, into the mainstream. Osteopathy and acupuncture are examples. Homeopathy has a strong following amongst doctors (and an equally vociferous medical opposition). The Alexander technique lacks much of an evidence base, but has sensible-sounding ideas about posture and voice training. Yoga and Transcendental Meditation are amongst a variety of Eastern-style philosophies that help patients relax (trials have shown them to be effective in lowering blood pressure, for example). Others, such as elimination diets and those to treat *Candida albicans*, are based on corrupted versions of Western science.

Lifestyle change

We are becoming increasingly aware of the effects of lifestyle on illness, and changes in lifestyle may provide a better remedy than medication. Some of the factors are listed below.

- Smoking remains a massive cause of ill-health of many kinds. Britain is doing relatively well compared to the rest of Europe, but the mortality and morbidity remain appalling.
- Alcohol may be a bigger problem than smoking. Alcohol-related problems cost an estimated £95 million to the Scottish NHS in 2001, and a billion pounds to Scotland as a whole in that period (Alcohol Misuse in Scotland: Trends and Costs. Final report Catalyst Health Economics 2001).
- Sexual activity: sexually transmitted diseases are increasing, including hepatitis B and acquired immune deficiency syndrome (AIDS).
- Sedentary lifestyles: we have become so used to sedentary lifestyles that very modest exercise can have enormous health gains. Cycling

for 40 minutes a day (in other words about 3 miles to work and back again) reduces the risk of ischaemic heart disease by nearly 50 per cent. Bone mass is increased more by exercise than by any other treatment of osteoporosis. Jogging, via endorphin release, is an effective treatment for mild and moderate depression.

- Work: working long hours under pressure puts a strain on relationships and may cause sleep and psychiatric problems. The physical working environment at the office may result in repetitive strain and back injuries, and worse at the factory. Changing working patterns may not be easy but may bring significant health benefits.
- Obesity: factors are often interrelated. Obesity relates to sedentary living and bad diets secondary to long working hours – and that includes middle-class fast food such as microwaveable tagliatelle, with its excess fat and salt (which enhances flavour at low cost to the manufacturer), just as much as burger and chip diets.

Is the drug effective?

Always consider whether there is evidence that the particular drug you choose is of proven benefit in the condition you propose to treat.

The rise of evidence-based medicine has made available to the GP a large and accessible body of evidence for the effectiveness of many treatments. This evidence is often used to provide guidelines and protocols for the management of a condition. Applying such guidelines in everyday practice is a major challenge of contemporary general practice. Guidelines do not negate the need for clinical judgement. Each patient's situation is different, and the challenge is to provide the best care for the individual patient based on the best available evidence.

Remember that indications for the treatment of any condition may differ with age, sex and other factors. For example, an elderly smoker with chronic obstructive pulmonary disease (COPD) who presents with influenza may very justifiably be given antibiotics to prevent secondary bacterial infection. There would be little reason to do the same for a fit 25 year old.

Is the drug safe?

Alarm point: never prescribe without considering the potential for adverse reactions and drug interactions.

Adverse reactions

All medications carry a risk of adverse reactions. These may be of several kinds. Rawlins and Thompson's (1977) useful classification of drug side effects included predictable (type A); idiosyncratic (type B); continuous reactions (type C) from long-term drug use, such as the tardive dyskinesias related to neuroleptic use; delayed reactions (type D), such as the potential for carcinogenesis from alkylating agents; and end-of-use reactions (type E) where problems arise on discontinuing therapy, such as withdrawal symptoms following discontinuation of benzodiazepines or addisonian symptoms after the withdrawal of steroids. You will meet patients who have experienced all of these reactions in general practice, but types A, B and E are particularly common. Also important is the wrong attribution of adverse reactions to medication; this is discussed in the next section.

Predictable reactions

Some side effects are entirely predictable as a consequence of the actions of the drug. For example, broad-spectrum antibiotics frequently produce diarrhoea in children and adults (5–30 per cent) through effects on normal bacterial flora (Editorial, 2002). In the debilitated, this can produce the life-threatening pseudomembranous colitis. I recently talked with parents whose 2-year-old child required admission and intravenous rehydration for antibiotic-related diarrhoea. The antibiotics were given for a simple URTI that was of likely viral origin.

Non-steroidal anti-inflammatory drugs (NSAIDs) are useful as painkillers in a range of situations, but are a major cause of upper gastrointestinal inflammation and bleeding, and elevate blood pressure through salt and water-retaining properties. Other drugs (such as paracetamol in combination or alone) are often equally effective.

Some drugs require more careful monitoring because of the risks of serious side effects (e.g. monitoring of prothrombin time during warfarin therapy or agranulocytosis with carbimazole).

Idiosyncratic reactions

Idiosyncratic reactions are not predictable, not dose related, and may be severe. Individual reactions are uncommon, and inevitably the doctor cannot be aware of all the many types and potential for idiosyncratic reactions of the drugs he or she uses. As elsewhere in general practice, prevention is much better than cure, reinforcing the importance of not prescribing drugs except when explicitly indicated.

Examples of idiosyncratic reactions include thrombocytopenia from quinine (commonly prescribed to the elderly for leg cramps) and Stevens–Johnson syndrome from sulphonamide antibiotics ('hidden' in combinations like co-trimoxazole, and in Flamazine cream, which is commonly used in treating burns and leg ulcers, from which systemic absorption can be high).

The *British National Formulary* (*BNF*) is the most useful everyday source of information about the reactions that may be associated with any particular drug or class of drugs.

GPs need a good working knowledge of the commoner predictable side effects of the drugs they use. This is another argument in favour of practice formularies. This offers the opportunity of better understanding of a more limited range of drugs.

The GP should always be aware that a patient's symptoms may result from drug side effects, and a thorough review of the patient's medication is an essential part of the patient's assessment. This medication may be unknown to the GP at the time of presentation. The possibility of a reaction from an OTC remedy or a new prescription from a recent hospital appointment must always be considered.

Serious side effects of established drugs and all side effects of newer drugs should be reported to the Committee on Safety of Medicines using the yellow card system.

End-of-use reactions

Withdrawal reactions from the discontinuation of a drug can produce a variety of symptoms. Benzodiazepine withdrawal, for example, may result in anxiety and muscle cramps, confusion, convulsions or frank psychiatric illness if not carefully managed. Abrupt withdrawal of long-term steroids will produce addisonian symptoms. A more common and insidious scenario is a patient who, some months after discontinuing steroids, develops an intercurrent infection and becomes unexpectedly ill. It may take a year or more for the adrenal glands to recover fully after steroid withdrawal, and the patient, while able to maintain a basal cortisol output, is unable to respond to the increased glucocorticoid needs brought about by the infection. The patient may present, not with classic addisonian symptoms, but merely as being unexpectedly unwell. Oral steroids need to be reintroduced to provide cover over this period and then quickly tailed off again.

Wrongly identified side effects

When patients report side effects of a medication, it is important to take a history of the alleged reaction and attempt to establish whether or not it was a true side effect. Many patients will tell you they are 'allergic to penicillin'; often, on further questioning, the drug turns out not to have been penicillin. The reaction may be that it 'made me feel sick' or 'gave me diarrhoea'. Assessing the likelihood of a reaction may prove very difficult: when a rash follows an antibiotic prescription it is often not clear whether it was due to the antibiotic or to the viral illness for which it was inappropriately given. This serves as a further warning against prescribing antibiotics when the indications are not clear. It is important to discuss with patients whether or not they should avoid that drug in future. Confirming that they may take penicillin when they initially believed themselves to be allergic to it may save their life at some time in the future.

Alarm point: when a patient tells you they are allergic to a medication, always explore fully what they mean and whether this is likely to be a true allergy.

Drug interactions

Interactions between drugs are common, are a frequent cause of morbidity and sometimes mortality and are often avoidable. The elderly are particularly at risk, often having multiple pathologies, and may be particularly sensitive to the effects of any medication (see the section on the prescribing for the elderly later in this chapter). Not all interactions are adverse. Synergistic effects of drugs in combination can be very useful, such as combining diuretics and angiotensin-converting enzyme (ACE) inhibitors for both heart failure and hypertension. Indeed, using lower doses of two drugs may be more therapeutically effective, while at the same time lowering the likelihood of dose-related side effects of the individual drugs. Interactions may be deliberately sought to offset the side effects of one drug with another; for instance, the potassium-leaching effects of furosemide are countered by potassium-sparing amiloride, while increasing the overall diuretic effect.

Drug interactions arise through a number of mechanisms. Those mechanisms particularly encountered in general practice settings are discussed below. The reader is encouraged to consult a textbook of pharmacology to gain a broader overview.

Drug interactions are classified as:

- pharmaceutical,
- pharmacodynamic, and
- pharmacokinetic.

We might add a further category of:

- 'pharmacoconfusion', where, as the number of medications increases, the chance of any being taken correctly decreases; this is perhaps the commonest and most important 'class' found in general practice.

Pharmaceutical reactions are rarely encountered by GPs. They occur when mixing drugs before they get to the patient; for example, diazepam when injected into an infusion bag precipitates out. Pharmacodynamic and pharmacokinetic reactions are discussed below.

Predictable (pharmacodynamic) interactions arise as a predictable consequence of the normal effects of the drugs. They are thus very common and frequently encountered in general practice. For instance, tricyclic antidepressants and alcohol both cause drowsiness. The effect of taking both is for one to augment the other. It is important to make a patient you are putting on tricyclics aware of this effect and its implications for safety, while driving for example. The NSAIDs are freely prescribed as analgesics, but their well-known salt and water-retaining properties will diminish the effect of diuretics and anti-hypertensives.

Pharmacokinetic interactions occur when one drug affects the plasma levels of another. These work through a number of mechanisms:

- *Absorption.* Interactions may occur through effects on drug absorption, for instance tetra-cyclines are chelated by aluminium (perhaps being taken by the patient as an OTC indigestion remedy) or milk (not a drug, but no less important as an interaction). Rifampicin-like medicines have an enzyme-inducing effect, and speed up the processing of some contraceptive hormones. This reduces the levels of the hormones in the blood and increases the potential for pregnancy.

- *Metabolism.* Drugs may stimulate or inhibit liver enzyme production, resulting in the enhanced or diminished breakdown of other drugs. Erythromycin inhibits enzymes metabolizing theophyllines; treating an acute exacerbation of COPD with this antibiotic could precipitate theophylline toxicity. Anticonvulsants induce the enzymes that metabolize oral contraceptives; the increased rate of breakdown of oestrogen and progestogen is predictable, and an effective response may therefore be to increase the strength of the pill – typically increasing the oestrogen component from 30 to 50 micrograms (μg).

- *Excretion.* The well-known potassium-leaching actions of loop and thiazide diuretics are often countered by combining them with a potassium-sparing diuretic such as spironolactone or amiloride. In this common example, the interaction is used to the patient's benefit. However, other interactions, such as the increased reabsorption of lithium when diuretics are given, will increase the blood levels and may produce serious toxicity.

GPs use a huge spectrum of drugs, both those they prescribe themselves and those prescribed initially by the hospital. If a patient is attending several clinics, the risk of adverse interactions multiplies, and the GP is best placed to overview the entire prescribing strategy. GPs need to be aware of the potential for interactions and actively monitor the overall prescribing pattern; they may be assisted by computer prescribing programs that can be set to warn automatically of potential interactions. Awareness of the potential for interactions, keeping up to date with new medications and vigilance with individual patients are crucial aspects of the GP's role.

Many medications are initiated in hospital and the GP subsequently takes responsibility for continuing to prescribe them. The importance of adequate and accurate communication between hospital and general practice and vice versa cannot be over-emphasized. Unfortunately, it is still commonplace for patients to be discharged from hospital with inadequate or no information. Similarly, many GP referrals do not contain adequate information about patients' medication, even though this can usually be readily obtained from the practice computer system.

'Pharmacoconfusion' and polypharmacy

Polypharmacy, defined as taking more than four drugs, is a major issue in prescribing. There is solid evidence that the more drugs are prescribed, the greater the likelihood of failure to take them correctly and to take less than the prescribed dose and multiple opportunities for interactions to occur. Classically this is a problem for the elderly with multiple pathologies requiring multiple drugs, increased sensitivity to those drugs and often impaired cognitive abilities to deal with the dosing regime. With more sophisticated therapies available in many areas such as HIV, cancer and transplants, the problem is not limited to the elderly. GPs coordinate the care for patients who may be seeing several different specialists. They have a particular responsibility to oversee the whole prescription package, reduce 'pharmacoconfusion' and remain alert to possible interactions.

Is therapy economical?

While many common drugs are relatively inexpensive, when this is multiplied across the whole NHS the costs can be enormous. In England, as at 2011, protein pump inhibitors cost from approximately £2 (generic omeprazole) to £20 (esomeprazole as branded 'Nexium') for a month's course. Altogether these cost the NHS around £10.5 million a year (Prescription Cost Analysis England 2010, The Health and Social Care Information Centre, 2011). It is therefore good practice to prescribe drugs by generic name rather than proprietary (brand) names. GPs are also encouraged to substitute a cheaper drug for a more expensive one in the same class where this is clinically as effective; for instance, omeprazole for esomeprazole, or simvastatin for atorvastatin. In the latter case atorvastatin is a more potent drug so is useful for those with more severe hypercholesterolaemia, however many drugs are 'me too' drugs which are minimally different versions of the same drug, developed by different drug companies to give them their own branded product. (Esomeprazole is a 'pro-drug' which is metabolized to the active omeprazole in the body.) Often there are no practical differences between different drugs in the same class and it makes economic sense to use the cheapest. Generic drugs are of the same quality as proprietary drugs and prescribing generically ensures that the cheapest preparation is dispensed. The important exception to this rule is with slow-release preparations, where different manufacturers' preparations have different release properties. These are discussed under 'Generic prescribing'.

Agreeing management with your patient

There is evidence that only a third of patients comply with recommended treatment; another third sometimes comply, and the remaining third do not comply at all (Fedder, 1982). Up to 20 per cent of patients do not take their prescriptions to be dispensed, and a sizeable proportion who do so do not subsequently take the drug (Fry, 1993). It has been estimated that, at most, only 50 per cent of people with chronic disease comply with their doctors' recommendations, irrespective of disease, treatment or age (Sackett and Snow, 1979; Dunbar-Jacob *et al.*, 2000).

Patients may choose not to take prescribed medication for a variety of reasons:

- Fear of taking a drug: 'It's not natural … messing up my body with chemicals.'
- Unconvinced about the need for medication: the asymptomatic hypertensive patient will be

understandably reluctant to engage in a lifetime of treatment with potential side effects.
- Concern about side effects (e.g. measles, mumps and rubella (MMR) vaccination and autism fears).
- Inconvenience: taking aerosol inhaler devices to school or work.
- Cost: significant in the UK, at £7.40 in England on 1 April 2011 per item, although many people (e.g. children, elderly people on social security benefits) are entitled to receive them free. As a result 80 per cent of prescriptions are not charged. The costs may be prohibitive in countries where the full cost has to be borne by the patient.
- Lack of confidence in the doctor: if patients feel their doctor has not understood their problem, they are less likely to comply with the suggested treatment.
- Stigma of illness: this may make diagnosis difficult to accept for the patient (e.g. depression or other psychiatric problems) and hence there is a reluctance to take the appropriate treatment.
- Risks outweigh benefits in the patient's eyes.
- Cultural values and health beliefs: patients' beliefs may be very different from the doctor's: 'drugs bring toxins into the body'.
- Complex drug regimens: multiple drugs, different dosing regimens may be hard to understand even though the patient attempts to do so.

Concordance: a negotiated approach to therapy

The extent to which patients conform to the doctor's plan is termed *compliance*. However, compliance is now seen as a very doctor-centred approach to therapy: it is about the doctor instructing the patient, who is expected to obey. This paternalistic view of therapy is thought to be part of the reason why compliance is so poor. A more recent and successful approach is to see therapy as a shared responsibility of patient and doctor, each of whom has a responsibility to understand the other's viewpoint (NCCSDO, 2005). This 'concordance' between doctor and patient over therapy is discussed below.

Often, such a discussion will be a very straightforward affair, with the patient keen to receive the medication and little discussion required. But sometimes detailed discussion and negotiation are required, for instance in starting a trial of high-dose oral steroids in a patient with suspected temporal arteritis who has well-founded concerns about the side effects of such medication.

In order to understand the patient's possible concerns about therapy, their views need to be actively sought. In the same way that in the consultation chapter we discussed the importance of eliciting patients' concerns, ideas and expectations concerning their illness, it is not difficult to see why this must be extended to patients' ideas concerning treatment. This can then be the basis for a sharing of views between doctor and patient, out of which a negotiated approach to therapy can come that is acceptable to the patient and doctor alike.

An approach to reaching concordance with a patient might run as follows:

■ The doctor presents the diagnosis and proposals for treatment.
■ The patient is encouraged to talk about his or her ideas, concerns and expectations regarding the diagnosis and proposed treatment.
■ The patient and doctor discuss their respective views of the illness and its treatment to reach a shared understanding.
■ Based on this shared understanding, a treatment plan is agreed.
■ The doctor gives clear instructions about the dose, frequency and duration of medication and checks the patient understands.
■ A plan is agreed to review progress.

Helping the patient take medication correctly

Besides discussing and negotiating therapy, there are a number of ways in which the doctor can help the patient to take medication correctly.

■ Give clear instructions and check the patient has understood them (perhaps by getting the patient to explain them back to you). It often helps to write them down – there is good evidence that patients remember very little of a consultation once they have left the room.
■ Prescribe as few medications as possible.
■ Keep the dosing schedule simple:
  – as few times a day as possible,
  – if using several drugs, the same regimen for each (e.g. all twice daily).

  – use combination tablets, 'polypills', where possible to simplify regimes (e.g. co-amilofruse).
■ Avoid drugs likely to produce side effects; discuss any likely side effects and what to do if these arise.
■ Stop drugs that are ineffective or no longer required.
■ Tell the patient how long they are expected to continue the medication.
■ Make use of the local pharmacist. Ensure your instructions to pharmacist are clear and encourage the patient to talk to the pharmacist to reinforce your instructions.

Reviewing your patients' progress and use of medication

Discussing medication use should be part of your regular review of your patients. Your review must be able to tell you the following:

■ *If the medication is having the desired effect*: This will come from your discussion with the patient, backed up by appropriate investigations. These investigations will take whatever form is appropriate (e.g. cardiovascular assessment in the patient with heart failure, reviewing the peak flow diary in the asthmatic patient or laboratory measurement of thyroid-stimulating hormone levels in the treated myxoedemic patient).
■ *Whether the medication is causing side effects*: Likely side effects should be enquired about explicitly. Patients may not realize that new symptoms represent side effects or may be reluctant to discuss them (such as the impotence produced by many anti-hypertensives).
■ *Whether the patient is taking the medication regularly*: Besides developing a relationship of trust with your patient, medication usage can be assessed by monitoring how often the patient collects prescriptions, which may suggest either over-use or under-use of medication. Prescribing software can give a rough indication of compliance by looking at how often repeat medication is collected. Measuring blood levels of drugs gives indirect evidence of compliance, for instance a fall in serum anticonvulsant levels may mean your patient is becoming forgetful about taking the tablets. All

these should be seen as the starting point for a discussion about compliance rather than eliciting a knee-jerk increase in dosage.

Prescribing for special groups

The 'special groups' of children and elderly are actually the commonest groups to be seen in general practice and each, in its own way, is particularly vulnerable to medication. GPs need to take particular care when prescribing for these patients.

Children

The questions of necessity, effectiveness and safety discussed above are of particular importance to this age group. The majority of children presenting in general practice have self-limiting illnesses for which simple supportive or symptomatic treatment only is required. Children are not merely small adults and may respond differently from adults to medication.

Making a firm diagnosis is difficult for a miserable child who is unable or unwilling to give a history or to be examined. Differentiating the genuinely sick child from the merely miserable is a critical skill. Sick children need careful assessment and sometimes reassessment by a GP colleague or paediatrician. Antibiotics are often given to such children 'just in case' of bacterial infection. There is some justification for this approach: the child is sick, the illness might be bacterial, the diagnosis may not be provable, or proving it may require unjustifiably invasive investigations, and the illness is potentially worse than the side effects of the antibiotics. The downside is that the risk of side effects remains and can on occasions be serious or rarely fatal. If the child develops new symptoms, such as a rash, it may be difficult to decide whether it is due to the drug or the illness. Labelling a child as allergic to a medication may have implications for the rest of their life.

Necessity

The majority of children seen in general practice have viral URTIs. There is no justification for treatment with antibiotics, even though there may be pressure from parents to provide them. There is no evidence that cough mixtures are effective. Miserable children with URTIs need rest, fluids and judicious doses of paracetamol or ibuprofen for fever and symptomatic relief (there is some evidence that ibuprofen is the better antipyretic and the longer duration of action is useful). Their carers need clear instructions about what new symptoms would concern you and if/when to return. Unexpectedly protracted illnesses produce parental concern, often manifested in an insistence on antibiotics; this will often not be appropriate. Serial URTIs, where one illness follows directly from another, are the commonest reason for a protracted illness. Asthma or post-nasal drip often follow a URTI and often present as a protracted and mainly nocturnal cough.

Effectiveness

Even those who present with likely bacterial infections are often not helped by antibiotics. For instance, there is little evidence that antibiotics change the history of otitis media; the majority of cases resolve spontaneously. Better public health means that progression to acute mastoiditis or chronic suppurative conditions that used to be common is now rare. Similarly, although pharyngitis is mainly viral, even the 40 per cent of cases that are bacterial are only marginally helped by antibiotics. One study demonstrated that giving antibiotics reduced the duration of symptoms by just 8 hours. Claims have been made that antibiotics prevent the progression of a minor illness to a more major one, for instance otitis media progressing to mastoiditis or sore throat to quinsy. The limited evidence available does not support this.

Safety

Safety is a major concern in prescribing for children. Children metabolize certain drugs differently from adults, their relative body proportion of fat is different (changing the drug's volume of distribution) and certain drugs behave in inexplicable ways (for instance, amphetamine is sedating in children and used to treat hyperactivity syndromes).

Relatively minor side effects with antibiotics, such as diarrhoea, may settle quickly, but, given the often-limited justification for prescribing them and the relatively minor conditions for which they may have been prescribed, it is difficult to justify this sort of prescribing. Moreover, occasionally children develop severe diarrhoea and dehydration, which may even be fatal in the case of antibiotic-related pseudomembranous colitis.

Calculating children's doses

Doses are often most accurately calculated from the child's surface area, itself estimated from nomograms relating to weight and height (Barrett *et al.*, 2002). More commonly dosage is calculated by body weight, which is less accurate and may give too large a dose in an obese child for example. The *BNF* gives dose ranges for children based on age. This imprecise approach is reasonable for 'ordinary' doses of 'safe' drugs given to 'normal' children and is suitable for most drugs given to children in general practice. However, if a high dose of a drug is required, if the therapeutic window is narrow (i.e. there is little leeway between therapeutic and toxic doses) or if the child is not of 'normal' height or weight, then more precise approaches must be adopted.

Concordance

Getting children to take the drug you have prescribed is fortunately delegated to the parents! The doctor can help by providing the drug in the most acceptable (or at any rate, least unacceptable) form to the child. Children are usually prescribed medication in liquid form, but may prefer tablets, so it is worth asking. If a dose of less than 5 mL is prescribed, an oral syringe must be supplied by the chemist; however, in practice, a syringe may be a far easier tool to use than the traditional teaspoon whatever the dose. A familiar form of the drug may be more acceptable, so the child may be persuaded to take proprietary 'Calpol' but not a strange-tasting generic paracetamol.

The elderly

Whereas 16 per cent of the population is over the age of 65, around 40–45 per cent of prescriptions are for this age group. The elderly are at particular risk from the effects of drugs and poor prescribing practices.

Elderly people in particular may:

- have multiple pathologies: elderly people often have several illnesses that may each require medication;

- be less able to cope: the patient's mental faculties may make him or her less able to cope with the drug regimen;
- have altered metabolism that may give rise to slower absorption, different distribution (for instance because of reduced serum albumin), and reduced excretion by the kidneys or metabolism by the liver. Generally, these factors tend to enhance the normal actions of a drug and increase the risk of dose-related adverse reactions.

A review of medicines as part of the National Service Framework (NSF) for Older People (Department of Health, 2001) identified a number of issues in prescribing particularly related to the elderly.

- *Adverse reactions could be prevented*: Between 5 and 17 per cent of hospital admissions are related to adverse reactions (Mannesse *et al.*, 2000).
- *Under-use of medications*: There is evidence that medications are under-used in areas such as stroke prevention, asthma and depression.
- *Polypharmacy*: Taking four or more medications is a particular risk factor for older people. There is clearly a relationship between polypharmacy and under-utilization of medication.
- *Poor use of repeat prescribing*: While automated repeat prescribing has many benefits, it needs careful monitoring to ensure medications are up to date and are being taken as intended. Perhaps 50 per cent of elderly people do not take their medications as intended (Royal Pharmaceutical Society of Great Britain, 1997). Inconsistent quantities prescribed on repeat prescriptions result in waste and confusion. It is estimated that 6–10 per cent of the total prescribing budget is wasted in this way (Davidson *et al.*, 1998).
- *Changes in medication after hospital discharge*: Many errors are made in medication following discharge from hospital. This partly relates to poor communication between primary and secondary care (see section on communication between primary and secondary care on page 134).
- *Inadequate dosage instructions on labels*: 'As directed' is unhelpful if the directions are not remembered.

■ *Carers*: Informal carers are often under-used and under-supported in helping elderly patients take medicine correctly and appropriately. In care homes, numerous problems have been identified, from continued prescription of unnecessary drugs and prescription of drugs for which no indication was recorded, to frank abuse, with residents being excessively sedated with inappropriate neuroleptics.

Principles for prescribing for the elderly are essentially the same as any principles for good prescribing, but need to be even more fastidiously observed.

■ Assess your patient and his or her medication carefully; do not rush to treatment.
■ Negotiate your proposed treatment carefully with the patient, ensuring he or she understands what is involved and is happy to comply.
■ Be realistic with the patient about what you can and cannot treat. Do not get drawn into chasing minor symptoms with drugs. Remember that depression is common in the elderly and often presents with physical rather than psychological symptoms.

Necessity

Only treat those conditions which are important, for which treatment can change the natural history or give relief from intolerable symptoms. These concerns may be particular to your elderly patients: for instance, there is no point in treating mild hypertension or raised cholesterol in an elderly individual who is unlikely to live long enough to benefit. Indeed, the side effects of the drugs may have serious consequences (e.g. falls related to anti-hypertensive use or confusion from sleeping tablets).

Effectiveness

Effective doses may be much lower in the elderly. Half the normal adult dose may be effective and is a sensible dose to start at.

Safety

Try to avoid medications with frequent side effects: these will be worse in your elderly patients. For example, NSAIDs are prescribed in vast quantities for mild osteoarthritis in the elderly; there is little evidence that they are more effective than simple paracetamol for mild disease and they are a major cause of gastrointestinal bleeding.

Concordance

The above principles on concordance and helping your patients take medication correctly are of particular importance to the elderly. The use of 'polypills' can be particularly helpful in simplifying a regime, with the important proviso that the required dose of each constituent drug is available in that particular combination.

For patients who have limited understanding or for a necessarily complicated regimen, the 'dosette' box can be very helpful (Figure 6.1). This is a box divided into sections for the days of the week and into subdivisions for morning, noon, afternoon and evening. The community pharmacist loads the box once a week and the patient then takes the contents of each section at the appropriate time each day. This is not foolproof: a dosette box was organized for a patient with learning difficulties and a complex drug regimen. The patient was delighted, swallowed the entire contents of the box on returning home and slept for 48 hours!

Review

Review your patient regularly, ensuring your treatment is doing what it is meant to, and be alert to side effects and adverse interactions. If your patient is also attending other clinics, review the prescription carefully after each visit in the context of the whole. As a GP, you need to overview the prescribing pattern, which can easily become confused if a number of clinics are involved. The NSF review recommends a detailed annual medication review or more often if the patient is at higher risk, i.e.:

■ taking multiple medications (more than four),
■ recently discharged from hospital,
■ living in a care home,
■ having known medicine-related problems,
■ following an adverse change of health (to identify potential drug contributors to the change).

'Brown bag' reviews

Get your patient to bring in all the medication he or she is currently taking. This allows you to assess

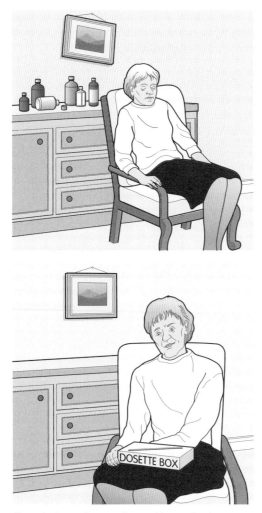

Figure 6.1 Improving compliance with complex drug regimens by the use of a dosette box.

the patient's understanding of what is being taken, any drugs you did not know about, drugs being taken incorrectly, outdated or obsolete medications hanging around in the cupboard and their spouse's drugs being taken in error or deliberately (my own parents share each other's painkillers) and potentially causing confusion. It has been suggested that community pharmacists could take on this role.

Generic prescribing

Most drugs have a generic name, usually an abbreviated version of their chemical name and a proprietary or trade name. For instance the beta-blocker metoprolol is available as non-proprietary metoprolol and under the trade names of Lopresor and Betaloc. Doctors are encouraged to prescribe generic formulations, not only for economic reasons but also to allow the pharmacist flexibility in purchasing drugs from a wider range of sources. It is also better practice for doctors to become familiar with one generic stem name rather than several trade names.

There are two exceptions to this. Certain modified-release preparations, such as some anti-epileptic drugs and calcium channel antagonists, have different bioavailabilities with different formulations. Such drugs should be prescribed by proprietary name. Some preparations contain several drugs and are known as *compound preparations*. It may be impracticable to write out all the constituents, and confusing for the pharmacist. In these cases it is permissible to use the trade name, for example with combined oral contraceptives. Recently, generic names have been developed for the commoner combinations, such as co-codamol (paracetamol and codeine) and co-amilofruse (amiloride and furosemide). Never be tempted to 'invent' generic names or abbreviate drug names on prescriptions: confusion and dispensing errors will result.

Prescribing support in primary care

To help GPs make appropriate and accurate prescribing decisions, a variety of sources of support are available to them. These can be broadly classified into paper, computer and human, and in different ways provide drug information and prescribing support to primary care.

Paper reference sources

The *BNF* is a condensed, practical textbook of the drugs currently available in Britain. It is, in effect, the drug handbook for the NHS and indicates which drugs may and may not be given on NHS prescriptions. It provides an invaluable brief overview of individual drugs and notes on approaches to the treatment of a wide variety of common conditions. For the student it is a tremendously useful summary of treatments and drug classes and you should aim to read it every time you come across an unfamiliar drug.

As part of its remit, the *BNF* lists every member of a class of drug (for instance it lists 16 beta-blockers and 14 NSAIDs), most of which have very similar actions. It is better for the individual doctor to become experienced with one or a few examples of each class of drug. Doctors working in groups (such as general practices) may find it useful to agree on which drugs they will choose to focus on. This is the basis for producing local practice formularies of agreed drugs that aim to promote rational, safe and cost-effective prescribing. Local formularies usually specify a limited choice of drugs to use in any particular condition, chosen for their effectiveness, safety and cost.

The choice of drugs can be linked to local protocols and guidelines, ensuring the most appropriate drug is available in any given situation. While this is a good foundation for rational and safe prescribing, it does not replace the need for clinical judgement. Guidelines give general advice that may not be appropriate to the particular circumstances of your patient. Departing from established guidelines should, however, be a conscious and carefully justified decision by the GP.

Costs can also be controlled by ensuring that after taking considerations of effectiveness into account, the formulary contains the cheapest acceptable preparations in that class. These will often be generic versions.

While general practice formularies allow GPs to initiate prescriptions from a limited and well-understood list, they often find themselves continuing prescriptions from other sources which are not within their chosen formulary. The GP has to decide whether it is in the patient's interests to change to a drug in their formulary or (more usually) to continue with the drug as originally prescribed.

The *Monthly Index of Medical Specialties* (*MIMS*) is a brief guide to medications produced by the drug industry and circulated to GPs. Being updated monthly, it contains details of new medications and other information that may not have reached the *BNF*.

A wide variety of other publications (many of them sponsored by drug companies) flood into the in-tray of the GP.

Computer-based sources

Web-based information has become ubiquitous since the last edition of this book. Both the *BNF* and *MIMS* are available electronically in forms easily accessible from the doctor's desk. With fast internet links available in most UK locations these are a quick and effective resource to use in the consultation.

Integrated prescribing support

Linkage of prescribing support information to practice prescribing systems gives automatic warnings of potential problems at the time of writing the prescription (Figure 6.2). To be effective these warnings must be specific and relevant – if every prescription warns the GP of theoretical but unlikely problems it will inevitably be ignored. These warning systems have become much more sophisticated over the last few years. In 2004 there were significant weaknesses in three-quarters of systems. Since then there has been considerable investment in this area.

Prescribing advisors

In the UK, primary care trusts have designated prescribing advisors who have specialized knowledge of drug and prescribing issues in primary care. Their role includes the development of prescribing policies in primary care and direct support of GPs in prescribing matters. Keeping down prescribing costs is an important aspect of their role.

Community pharmacists

These professionals are highly trained and knowledgeable about drug matters and an excellent source of information. Further information on

---

Practical Exercise

❑ Find out what sources of information on prescribing are available in your practice. Ask your GP tutor and practice manager to help you.
❑ Is there a practice formulary? Is it used?
❑ Consider with your GP tutor the advantages and disadvantages of a practice drug formulary.

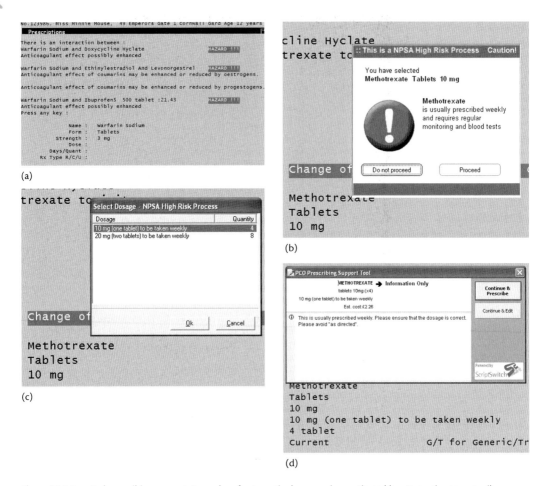

Figure 6.2 Integrated prescribing support. Examples of automatic drug warnings activated by attempting to prescribe a drug. (a) On attempting to prescribe warfarin, the computer identifies potential interactions with existing patient medications (doxycycline and oestrogen/progestagen) and gives specific information about potential problems. (b) Writing up methotrexate – potentially very dangerous if wrongly prescribed or if prescribed at the wrong dose or frequency – brings up specific warnings (c, d) and then guides the prescriber through the prescribing process step by step.

community pharmacists can be found later in this chapter.

Writing a prescription

A prescription is a written instruction to a pharmacist to dispense a drug. Historically, prescriptions were only written by doctors; more recently, nurses with specialist training are now also allowed to prescribe from a limited list. Only registered doctors can write general practice prescriptions – so 1st year foundation doctors are not allowed to do so. The legal responsibility for the prescription lies with the doctor who signs it. A

prescription is therefore a legal document. NHS prescriptions are issued from general practice on a form known as an FP10. When writing a prescription, you should follow the guidelines set out by the Department of Health, which you will find in the *BNF*. These are summarized under 'How to write a prescription' below.

Prescribing by computer

Most prescriptions in general practice are computer generated. The main exception to this is when the doctor is visiting patients at home. Always use computer-generated prescriptions if possible, first to ensure the patient's drug record is integrated with the rest of their notes, and second because it is significantly safer to do so. The reasons are listed below. Electronic prescribing has been estimated to reduce prescription errors by 60 per cent. However the remaining 40 per cent is a very significant problem. An evaluation of drug warnings given by practice prescribing systems in 2004 showed 'about three quarters had clinically important deficiencies', although systems have become significantly more sophisticated since then (Ferner, 2004). Thus computers, although they reduce prescribing errors, do not remove the need for skill or vigilance by the prescriber and are only as good as the drug and patient information stored in the computer's database.

Prescribing by computer has a number of advantages (Figures 6.3 to 6.5):

- Prescribing is from a database of recognized drugs in recognized doses, improving drug choice and dose accuracy.
- The computer will not allow the prescription until all key information has been included.
- The computer automatically adds the prescription to the patient's record.
- The prescription data are stored in a form that can be readily audited.
- The computer automatically includes correct patient details (name, age and address).
- The output is a printed and therefore legible prescription.
- Computers can semi-automatically produce generic prescriptions and so increase generic prescribing.
- Some systems provide immediate warnings of potential adverse reactions based on past drug histories stored on the system, and adverse interactions with other drugs the patient is taking.
- Computers can be set to produce repeat prescriptions, which can be produced by practice staff (though all have to be approved and signed by a doctor) (see 'Repeat prescribing' below).
- Computers provide an accurate printed record of repeat medications for the patient.

How to write a prescription

Writing a prescription by hand is a useful exercise. Starting from a more or less blank sheet of

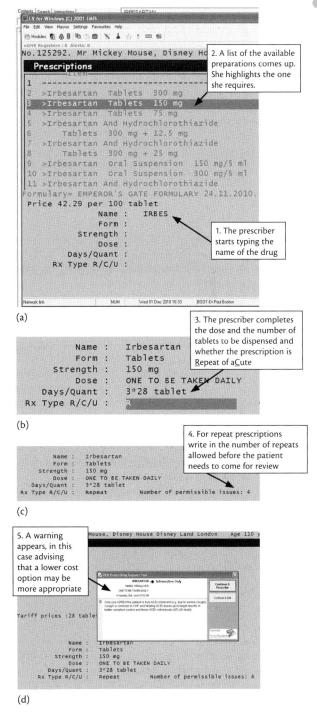

Figure 6.3 Writing a prescription by computer. These screenshots are taken from the EMIS LV computer system which is a popular GP system despite its old-fashioned non-Windows interface.

paper is a good way of testing whether you have understood the principles of safe prescribing. In hospital practice, admission drug charts and other prescriptions are still handwritten. Handwriting prescriptions is a crucial skill for you to acquire for your foundation posts. The principles below apply to all kinds of prescription whether in hospital or primary care.

A prescription should be written legibly in ink or other indelible substance and should include the following (see Figure 6.4):

■ *The name and address of the patient.* Always confirm the patient's address. A wrong address could result in the patient being untraceable which, in the event of a prescribing, dispensing or collection error, could have disastrous consequences.

■ *The patient's age* (a legal requirement in children under 12 years).

■ *The drug name.* Use the generic name unless there are good reasons not to (see 'Generic prescribing' above).

■ *The drug formulation*, e.g. capsules, tablets, suppositories, syrup, ampoules, etc.

■ *The drug dosage*:
  – quantities of one gram or more should be written as 1 g, 2 g, etc.;
  – quantities less than one gram should be written in milligrams, as 1 mg, 2 mg, etc.;
  – quantities less than one milligram should be written in micrograms, e.g. 50 micrograms (*'micrograms' should not be abbreviated*);
  – decimal points should be avoided; when this is not possible, the decimal point should be preceded by zero, e.g. 0.5 mg;
  – with liquid preparations, millilitre, ml or mL is used, e.g. 5 ml (and not cubic centimetre or cc).

■ *The dose frequency*, e.g. three times daily or eight hourly. You will sometimes see Latin abbreviations used on prescriptions, e.g. b.d., t.d.s. (see the back page of the *BNF* for more), but English is preferred.

■ *The number of days' treatment or the total quantity to be dispensed.* There is a box for this on the FP10, but if several items with different lengths of treatment are to be prescribed, specify each separately.

■ *Special advice about how to take the drug*, e.g. whether it should be taken before food, as with a tetracycline, or after food, as with a NSAID, or at night, for hypnotics. The pharmacist may add precautionary warnings to your own instructions on the drug name label.

■ *Limit the number of items to three* on any prescription form. The pharmacist will dispense more if included, but the more congested the prescription, the greater the risk of error.

■ *The prescriber's signature and date.*

■ *The name and address of the GP* and the *doctor's prescribing number* will normally be pre-printed at the bottom of the prescription, but must be added if absent.

Repeat prescribing

Over 80 per cent of prescriptions issued in the UK are 'repeats' (Harris and Dajda, 1996). In repeat prescribing, the GP makes a decision that a particular drug needs to be continued long term; the patient is then allowed to request further supplies without needing to see the doctor each time. Usually the system is computerized and the patient has a list of the drugs allowed, and the length of time, or number of repeats they can request before medical review. Requests are handed to the reception staff, who use the computer database to generate a computer prescription if the request meets the set criteria (Figure 6.5). The doctor then checks and signs the script, which is then collected by the patient. If the patient's request does not meet these criteria the doctor will usually review the request and decide whether to ask the patient to come for review.

Repeat prescribing can save time for patients and doctors, but unchecked leads to problems. Patients may fail to be reviewed regularly, their underlying disease not being monitored, drugs being continued when no longer needed, side effects being missed or compliance not being assessed. It is therefore important to ensure that effective review systems are built into any repeat prescription system, such that each patient is only allowed a certain number of repeats before being reviewed by the doctor. This can be a cause of friction between patient and receptionist, where

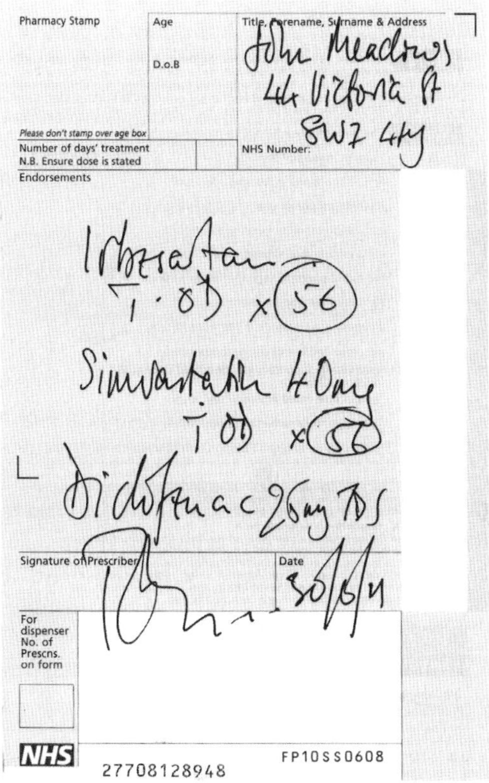

Pharmacy Stamp | Age | Title, Forename, Surname & Address

D.o.B

John Meadows
44 Victoria St
SW7 4HJ

Please don't stamp over age box

Number of days' treatment
N.B. Ensure dose is stated

NHS Number:

Endorsements

Irbesartan
1 OD x(56)
Simvastatin 40mg
1 OD x(56)
Diclofenac 25mg TDS

Signature of Prescriber | Date 30/6/11

For dispenser No. of Prescns. on form

NHS 27708128948 FP10SS0608

Figure 6.4 Handwritten Prescription. Most GPs prescribe acutely using computers. This integrates medication with the patient record, reduces risk of error and allows medication to be audited. Handwritten prescriptions are still used, for instance on home visits. Doctors' bad handwriting may be a weak joke, but legibility issues can and do result in dispensing errors. Prescriber mistakes and omissions (here failing to put the strength of irbesartan and the quantity of diclofenac) raise real risks for patients, which are largely avoided with computerised prescribing.

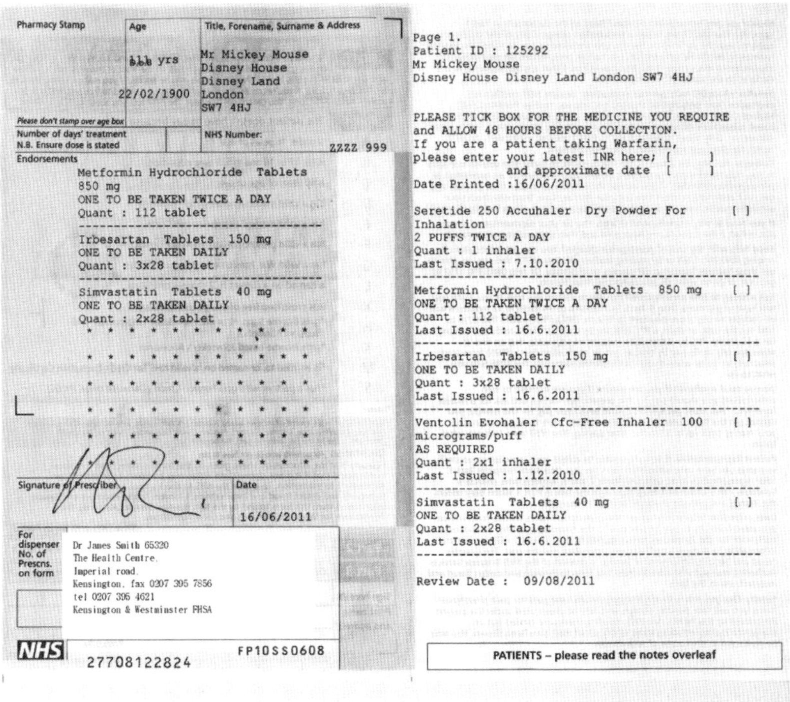

Pharmacy Stamp | Age | Title, Forename, Surname & Address

111 yrs
22/02/1900

Mr Mickey Mouse
Disney House
Disney Land
London
SW7 4HJ

Please don't stamp over age box

Number of days' treatment
N.B. Ensure dose is stated

NHS Number: ZZZZ 999

Endorsements

Metformin Hydrochloride Tablets
850 mg
ONE TO BE TAKEN TWICE A DAY
Quant : 112 tablet

Irbesartan Tablets 150 mg
ONE TO BE TAKEN DAILY
Quant : 3x28 tablet

Simvastatin Tablets 40 mg
ONE TO BE TAKEN DAILY
Quant : 2x28 tablet

Signature of Prescriber | Date 16/06/2011

For dispenser No. of Prescns. on form

Dr James Smith 65320
The Health Centre,
Imperial road,
Kensington, fax 0207 395 7856
tel 0207 395 4621
Kensington & Westminster FHSA

NHS 27708122824 FP10SS0608

Page 1.
Patient ID : 125292
Mr Mickey Mouse
Disney House Disney Land London SW7 4HJ

PLEASE TICK BOX FOR THE MEDICINE YOU REQUIRE
and ALLOW 48 HOURS BEFORE COLLECTION.
If you are a patient taking Warfarin,
please enter your latest INR here; [ ]
and approximate date [ ]
Date Printed :16/06/2011

Seretide 250 Accuhaler Dry Powder For Inhalation [ ]
2 PUFFS TWICE A DAY
Quant : 1 inhaler
Last Issued : 7.10.2010

Metformin Hydrochloride Tablets 850 mg [ ]
ONE TO BE TAKEN TWICE A DAY
Quant : 112 tablet
Last Issued : 16.6.2011

Irbesartan Tablets 150 mg [ ]
ONE TO BE TAKEN DAILY
Quant : 3x28 tablet
Last Issued : 16.6.2011

Ventolin Evohaler Cfc-Free Inhaler 100 micrograms/puff [ ]
AS REQUIRED
Quant : 2x1 inhaler
Last Issued : 1.12.2010

Simvastatin Tablets 40 mg [ ]
ONE TO BE TAKEN DAILY
Quant : 2x28 tablet
Last Issued : 16.6.2011

Review Date : 09/08/2011

PATIENTS – please read the notes overleaf

Figure 6.5 Computer generated repeat prescription. This shows a repeat prescription, which is produced alongside a form for the patient to use to request their next supply. This is convenient for the patient and time saving for the doctor, but has to be part of a well organised system that reviews the patient at regular intervals to ensure medication remains appropriate.

the patient feels obstacles are being put in the way of them receiving their medication. But it is an important backstop to ensure the patient is being adequately reviewed and prescriptions monitored.

Any repeat prescribing system (computer or manual) should:

- provide only the medications and doses agreed with the doctor;
- monitor patient compliance by providing a warning if patients are taking too much or too little of their medication (by giving a warning if the prescription is collected before or after it is due);
- not allow a prescription to be produced if the regular review of the patient has not taken place;
- be flexible: a patient should not be deprived of treatment because he or she has missed an appointment, but any deviations from the agreed protocol must be with the doctor's permission and appropriate review agreed.

Practical Exercise

Find out about the repeat prescribing system in your practice. Ask one of the reception staff to explain the system to you. Consider the advantages and disadvantages of repeat prescribing and discuss these with your GP tutor.

Abuse of drugs and controlled drugs

While drug abuse is a major problem in society, very few illegal drugs derive from pharmaceutical or healthcare sources. Nevertheless, stringent precautions are taken to ensure that potential drugs of abuse are not accessible illegally.

These precautions include the physical security of the practice and legal requirements to store drugs securely, and controls over the prescribing of certain potential drugs of abuse.

Many GPs in inner cities, where drug problems are widespread, have an interest in addiction management and take an active part in harm reduction programmes and the management of addiction.

Prescribing controlled drugs

In order to control the availability of particular drugs, the various Misuse of Drugs Acts specify certain drugs as 'controlled drugs', to which particular prescribing requirements apply.

Prescriptions must include:

- the patient's name and address,
- the form and strength of the preparation,
- the total quantity of the preparation in both words and figures,
- the dose (e.g. one tablet three times a day),
- the date and prescriber's signature.

These requirements apply to schedule 2 and 3 drugs, which include the morphine derivatives cocaine and amfetamine. Schedule 3 includes the barbiturates, which are now little used and to which the above rules also apply. Benzodiazepines are (somewhat surprisingly) controlled drugs in schedule 4 but no special prescribing requirements apply. Schedule 1 contains drugs such as LSD and cannabis, which are not used medicinally and so cannot be prescribed.

The doctor's bag

Usually GPs prescribe, but are not allowed to dispense medications. The exceptions to this are drugs for emergency and on-call use, and in some rural practices that dispense all their patients' drugs (see below). GPs on call have to treat emergencies and urgent problems and are permitted to carry and dispense appropriate drugs in order to do so. They also carry small quantities of basic drugs that they are allowed to dispense to patients to avoid delay in starting medications at night and other times when community pharmacies are closed. This is particularly important in rural areas, where the pharmacies and hospital resources may be at some distance. It carries dangers in urban areas, where doctors are at risk of being assaulted by drug users trying to obtain supplies.

Dispensing practices

In the UK, practices are allowed to dispense drugs for those patients on their practice list who live more than a mile from a pharmacy. To make this worthwhile for a practice, it needs to apply to a sizeable proportion of patients and usually this is only the case in rural practices. Dispensing practices act as pharmacies, buying drugs in, dispensing them and claiming payment from the NHS. This is a useful service for patients and generates income for the practice. Possible drawbacks are the need for extra security in the practice if stocks of drugs are kept on the premises and the need for specialized knowledge on the part of the GP. The practice may employ a pharmacist or trained dispenser.

Prescribing by nurses in practice

Nurse practitioners are trained to diagnose and treat a range of ailments. They are allowed to prescribe a limited range of medications on their own initiative, including emollient creams, nicotine preparations and some aperients. A full list can be found in the *BNF*.

The role of the community pharmacist

Community pharmacies (usually known to the public as 'the chemist') dispense the majority of the drugs prescribed in general practice as well as 'over-the-counter' (OTC) remedies, as discussed in the next section.

Community pharmacists are highly trained and knowledgeable about drug matters, but are currently under-utilized in primary care. In the UK there is a move towards extending the role of community pharmacists and integrating them into the primary healthcare team.

Potential areas of collaboration between pharmacists and GPs include (Bradley *et al.*, 1997):

- repeat prescription review,
- total medication 'brown bag' review (where the patient brings all medication, prescribed or not, for review),
- Prescribing, Analyses and Cost (PACT) data analysis (see later in chapter),
- development of practice formularies,
- development of prescribing policies, e.g. for antibiotics,
- prescribing audits.

Such joint working could benefit GPs, pharmacists and patients.

Community pharmacists are also an important source of advice to the general public on health issues generally and on the treatment of minor ailments in particular. Community pharmacists are trained to advise on minor illnesses and to recommend non-prescription medications. A pharmacist who is concerned that the illness is more serious or beyond his or her abilities to advise you will recommend the patient attends their GP.

Practical Exercise

Local pharmacists have an important role to play in the primary healthcare team. In addition to dispensing prescribed drugs, they sell drugs 'over the counter' and give advice on health and drug matters.
- Ask your GP tutor to arrange for you to spend some time in a local pharmacy.
- Find out about the role pharmacists play and their training.
- Observe how prescriptions are dispensed.
- What kinds of advice do pharmacists give patients?
- Are there rules governing the sale of OTC drugs?

Over-the-counter medication

For every prescription medicine consumed there is probably at least one non-prescription medicine taken. In the UK, the Medicines Control Agency is responsible for classifying drugs as prescription only (PoM), pharmacy only (P) – sold only in pharmacies under the supervision of a registered pharmacist but without the need for a prescription – or general sales list (GSL) – available from a wide range of retailers (e.g. supermarkets) and including cough mixtures, throat pastilles and indigestion remedies.

Recent national and international developments have led to many drugs previously designated as prescription only being reclassified as pharmacy only and thus available 'over the counter'; examples include antihistamines, hydrocortisone cream, H_2 blockers for dyspepsia, 'morning after' contraceptive pills, and small quantities of analgesics such as paracetamol and ibuprofen. Criteria for such a change include the need for a proven safety record, low toxicity in overdose and use for the treatment of minor self-limiting conditions.

Potential advantages of such an increase in OTC preparations include promoting individuals to take more responsibility for their own health, decreasing the need for GP appointments (less inconvenience for the patient and saving time for GPs), less financial cost to patients (often OTC preparations are cheaper than the prescription charge) and removing some of the financial burden for the NHS. Potential disadvantages include the fostering of a 'pill for every ill' mentality among the public, an increased risk of interactions and side effects (some OTC preparations can have serious side effects – Clark *et al.*, 2001), less feedback to the regulatory authorities on adverse drug reactions, patients taking the wrong preparation or in the wrong way, and patients self-medicating for a serious condition requiring medical attention (Bradley and Bond, 1995). Taking proton pump inhibitors (PPIs) or H_2 blockers for undiagnosed abdominal pain, or taking OTC statins (which are sold OTC in low doses) carry real risks of under-diagnosing or inappropriately managing potentially serious medical problems.

Doctors need to take into account any non-prescription medicines their patients may be taking (the *OTC Directory* lists 95 per cent of the market); OTC preparations can interact with prescribed drugs and cause adverse drug reactions.

Communicating about medications between primary and secondary care

Sometimes it seems that the only things reliably transferred between primary and secondary care are the patients themselves! Poor communications have a deleterious effect on care generally and, for medication, may be disastrous. Unintentional changes in medication following discharge from hospital to primary care have been identified in half the patients discharged (Duffin *et al.*, 1998).

Many medications are initiated by the hospital, and the GP subsequently takes responsibility for continuing to prescribe them. Unfortunately, it is still commonplace for patients to be discharged from hospital with inadequate or no information. Similarly, many GP referrals do not contain adequate information on the patient's medication, even though this can usually be readily obtained from the practice computer system.

As a student who will soon enough be a foundation doctor, you can have a major impact in this area by providing accurate discharge notifications or summaries. An accurate summary of medication is often the most important part.

A discharge notification should be legible and prompt (often, handing it to the patient at discharge is the best way of ensuring the GP receives it). The medication details are best written as a prescription (indeed, in most trusts the medication details are also used as prescription instructions to the hospital pharmacy). Make sure you:

- write legibly;
- state the duration of treatment for each drug (i.e. is this a course of treatment of limited duration, like an antibiotic, or is it intended for long-term use, like an antihypertensive?);
- stop any medications not needed out of hospital (such as night sedation, which may have been necessary in a noisy ward);
- include the consultant's name and contact details in case of uncertainties;
- do it now (most hospitals only give a two-week supply of discharge medications – late notifications cause delays and errors).

Alarm point: As a foundation doctor you can have a major effect on your patient's health by:

- taking a careful drug history on admission and writing up admission drugs correctly (up to 50 per cent of errors in studies);
- communicating promptly and clearly with the GP via the discharge notification (up to 50 per cent error (again) transcribing the hospital's intention to the GP prescribing record).

Prescribing costs and monitoring

In the UK, as of 2011, primary care trusts set budgets for prescribing costs for individual general practices. Factors taken into account when setting these budgets include historical prescribing patterns, average prescribing costs locally, list size and age profile, and special factors identified by the practice or primary care trust. Practices are encouraged to stay within, or save on, their budget by incentives such as bonus amounts that can be used in other areas (e.g. service development). In addition, sanctions may be applied in the case of an over-spend. Detailed information on prescribing in primary care is available in the form of PACT data (similar systems exist in Scotland and Wales). PACT data contain information on prescribing costs, the number of items prescribed and the level of generic prescribing at individual GP level, health authority and national level. Unfortunately, PACT data cannot be linked with demographic or clinical patient information.

They can be used by the NHS to set prescribing budgets for health authorities, by health authorities and primary care trusts to set and monitor GP prescribing budgets, by health service researchers and by individual GPs to audit and improve their prescribing (Majeed *et al.*, 1997). GPs receive quarterly PACT reports that include a comparison with local and national averages.

Practical Exercise

Ask your GP tutor to go through his or her PACT data with you. (If you are studying outside the UK, find out if similar data exist locally.) What are the benefits and limits of such data?

SUMMARY POINTS

To conclude, the most important messages in this chapter are as follows:

- The scale of prescribing is large, costs are high and drugs have both beneficial and harmful effects; you must therefore prescribe effectively and safely.
- In order for the drugs that you prescribe to be taken by the patient, agreement must be reached with the patients that the drugs are necessary, the patient needs to understand what the drugs do and how to take them correctly, and the patient's use of the medication and progress must be reviewed regularly.
- Children and the elderly are particularly vulnerable to medication, and care needs to be taken when prescribing for these patients.
- Paper references and computer-based prescribing sources, prescribing advisors and community pharmacists are all helpful in providing support for prescribing.

References

Barrett, T., Lander, A. and Diwaker, V. 2002: *A paediatric vade-mecum*, 14th edn. London: Arnold.

Bradley, C. and Bond, C. 1995: Increasing the number of drugs available over the counter: arguments for and against. *British Journal of General Practice* 45, 553–6.

Bradley, C., Taylor, R. and Blenkinsopp, A. 1997: Primary care – opportunities and threats: developing prescribing in primary care. *British Medical Journal* 314, 744–7.

British National Formulary 2003. London: The British Medical Association and the Royal Pharmaceutical Society of Great Britain.

Clark, D., Layton, D. and Shakir, S. 2001: Monitoring the safety of over the counter drugs. *British Medical Journal* 323, 706–7.

Davidson, W., Collett, J.H., Jackson, C. and Rees, J.A. 1998: An analysis of the quality and cost of repeat prescriptions. *Pharmacology Journal* 260, 458–60.

Department of Health 2001: *Medicines for older people: implementing medicines-related aspects of the NSF for Older People 2001*. London: Department of Health. Also available at www.doh.gov.uk/nsf/olderpeople/pdfs/medicinesbooklet.pdf

Duffin, J., Norwood, J. and Blenkinsopp, A. 1998: An investigation into medication changes initiated in general practice after patients are discharged from hospital. *Pharmacology Journal* 261 (Suppl.), R32.

Dunbar-Jacob, J., Erlen, J., Schlenk, E., Ryan, C., Sereika, S. and Diswell, W. 2000: Adherence in chronic disease. *Annual Review of Nursing Research* 18, 48–90.

Editorial 2002: Managing antibiotic-associated diarrhoea. *British Medical Journal* 324, 1345–6.

Fedder, D.O. 1982: Managing medication and compliance: physician–pharmacist–patient interaction. *Journal of the American Geriatric Society* 30, S113–17.

Ferner, R.E. 2004: Computer aided prescribing leaves holes in the safety net. *British Medical Journal* 328, 1172–3.

Fry, J. 1993: *General practice: the facts*. Oxford: Radcliffe Medical Press.

Harris CM, Dajda R. 1996: The scale of repeat prescribing. *British Journal of General Practice* 46, 649–53.

Kohn, R. and White, K. 1976: *Health care*. Oxford: Oxford University Press.

Majeed, A., Evans, N. and Head, P. 1997: What can PACT tell us about prescribing in general practice? *British Medical Journal* 315, 1515–19.

Mannesse, C.K., Derkx, F.H., de Ridder, M.A., Man in't Veld, A.J. and van der Cammen, T.J. 2000: Contribution of adverse drug reactions to hospital admission of older patients. *Age and Ageing* 29, 35–9.

NCCSDO (National Co-ordinating Centre for NHS Service Delivery and Organisation R & D) 2005: *Concordance, adherence and compliance in medicine taking*. www.medslearning.leeds.ac.uk/pages/documents/useful_docs/76-final-report%5B1%5D.pdf (accessed May 2011).

Palmer, K.T. 1998: *Notes for the MRCGP*, 3rd edn. Oxford: Blackwell Science.

Rawlins, M.D. and Thompson, J.W. 1977: *Pathogenesis of adverse drug reactions*, 2nd edn. Oxford: Oxford University Press.

Royal Pharmaceutical Society of Great Britain 1997: *From compliance to concordance – achieving partnership in medicine-taking*. London: RPSGB.

Sackett, D.L. and Snow, J.C. 1979: The magnitude of compliance and non-compliance. In: Haynes, R.B. and Sackett, D.L. (eds) *Compliance in health care*. Baltimore: Johns Hopkins University Press, 11–22.

York Health Economics Consortium 2010: *Evaluation of the scale, causes and costs of waste medicines. Final report*. London: YHEC/School of Pharmacy, University of London. www.pharmacy.ac.uk/fileadmin/documents/News/Evaluation_of_NHS_Medicines_Waste__web_publication_version.pdf (accessed May 2011).

Further reading

British National Formulary. London: British Medical Association and the Royal Pharmaceutical Society of Great Britain.

This is an invaluable source of information on prescribing. Your medical school may arrange for you to receive your own copy; use it frequently. It is also available on CD-ROM and online at www.bnf.org/
Drug and Therapeutics Bulletins. London: Which? Ltd.
MeReC Bulletins. Liverpool: Medicines Resource Centre.

These organizations publish monthly bulletins summarizing prescribing information on various topics. www.concordance.org

This website discusses a variety of issues related to concordance and compliance.

Acknowledgements

Thank you to Dr Joanna Collerton who was co-author in previous editions.

SINGLE BEST ANSWER QUESTIONS

6.1 A thyrotoxic patient develops a sore throat several weeks after starting carbimazole. This is an example of:

a) A predictable reaction
b) An idiosyncratic reaction
c) A continuous reaction
d) A delayed reaction
e) An end-of-use reaction.

6.2 Patients are most likely to take their prescribed treatment:

a) If the doctor stresses the importance to them
b) If the doctor makes the patient repeat back the instructions
c) If the doctor and patient reach a shared understanding of the problem and its treatment
d) Adopting a simple 'breakfast, lunch and dinner' dosing regime
e) The doctor showing empathy and consideration when prescribing.

6.3 When prescribing for the elderly:

a) Standard doses of drugs should normally be used
b) More than six drugs constitutes polypharmacy

c) Avoid fixed combinations of drugs
d) Recruit relatives or other carers to aid compliance
e) Community pharmacists can be recruited to ensure compliance.

6.4 A legal prescription:

a) Must state the patient's age
b) Avoid abbreviations such as mg for milligrammes
c) Microgrammes may be written as 'mcg'
d) Latin dosage abbreviations are not permitted
e) May include additional written advice about how to take the drug.

6.5 When you discharge a patient from hospital as a foundation doctor:

a) Write to the GP only when the outstanding tests are available
b) Briefly list each medication (GPs have no time for long communications)
c) Let the GP decide which medications to stop and which to continue
d) Tell the patient to arrange an appointment in one month to review medication
e) Always give the consultant's name and contact details on every discharge note.

CHAPTER

7

COMMON ILLNESSES IN GENERAL PRACTICE

- What do people do when they feel unwell?
- Which types of illnesses present to general practice in the UK?
- Key general practice presentations for medical students
- How to find out more about particular illnesses
- Red flag symptoms
- Summary points
- References
- Further reading
- Single best answer questions

Only a small proportion of symptoms experienced by the general population are presented to a healthcare practitioner. This chapter considers the factors that influence the decision to consult and the types of conditions seen in general practice. A framework for aiding learning about medical conditions is presented.

LEARNING OBJECTIVES

By the end of this chapter you will be able to:

- understand the reasons why patients bring problems to their general practitioner;
- list the types of conditions that present to general practice in the UK;
- list the commonest general practice conditions for student learning;
- seek further information about a particular condition and know how best to structure that information to aid learning;
- search for red flag symptoms (symptoms which indicate more serious underlying pathology) amongst the multitude of common symptoms which people bring to their GP.

What do people do when they feel unwell?

Symptoms are common. During the course of a week, the average adult experiences one or two symptoms. The commonest of these are musculoskeletal problems, headaches and viral upper respiratory tract symptoms. Indeed, it is rare for people not to experience symptoms. In a study by Wadsworth *et al.* (1971), 95 per cent of a randomly selected sample of 2153 London adults experienced symptoms in a 14-day period. Figure 7.1 shows the proportion of the general population who suffer from a selection of common problems in a year. As you can see, the majority

of the population experience such problems each year. Fortunately, not all of these are brought to general practice.

When an individual feels unwell, they may choose to:

- ignore the symptoms;
- 'self-care', i.e. to cope with the symptoms themselves or to seek help from friends or relatives (the lay referral system); self-care may take the form of no action, home remedies (e.g. honey and lemon for a cough) or 'over-the-counter' remedies (e.g. cough linctus);
- consult a traditional healthcare professional such as a GP or practice nurse;

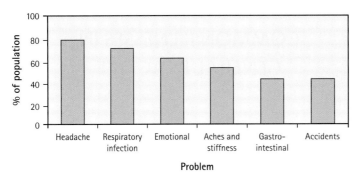

Figure 7.1 The annual occurrence of common problems in the general population. From Fry, J. and Sandler, G. 1993: *Common diseases: their nature, prevalence, and care*, 5th edn. Newbury: Petroc Press, p. 7. Reproduced with kind permission from Petroc Press.

■ consult a practitioner of alternative medicine such as an aromatherapist or osteopath (Armstrong, 2002).

Practical Exercise

The objectives of this exercise are to look at the actions people take when they experience common symptoms and to consider the factors that influence the decision to seek medical advice.

1. Choose a common symptom, e.g. headache, cough, nausea, indigestion.
2. Design a short questionnaire aiming to explore the objectives above.
3. Arrange with your GP tutor to interview a sample of subjects. The easiest way to do this is to interview patients in the doctor's waiting room.
4. Introduce yourself to each patient and obtain their permission for a short interview. If possible, find a room where you can have a confidential conversation. Patients will be worried about missing their turn with the doctor, so make arrangements with the receptionist to ensure this does not happen; if necessary, complete your interview after their appointment.
5. Pilot your questionnaire and make any necessary adaptations.
6. Interview at least ten people.
7. Review their responses.
8. Discuss your findings with your GP tutor. In particular, discuss why different symptoms might result in different decisions about how to respond.

(After Graham and Seabrook, 1995)

In the majority of instances, people opt to ignore their symptoms or prefer to self-care. In the UK, possibly as few as 2.7 per cent (1 in 37) of all symptoms result in seeking help from a healthcare professional (Morrell and Wale, 1976). In other research based on a different methodology and concentrating on better defined symptoms, only 20 per cent of these symptoms reached general practice, 79 per cent were dealt with by self-care and the remaining 1 per cent presented directly to hospital (Fry, 1978). This is illustrated by a pie chart in Figure 7.2. The term 'the clinical iceberg' refers to the high proportion of symptoms dealt with outside formal healthcare. Importantly, it is an 'iceberg' rather than a linear 'column', so that just a small reduction in the threshold for consulting with a GP will result in a large increase in the number of patients booking appointments.

The ways in which people react when they experience symptoms form part of their *illness*

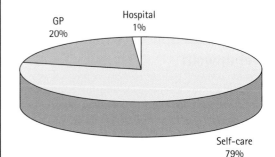

Figure 7.2 Symptoms experienced by the general population: proportion of symptoms cared for at self-care, general practice and hospital levels. From Fry, J. 1978: *A New Approach to Medicine: Principles and Priorities in Health Care*. Lancaster: MTP Press, p. 40 (information from Logan and Brooke, 1957; Jefferys *et al.*, 1960; Wadsworth *et al.*, 1971; Dunnell and Cartwright, 1972). Reproduced by kind permission from MTP Press.

behaviour. This can be defined as 'the ways in which given symptoms may be differentially perceived, evaluated and acted upon (or not acted upon) by different kinds of persons' (Mechanic, 1962).

A helpful way of understanding an individual's illness behaviour is to consider the Health Belief Model (Rosenstock, 1966; Becker and Maiman, 1975). This proposes that individuals differ in the way they perceive:

- *their susceptibility and vulnerability to illness*: those who believe themselves to be more vulnerable are more likely to seek medical attention;
- *the severity of their symptoms*: in general, symptoms more likely to be perceived as serious include unusual symptoms, those with an acute onset and those associated with visible signs, although there is great variation amongst individuals; symptoms perceived as serious are more likely to be brought to the attention of a healthcare professional;
- *the costs of health-seeking behaviour*: possible costs include the inconvenience of attending surgery, a potential lack of sympathy from the doctor and the financial cost of a prescription;
- *the benefits of health-seeking behaviour*: possible benefits include obtaining therapy to cure symptoms and legitimization of an illness by obtaining a sick certificate.

Certain triggers to the timing of consultations with healthcare professionals have been identified (Zola, 1973):

- the occurrence of an interpersonal crisis;
- the perceived interference with social or personal relations;
- sanctioning or pressure from family or friends;
- the perceived interference with vocational or physical activity;
- the setting of a deadline ('If I'm not better by Monday ... ').

In any consultation, it is important to consider not only why that person has presented, but also why at that particular time. Zola (1973) found that if doctors paid insufficient attention to the specific triggers prompting an individual to seek help, that person was less likely to comply with treatment. (More about this in Chapter 8 on psy-chological issues in general practice.) The perceptive GP approaches these consultations with the question, 'Why now?'

Case Study 7.1

Mr J, a 45-year-old business man, develops acute back pain following a long car journey. He is usually fit and well and does not like to think of himself as ill. Initially, he tries to ignore the pain, but when it starts to affect his sleep he takes some paracetamol. However, the pain persists and begins to interfere with his work. He mentions it to a friend who has had similar problems in the past. His friend recalls that his GP was unable to cure his symptoms, so he went to an osteopath instead. Although expensive, this proved very effective. Mr J decides to follow his friend's example and consults an osteopath.

Thinking and Discussion Point

Reflect on Case study 7.1; can you identify any aspects of the Health Belief Model or Zola's triggers in Mr J's behaviour?

The annual consultation rate (the average number of times a patient consults with a GP practice per year) has been rising rapidly in the last ten years. In 1995, the UK average was 3.9 consultations each year, rising to 5.5 consultations each year in 2008/9 (The Information Centre, 2008). These figures refer to all contacts with the practice and include GP, nurse and other primary healthcare team appointments; they also include home visits and telephone consultations. The pattern of attendance has also changed with the proportion of consultations carried out by practice nurses rising from 21 to 34 per cent over the same period. Changes have taken place in the mode of consultation. Back in 1995, 86 per cent were conducted in the GP surgery, 9 per cent were home visits and 3 per cent were telephone consultations. By 2006, 84 per cent were conducted in the GP surgery, home visits had fallen to 4 per cent and telephone consultations had grown to 10 per cent of all consultations. It is likely that the trend toward telephone consultations will continue.

Thinking and Discussion Point

Having read about the changes in consultation patterns, it might be worth spending some time trying to list a series of possible reasons for these changes. Remember that society is changing, as are the structures of general practice.

Factors affecting consultation rates include the following (Campbell and Roland, 1996):

- *Age*: The elderly and children are more likely to consult than young adults or the middle aged.
- *Sex*: Women are more likely to consult than men, partly because of their use of obstetric and contraception services and partly because they have higher rates of illness.
- *Social class*: Individuals in lower social classes have greater morbidity and mortality than those in higher social classes and consult more frequently. However, such individuals still make less use of health services than would be expected on the basis of their poorer health.
- *Ethnicity*: In the UK, consultation rates vary among different ethnic groups, e.g. Asians and Afro-Caribbeans consult more frequently than white populations. This is thought to be due partly to increased morbidity and partly to differences in illness behaviour.
- *Social networks*: The existence of a good social support network is associated with a lower consultation rate. This appears to be due a combination of improved health and a better ability to cope with problems in those who are well supported.
- *Accessibility of healthcare*: An individual is more likely to consult if the surgery is nearby and appointments are easy to obtain.

In summary, the presence of a symptom is not the only determinant of whether an individual decides to consult. The way in which the person evaluates that symptom affects the action he or she takes, and this is profoundly affected by psychosocial factors, including cultural and family influences. There seems to be little correlation between a person's decision to consult and either the true seriousness of the condition or the doctor's perception of the need to consult. The consultation paradox is that many people fail to present despite suffering from serious disease (Last, 1963), and yet at the same time, many consult with what GPs consider to be trivial or minor complaints (Cartwright and Anderson, 1981).

Thinking and Discussion Point

Consider your interview sample; what actions did your interviewees take when they experienced symptoms and what factors influenced their decisions to seek medical advice? Can you identify any of the factors mentioned in this section?

Which types of illnesses present to general practice in the UK?

The illnesses seen in general practice differ in severity and type from those seen in hospitals. Data on the disease groups and the specific minor, chronic and major conditions commonly presenting to general practice in the UK are summarized in this section. The source of much of this data is the Fourth National Study of Morbidity Statistics from General Practice 1991–1992 (McCormick *et al.*, 1995), in which consultations in 60 general practices across England and Wales were analysed, representing a 1 per cent sample of the population. Unfortunately, this national study has not been repeated since completion in 1992.

Tables 7.1–7.4 summarize two key statistics for a range of conditions commonly seen in general practice:

- the percentage of a practice population who consult at least once a year with each condition;
- the number of cases an average GP (list size 2000) would expect to see in a year.

Table 7.1 shows the disease groups that commonly present to general practice: respiratory, nervous system, skin, musculoskeletal, injury and poisoning, and infections.

In addition to considering the disease groups that present to general practice, it is also useful to classify conditions as minor, chronic or major.

Table 7.1 Common disease groups presenting to general practice

Disease group	Percentage of practice population consulting in 1 year	Number of cases seen by average GP in 1 year
Respiratory	30	600
Nervous system (including eyes and ears)	17	340
Skin	15	300
Musculoskeletal	15	300
Injury/poisoning	15	300
Infections	14	280
Genitourinary (excluding obstetric)	11	220
Gastrointestinal	9	180
Cardiovascular	9	180
Psychiatric	7	140
Endocrine/metabolic	4	80
Non-specific symptoms and signs	15	300

From McCormick, A., Fleming, D. and Charlton, J. 1995: *Morbidity statistics from general practice: fourth national study 1991–1992.* Crown copyright 1995. National Statistics Crown copyright material is reproduced with the permission of the Controller of HMSO.

Minor conditions are defined as self-limiting, *chronic* as lasting more than six months, and *major* as acute and potentially life threatening. Figure 7.3 shows the proportions of illnesses presenting to general practice classified in this way, and illustrates that the majority of conditions are minor or chronic, with a smaller proportion of major conditions.

Fifty-two per cent of all illness presenting to general practice can be classified as minor or self-limiting. Table 7.2 shows the most common minor conditions.

Thirty-three per cent of illnesses presenting to general practice may be classified as chronic. Table 7.3 shows the most common chronic conditions. (See more in Chapter 9 on chronic illness and its management in general practice.)

Fifteen per cent of conditions presenting to general practice may be classified as major. Table 7.4 shows the most common major conditions.

The National Morbidity Studies provide valuable information concerning those conditions presenting to general practice. However, it is important to remember that the data refer only to those patients who consulted either a GP or a practice nurse. They give no indication of disease rates among individuals who do not attend general practice because they are not registered with a practice or they self-care or go direct to hospital. The data cannot, therefore, be used to estimate the true incidence or prevalence of diseases in the community as a whole.

National Morbidity Study data have been published on the specific diseases seen in general practice. However, many consultations involve a confusing mass of physical or psychological symp-

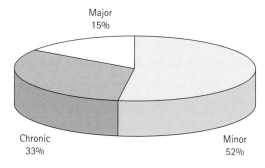

Figure 7.3 Grades of disease presenting to general practice. From Fry, J. and Sandler, G. 1993: *Common diseases: their nature, prevalence, and care,* 5th edn. Newbury: Petroc Press, p. 27. Reproduced by kind permission from Petroc Press.

Table 7.2 Specific minor conditions presenting to general practice

Condition	Percentage of practice population consulting in 1 year	Number of cases seen by average GP in 1 year
Acute throat infections	8	160
Psycho-emotional	7	140
Backache	6	120
Eczema	5	100
Acute otitis media	5	100
External ear problems (mainly wax and otitis externa)	4	80
Hay fever	3	60
Dyspepsia	2	40
Headache	2	40
Dizzy spells	1.5	30
Constipation	1	20
Piles	1	20
Varicose veins	0.9	18

From McCormick, A., Fleming, D. and Charlton, J. 1995: *Morbidity statistics from general practice: fourth national study 1991–1992.* Crown copyright 1995. National Statistics Crown copyright material is reproduced with the permission of the Controller of HMSO. Also from Fry, J. 1993: *General practice: the facts.* Oxford: Radcliffe Medical Press, p. 25. Reproduced with kind permission of Radcliffe Medical Press.

toms which students (and GPs) find difficult to classify as a particular disease. In addition, many general practice consultations do not deal with disease alone. Social issues such as poverty, unemployment, homelessness and divorce influence the health of a population, and it has been estimated that one-third of general practice consultations involve such social issues (Fry and Sandler, 1993). Twenty per cent of consultations deal with preventative and health promotion activities such as cervical smears, immunizations and travel advice (Fry and Sandler, 1993).

Over time, the balance between the different types of GP consultation has shifted. In the decade leading up to 2001, there was a general decline in acute infectious diseases and accidents (Fleming *et al.*, 2005). These facts illustrate the concept of the 'threshold to consultation'. This concept describes the *tipping point* when a person decides to book an appointment at their general practice and seek the help of a health professional. There is no good reason to assume that the community incidence of infections and accidents has declined over the preceding decade

and almost certainly, people with these problems are resorting to self-management strategies, reinforced by health education campaigns run by the government and by GPs themselves. The declining proportion of consultations for these conditions is therefore likely to represent a raised threshold to consultation such that only patients with more serious infections or accidents see their GP or practice nurse. Rising Accident and Emergency Department attendance rates suggest that at least some patients with these clinical presentations bypass primary care altogether and obtain help directly from the hospital. The same survey found that most chronic diseases ('long-term conditions') increased as a proportion of all consultations, particularly consultations relating to hypertension and diabetes; the exception was asthma which had declined as a reason for consultation. The consultation rate for most 'mental disorders' was largely steady over the decade of study although consultations for the major psychoses increased. The prevalence of skin disorders and musculoskeletal conditions remained almost constant.

Table 7.3 Specific chronic conditions presenting to general practice

Condition	Percentage of practice population consulting in 1 year	Number of cases seen by average GP in 1 year
Respiratory		
Asthma	4.3	86
Chronic obstructive airways disease	1.2	24
Cardiovascular		
Hypertension	4.2	84
Ischaemic heart disease	1.7	34
Musculoskeletal		
Backache	4	80
Osteoarthritis	3	60
Endocrine		
Diabetes mellitus	1.1	22
Thyroid disorders	0.7	14
Gastrointestinal		
Irritable bowel syndrome	1	20
Peptic ulcer	0.5	10
Inflammatory bowel disease	0.3	6
Diverticular disease	0.2	4
Neurological		
Cerebrovascular disease (after-effects)	1	20
Epilepsy	0.4	8
Parkinson's disease	0.2	4
Multiple sclerosis	0.1	2

From McCormick, A., Fleming, D. and Charlton, J. 1995: *Morbidity statistics from general practice: fourth national study 1991–1992.* Crown copyright 1995. National Statistics Crown copyright material is reproduced with the permission of the Controller of HMSO. Also from Fry, J. 1993: *General practice: the facts.* Oxford: Radcliffe Medical Press, p. 26. Reproduced with kind permission of Radcliffe Medical Press.

Table 7.4 Specific major conditions presenting to general practice

Condition	Percentage of practice population consulting in 1 year	Number of cases seen by average GP in 1 year
Acute chest infection	7.5	150
Severe depression	0.6	12
Acute myocardial infarction	0.3	6
Acute cerebrovascular accident	0.3	6
Acute abdomen	0.3	6

From McCormick, A., Fleming, D. and Charlton, J. 1995: *Morbidity statistics from general practice: fourth national study 1991–1992.* Crown copyright 1995. National Statistics Crown copyright material is reproduced with the permission of the Controller of HMSO. Also from Fry, J. 1993: *General practice: the facts.* Oxford: Radcliffe Medical Press, p. 27. Reproduced with kind permission of Radcliffe Medical Press.

Thinking and Discussion Point

There may be many reasons why GP consultations now feature less acute illness and more chronic disease. Can you think why this shift may have occurred?

Practical Exercise

The following exercises may be carried out within a routine surgery. Discuss the issues involved with your GP tutor in advance and decide on the best way of recording and interpreting the information you obtain.

1. Interview a selection of patients prior to their consultation with the doctor. Attempt to identify the reason why each patient has come to the GP and what they hope to gain from their consultation (this may not be as straightforward as it sounds).
2. Sit in on these patients' consultations with the doctor. Observe the consultation; does the GP obtain the same information as you did?
3. Following each consultation, discuss the issues raised with the GP. Compare your analysis of the perceived reasons for each consultation with those of the GP tutor.
   Not infrequently, there is a discrepancy between the reason a doctor thinks a patient has consulted and why the patient has actually consulted. What influences may this have on patient care?
4. Classify the conditions presenting into minor, chronic or major. Compare your results with the figures given in this chapter.
5. Consider how many consultations have a social agenda.

Key general practice presentations for medical students

As you will have realized, any disease may present to general practice, and it can be dif-

ficult for students to know which conditions to focus on during their general practice module. As a guide, you should read up about those conditions you come across during your GP attachment; it is easier to recall information about a condition if you can relate it to a particular patient. In particular, reflect on how the presentation, diagnosis and management of each condition differ between the general practice and hospital settings. The Royal College of General Practitioners has published a Core Curriculum for the postgraduate training of GPs. This consists of 15 components which are presented below as a starting point for your own learning (Royal College of General Practitioners, 2007).

1. *Being a GP*: This covers issues concerning the role of the GP as a health professional and as a generalist within the context of primary care.
2. *The consultation*: This covers issues about the dynamics of consulting, the components of the consultation and promoting patient-centred care.
3. *Personal and professional responsibilities*: This covers clinical governance, patient safety, ethics, promoting equality, evidence-based practice, research and education.
4. *Management*: This covers practice management and also the use of IT in primary care.
5. *Healthy people*: This covers health promotion and the prevention of disease.
6. *Genetics in primary care.*
7. *Care of acutely ill people.*
8. *Care of children and young people.*
9. *Care of older adults.*
10. *Gender-specific health issues.*
11. *Sexual health.*
12. *Care of people with cancer and palliative care.*
13. *Care of people with mental health problems.*
14. *Care of people with learning disabilities.*
15. *Clinical management*: This covers the management of specific conditions, based on a systems approach, e.g. cardiovascular problems, digestive problems, respiratory problems, etc.

How to find out more about particular illnesses

A full description of common general practice conditions is beyond the scope of this book, so where should you look for further information? A good starting point is to identify the subject matter, for example general medicine, obstetrics or paediatrics, and then consult the standard student textbook on that subject recommended by your medical school. However, many minor conditions are poorly covered in standard medical books, so you will also need access to a specialized general practice text; this will provide information on the presentation and management of key conditions with a specific primary care focus (see examples in the further reading list at the end of this chapter). Note, however, that the information contained in textbooks is frequently out of date, especially with regard to up-to-date therapy, and you may need to consult the current research literature on the topic. The section on evidence-based medicine in Chapter 5 on diagnosis and management provides guidance on how to do this.

Most medical students are overwhelmed by the amount of information they are expected to remember about a bewildering array of different conditions. It is helpful to structure this information under various subheadings, to aid learning and recall, both in examination settings and when practising as a doctor. The following scheme is a starting point for you to adapt for your own use.

1. Definition.
2. Epidemiology (incidence and prevalence; age, gender, geographical, social class variations).
3. Aetiology and risk factors.
4. Basic science (what aspects of pathology, physiology, anatomy, etc. are relevant?).
5. Clinical features (typical symptoms and signs).
6. Investigations (which to request and what results to expect).
7. Differential diagnosis (what other conditions may present in a similar way and how can you differentiate between them).
8. Management (remember to think more widely than drug therapy).
9. Prognosis.

Now consider how this scheme can be applied to acute otitis media.

1. Definition: acute inflammation of the middle ear.
2. Epidemiology: very common – 5 per cent of a practice population will consult in 1 year (30 per cent of children under 3 years) and 50 per cent of children under the age of 10 are affected at some time; rare in adults. The average GP will see 100 cases per year (equates to 1.5 million cases annually in England and Wales).
3. Aetiology: most commonly follows an upper respiratory tract infection. The commonest bacterial pathogens are *Haemophilus influenzae*, *Streptococcus pneumoniae* and *Moraxella catarrhalis*, but most cases are viral in aetiology.
4. Risk factors: eustachian tube dysfunction, e.g. short tube (children), obstructed tube (adenoids, allergy) and unresolved middle ear effusions.
5. Basic science: further detail not necessary in this case.
6. Clinical features: symptoms include earache, fever, irritability, aural discharge and deafness; signs include pyrexia, a red, bulging tympanic membrane and discharge. Common presentations include an infant with fever and irritability and a young child with earache, fever and deafness.

7. Investigations: seldom performed; culture of aural discharge, where present, in refractory cases.

8. Differential diagnosis: other causes of otalgia (e.g. eustachian tube dysfunction, glue ear, otitis externa, dental pain) and other childhood infections.

9. Management: education (as to the nature of the condition and its natural course) and reassurance of parents and child, together with analgesia and temperature control are the main aims of care. The role of antibiotics is a subject of much debate. Antibiotic use for acute otitis media varies from 31 per cent of cases in the Netherlands to 98 per cent of cases in the USA and Australia. A Cochrane Review (Glasziou et al., 2003) confirmed the effects of antibiotics in children with otitis media to be modest: 16 patients have to be treated in order to prevent one from suffering ear pain (a 'number needed to treat', or NNT, of 16). Their use is not without problems in terms of side effects, antibiotic resistance and financial cost: 1 in 24 children experienced side effects from antibiotics. Meta-analysis of a subset of the trials included in this Review suggested that antibiotics were of most use in children under 2 years of age with bilateral otitis media, or those with otitis media and an ear discharge. A more appropriate approach might be to reserve antibiotics for those at highest risk, based on these criteria, and to watch and wait for the majority, while offering management of pain and fever at the same time. If antibiotics are prescribed, the usual choice is amoxycillin (5-day course). Patients should be instructed to return if symptoms persist, and all cases of perforation should be followed up to ensure healing occurs.

10. Prognosis: resolution over 2–3 days is usual (80 per cent of cases). The drum may remain dull red or pink and deafness may persist for 2–3 weeks. In some cases, the tympanic membrane perforates, leading to discharge and resolution of the pain; the perforation will heal spontaneously in the majority of cases. The most important risk factors for poor outcome are young age and attend-ance at a day-care facility. Other risk factors include white race, male sex and a history of enlarged adenoids, tonsillitis or asthma. The role of environmental tobacco smoke is controversial. Forty per cent of cases will recur within 12 months; those with unresolved middle ear infections are particularly prone. Recurrences tend to cease after the age of 8 years. Complications such as mastoiditis and cerebral abscess are very rare in developed countries.

There is more about this in Chapter 5 on the diagnosis and management of acute illnesses in general practice.

Practical Exercise

Use the suggested scheme to learn more about a particular medical condition.

1. Choose a condition about which you know little or nothing, based on a patient encounter during your general practice attachment.
2. Research this topic and try to organize your learning using the scheme detailed above.
3. Consider how the information you gain applies to the patient you saw.
4. Arrange a time when you can present the information to your GP tutor and, perhaps, an audience of practice staff.
5. The next time you see a patient with this condition, consider how you can apply your knowledge to understand his or her problems better.

Red flag symptoms

The discussion so far may have suggested that common symptoms are synonymous with minor symptoms, and that they usually do not reach the GP. On the other hand, it might be assumed that symptoms of potentially more serious pathology would almost invariably present to the GP. However, this is not the case. Potentially serious symptoms sit alongside those of very little significance. This is one of the greatest skills of the primary care generalist – to be able to sift through symptoms and determine those patients who might be suffering from a more serious condition. The GP with too high an index of suspicion will have an excessively high rate of investigation and referral to secondary care specialists; the one with too low an index of suspicion may miss serious pathology.

Symptoms that might indicate more serious underlying pathology are termed 'red flag' symptoms. Sometimes patients present with red flag symptoms and sometimes they have to be elicited by direct questioning. Each of the body systems has its own red flags. For example, the overwhelming majority of headaches are functional or stress related. However, the presence of morning headaches which wear off by the middle of the morning and which respond well to analgesia, particularly if the headaches are of recent onset, might suggest an underlying brain tumour. Similarly, most febrile children are likely to have a self-limiting viral illness but the presence of a raised respiratory rate, drowsiness, confusion, cold hands and feet, a rash or vomiting may all suggest an underlying septicaemia and the need for urgent referral and treatment with intravenous antibiotics.

Not all potential red flag symptoms even reach the GP. Rectal bleeding may be the presenting symptom of a relatively innocent pathology such as haemorrhoids, or may be the first indication of the development of a rectal cancer. In spite of the potentially alarming nature of this symptom, fewer than half of adults experiencing this symptom present to their GP (Jones and Tait, 1995). The consequences of ignoring or self-care might, in these circumstances, result in delayed diagnosis and reduce the chances of cancer survival.

One new area of research is to try to put predictive values on different symptoms in order to determine the likelihood of underlying serious disease. Until recently, we knew the importance of eliciting red flag symptoms but not the proportion of patients with any given red flag symptom who could be expected to have serious pathology. Increasingly, research is providing data from which estimates can be based on the likelihood of serious disease. For example, an adult with dysphagia has a 5.7 per cent chance of an underlying carcinoma of the oesophagus if male or 2.4 per cent if female; these positive predictive values are further modified by age, such that men aged 65–74 years with dysphagia had a 9.0 per cent chance of cancer (Jones et al., 2007).

A more recent study has sifted through the different presenting symptoms for cancers in general, and has created a list of eight symptoms and signs which are above a 5 per cent threshold for predicting cancer (positive predictive threshold) (Shapley et al., 2010). These eight symptoms are:

- Rectal bleeding: both sexes, age ≥75 years
- Iron-deficiency anaemia:
  - Hb ≤12 g/dL: male, age ≥60 years
  - Hb ≤11 g/dL: female, age ≥70 years
  - Hb ≤9 g/dL: female, age ≥60 years
- Haematuria: both sexes, age ≥60 years
- Rectal examination: malignant feeling prostate, male, age ≥40 years
- Haemoptysis: male, age ≥55 years; female, age ≥65 years
- Dysphagia: male, age ≥55 years
- Breast lump: female, age ≥20 years
- Postmenopausal bleeding: female, age 75–84 years.

Case Study 7.2

Now consider the same patient presented as Case study 7.1, above. He is aged 45 years and has acute back pain. The pain did not settle with osteopathic treatment. It started to wake him up at night and became unremitting. Although generally fit and well, he had begun to get aches and pains in other sites, particularly over the ribs. Over the last month, he had been feeling increasingly tired and his friends at work said that he looked pale.

Thinking and Discussion Point

Reflect on Case study 7.2; can you think of other possible underlying causes for this patient's back pain? How would you go about disentangling these possible causes?

SUMMARY POINTS

To conclude, the most important messages of this chapter are as follows.

- Probably under 3 per cent of symptoms experienced by the general population are presented to a GP; the majority are dealt with by sufferers or their families. The presence of a symptom is not the only determinant of whether an individual decides to seek medical help. The way in which they evaluate that symptom affects the action they take and is profoundly affected by psychosocial factors, including cultural and family influences.
- About 80 per cent of a practice population will consult a GP or practice nurse at least once a year, with an average consultation rate of 5.5 per person registered.
- The illnesses seen in general practice differ in severity and type from those seen in hospital. In general practice, most conditions are minor or chronic: 52 per cent of all illness presenting to general practice can be classified as minor, 33 per cent as chronic and 15 per cent as major.
- The most common minor conditions presenting to general practice are acute throat infection, psycho-emotional disorder, backache, eczema and ear disorders.
- The most common chronic conditions are asthma, chronic obstructive airways disease, hypertension, backache, osteoarthritis, ischaemic heart disease and diabetes mellitus.
- The most common major conditions are acute chest infection, depression, myocardial infarction, cerebrovascular accident and acute abdomen.
- Social factors influence the health of the population and play a role in 33 per cent of consultations. Health promotion and preventative activities take place in 20 per cent of consultations.
- Knowing where to seek further information about a particular condition and how best to structure that information are important aids to learning.

(UK data)

References

Armstrong, D. 2002: *Outline of sociology as applied to medicine*, 5th edn. London: Arnold.

Becker, M. and Maiman, L. 1975: Sociobehavioural determinants of compliance with health and medical care recommendations. *Medical Care* 13, 10–24.

Campbell, S. and Roland, M. 1996: Why do people consult the doctor? *Family Practice* 13, 75–83.

Cartwright, A. and Anderson, R. 1981: *General practice revisited: a second study of patients and their doctors.* London: Tavistock.

Dunnell, K. and Cartwright, A. 1972: *Medicine Takers, Prescribers and Hoarders.* London: Routledge and Kegan Paul.

Fleming, D., Cross, K.W. and Barley, M.A. 2005: Recent changes in the prevalence of diseases presenting for health care. *British Journal of Clinical Practice* 55, 589–95.

Fry, J. 1978: *A New Approach to Medicine: Principles and Priorities in Health Care.* Lancaster: MTP Press.

Fry, J. 1993: *General practice: the facts.* Oxford: Radcliffe Medical Press.

Fry, J. and Sandler, G. 1993: *Common diseases: their nature, prevalence, and care*, 5th edn. Newbury: Petroc Press.

Glasziou, P., Del Mar, C., Sanders, S. and Hayem, M. Antibiotics for acute otitis media in children (Cochrane Review). In: *The Cochrane Library*, Issue 2, 2003. Oxford: Update Software. The Cochrane Library can be accessed free of charge through the National Electronic Library for Health at www.nelh.nhs.uk

Graham, H. and Seabrook, M. 1995: Structured learning packs for independent learning in the community. *Medical Education* 29, 61–5.

Jefferys, M., Brotherston, J.H., Cartwright, A. 1960: Consumption of medicines on a working-class housing estate. *British Journal of Preventive and Social Medicine* 14, 64–76.

Jones, R. and Tait, C.L. 1995: The gastrointestinal side effects of non-steroidal anti-inflammatory drugs: a community based study. *British Journal of Clinical Practice* 49, 67–70.

Jones, R., Latinovic, R., Charlton, J. and Gulliford, M. 2007: Alarm symptoms in early diagnosis of cancer in primary care: cohort study using General Practice Research Database. *British Medical Journal* 334, 1040.

Last, J. 1963: The clinical iceberg: completing the clinical picture in general practice. *Lancet* 2, 28–30.

Logan, W.P.D. and Brooke, E. 1957: *Survey of sickness, 1943–1952.* London: HMSO.

Mechanic, D. 1962: The concept of illness behaviour. *Journal of Chronic Diseases* 15, 189–94.

McCormick, A., Fleming, D. and Charlton, J. 1995: *Morbidity statistics from general practice: Fourth National Study 1991–1992.* London: HMSO.

Morrell, D. and Wale, C. 1976: Symptoms perceived and recorded by patients. *Journal of the Royal College of General Practitioners* 26, 398–403.

Rosenstock, I. 1966: Why people use health services. *Milbank Memorial Fund Quarterly* 44(3), Suppl., 94–127.

Royal College of General Practitioners. 2007: *Being a general practitioner. Curriculum Statement 1.* London: RCGP.

Shapley, M., Mansell, G., Jordan, J. and Jordan, K. 2010: Positive predictive values of ≥5% in primary care for cancer: systematic review. *British Journal of General Practice* 60, 366–77.

The Information Centre 2008: *Trends in consultation rates in general practice 1995 to 2007: Analysis of the QResearch database.* Leeds: The Information Centre.

Wadsworth, M., Butterfield, W. and Blaney, R. 1971: *Health and sickness: the choice of treatment: perception of illness and choice of treatment in an urban community.* London: Tavistock.

Zola, I. 1973: Pathways to the doctor: from person to patient. *Social Science and Medicine* 7, 677–89.

Further reading

Armstrong, D. 1995: *An outline of sociology as applied to medicine,* 4th edn. London: Arnold.
A good introduction to medical sociology that contains further information concerning illness behaviour.

Campbell, S. and Roland, M. 1996: Why do people consult the doctor? *Family Practice* 13, 75–83.
A helpful review article that summarizes the reasons why people seek professional medical help.

Fry, J. and Sandler, G. 1993: *Common diseases: their nature, prevalence, and care.* Newbury: Petroc Press.
A useful book that contains fairly detailed information about diseases commonly seen in general practice, including those poorly covered in standard medical texts.

Jones, R. (ed.) 2003: *Oxford textbook of primary medical care.* Oxford: Oxford University Press.
A two-volume text, the second of which, the clinical volume, covers in depth all the medical problems commonly seen in general practice worldwide.

Mead, M. and Patterson, H. 1999: *Tutorials in general practice,* 3rd edn. Edinburgh: Churchill Livingstone.
An illuminating selection of case studies focusing on problems commonly seen in general practice.

Murtagh, J. 1999: *General practice,* 2nd edn. Australia: McGraw-Hill Health Professions Division.
A useful reference source that presents a systematic review of patient assessment and management strategies for common conditions in general practice.

Taylor, R.J., McAvoy, B.R. and O'Dowd, T. 2003: *General practice medicine.* Edinburgh: Churchill Livingstone.
An illustrated text that outlines common illnesses seen in general practice.

SINGLE BEST ANSWER QUESTIONS

7.1 Common symptoms can best be defined as:

a) Minor symptoms
b) Symptoms which patients should not really trouble the doctor with
c) Symptoms which occur frequently in the general population
d) Symptoms which are easy for the doctor to deal with
e) Symptoms of common diseases.

7.2 A 66-year-old man comes to see you with a headache. What do you think the most likely diagnosis is going to be?

a) A brain tumour
b) Temporal arteritis
c) New onset migraine
d) Depression
e) Sinusitis.

7.3 Patients with a 'serious symptom':

a) Always go to their GP as a matter of urgency
b) Often delay attending their GP through fear of possible unpleasant disease
c) Often ignore their symptoms
d) Usually attempt self-treatment and only attend their GP if this fails
e) Look it up on the internet.

7.4 A 40-year-old obese man tells you that he commonly experiences feelings of indigestion, felt mostly over the sternum. What is the most important thing you should you do in this situation?

a) Offer to prescribe some Gaviscon
b) Encourage him to go to the pharmacist and get an over-the-counter medication
c) Take a full medical history including 'systems' questions covering GI, chest and cardiovascular system symptoms
d) Ask him 'why now?'
e) Encourage him to lose weight.

7.5 You have just seen a 35-year-old man with recurrent abdominal pain for 4 years. He has had every single investigation under the sun but still gets disabling bouts of pain which have resulted in a lot of time off work. He is not too impressed with all the previous doctors who have tried and failed to cure his pain. Your best management option is to:

a) Explore his underlying concerns
b) Offer reassurance
c) Prescribe stronger painkillers
d) Think of an investigation which hasn't been thought of by the previous doctors
e) Arrange for a laparotomy.

8

PSYCHOLOGICAL ISSUES IN GENERAL PRACTICE

- Why are psychological issues so important?
- The biopsychosocial model
- Why are psychological issues so important in primary care?
- Red flag symptoms
- Assessing mental state
- Adjusting to life changes
- Mad, bad or sad? The debate about mental health
- Classification and assessment: how do we make sense of it all?

- Practical questions in classification
- Dangerousness
- Symptoms and circumstances
- Who can help provide help and how?
- Systems and frameworks
- Effects on the professions: the way forward
- Summary points
- References
- Further reading
- Single best answer questions

Psychological issues are important in all encounters between a doctor and a patient, and the ability to comprehend, assess and manage these, in partnership with the patient, is a basic medical skill. General practice is the place where emotional issues may be identified and managed. The doctor's psychological responses and state of mind may be as important as those of the patient.

LEARNING OBJECTIVES

By the end of this chapter, you will be able to:

- describe the importance of psychological issues in primary medical care;
- describe the ways in which patients may present with these issues, and how they can be assessed;
- outline the common ways in which personal, family, social or cultural factors may influence presentation or outcome;
- outline the possible responses that can be offered, and by whom;
- give an account of the way in which doctors and other members of the team may be affected by this work, and how it can be managed;

Why are psychological issues so important?

A common but now outmoded model of medical care assumes that a *patient* has a *physical disease* and comes to a *doctor* for it to be *cured*. The new professional model challenges each of the emphasized concepts, so let us look at these in turn.

Thinking and Discussion Point

Look at the opening statement of the paragraph opposite and see how many of the ideas in it you would consider 'outmoded' in general practice and primary medical care

Becoming a 'patient'

The first point at which a person meets the health service is primary care, and this is often (but not exclusively) in general practice. However, people may not see themselves as patients, or accept the idea (even if the doctor or others see it as necessary), and may wish to think long and hard about the consequences of this new 'role'.

Case Study 8.1

A young couple presented to the general practitioner (GP) in evening surgery. The woman explained that she had brought her partner in because she had become very upset and depressed on their holiday together. She had thought she was pregnant, but had had a period while they were away. They had been trying to have a baby for 2 years. When the doctor talked about both their backgrounds, the man looked alarmed: 'Don't bring me into this doctor – there's nothing wrong with me.'

Thinking and Discussion Point

- Make a note of your reactions to Case study 8.1.
- Taking each of the three people involved in turn, what would they be feeling and what would they want to achieve? If the feeling is standing in the way of their reaching their goals, what can be done to change things?

'Physical'

Although doctors are often distinguished by their concerns for bodies, the mind is also part of that body. The split between mind and body (represented, to be fair, by our title) seems increasingly unhelpful in professional work. We recognize the existence and state of our own body by using our senses, and these are collected and coordinated by the brain or mind. For instance, a pain cannot be seen: however physical its origin, it is perceived and responded to initially by the mind. Equally, many of the ways in which we establish mental states, even our own, are expressed by the body, such as weight loss, sweating, crying, shouting.

Case Study 8.2

A middle-aged executive presented to her doctor feeling tired, but not prepared to say much else about herself. Her doctor checked her and found nothing physically wrong. He reassured her, but a week later the patient committed suicide with paracetamol.

Thinking and Discussion Point

With reference to Case study 8.2:
- What are your reactions to this case?
- Could the doctor have done anything to prevent the patient's death and, if so, what and how?

'Disease'

This is one of the words that many people (including doctors, surprisingly) use imprecisely. It is usually used for an objectively recognizable condition, often in contrast to an illness. Illness is usually used to describe a set of feelings which someone recognizes (subjectively) and can tell the doctor about, but which sometimes cannot be defined objectively by examinations or tests. It is subjective feelings or symptoms that usually bring people first to a health professional; that person may be able to find objective signs or measure something, but he or she equally may not, and if not the condition will still be as real to the patient and requiring medical attention. In addition a doctor's validation of the illness ('yes this is something that should occupy my time') is the first part of the route into care, and may have implications for society as a whole, like receiving financial support from state or insurance company. Doctors may be pressed to give them a label, but there is work suggesting that labelling the condition too early or too firmly may be a mistake. Medical labels may be very sticky.

Patient comment

'I used to be schizophrenic in north London, doctor, but now down here I'm bipolar and it makes a lot of difference.' What sort difference do you think it would make?

Case Study 8.3

A young man came in on Saturday morning with a headache. He was a bouncer in a nightclub but said he had not been drinking much the night before. In the silence that the doctor allowed to develop after this, the patient explained that he was going to court on Monday to defend himself on an assault charge, and was unable to think clearly because of the headache.

Thinking and Discussion Point

Does the man in Case study 8.3 have a disease or an illness and, if so, what? If not, what else might be wrong which a doctor could help with?

'Doctor'

You will have seen that many people other than doctors make contact with patients, especially in primary care, and share the processes of assessment and management.

Case Study 8.4

The receptionist came in to explain to the doctor how he had been talking to the next patient due to see her and that the patient was extremely upset about her son, who was going through a difficult time. The receptionist felt this knowledge would help the doctor to get to the point of the patient's visit. When the patient came in, the doctor mentioned that she knew something about the family problems. 'Oh thank you, doctor, but I've talked to that nice man on the front desk all about that. I've come to see you about these horrible varicose veins.'

Thinking and Discussion Point

Consider for a moment the personal and professional skills that might be needed to deal with the different case studies you have read in this chapter so far. Which of these skills particularly should a doctor have, and do you feel confident that you are already or could be skilled in this way? If not, who in your learning environment would help you?

'Cured'

Maybe we all wanted to be doctors in order to help people get better. Many conditions get better by themselves ('self-limiting') and some, like diabetes, are to be managed over the long term.

Student comment/tutor response

Student: 'I've just come from intensive care looking after patients with heart attacks, but there don't seem to be many people we can cure here.'
Tutor: 'Can you cure a heart attack?'

Thinking and Discussion Point

What do you think about this interchange between student and tutor, particularly when it comes to psychological issues?

The biopsychosocial model

Medical work embraces all sides of illness and disease, which include the social and psychological as well as the physical (the biopsychosocial model); takes as much notice of what the patient says as of what the professional observes; considers factors which influence professional judgement as well as the sick person's presentation; considers prevention and long-term care even in acute situations; and sees medical work as a team enterprise. Focusing on psychological issues means that we shall want to know about feelings and emotional issues as much as about madness, and that we should be prepared to look at ourselves as professionals (how we view our work, our relationship with our patients, the effect we have on them and they have on us, and so on) and as members of a group. Before examining psychological issues specifically in primary care, it would be worth thinking through the implications of the biopsychosocial model for yourself and your training.

Thinking and Discussion Point

- Do you agree that the above describes medical work? If not, why not?
- Are there dangers that doctors might have too wide a role? What limits have to be set to doctors' responsibilities?

Thinking and Discussion Point continued

> If you are already aiming for a particular type of doctoring (if you want to be a neurosurgeon or a parasitologist, for example), what are the implications of this discussion for your chosen area of work?

Why are psychological issues so important in primary care?

Preventing preventable deaths is one of the prime tasks of all doctors. An important cause of death in many societies is serious depression that may result in suicide. Other causes of death include violence and road traffic accidents. Alcoholism and drug misuse enters this list both in its own right and as a risk factor in precipitating any of the above three. Although doctors have potential duties alongside many other agencies in this respect, Case study 8.2 demonstrates that some desperately distressed people first visit their GP – some studies have suggested this is a common pattern (Matthews *et al.*, 1994). So intervention at this time might be considered important, even if only a small percentage of people at risk were influenced, or even if the work was not completely effective.

Being upset emotionally – anxious or depressed – is a normal human response, but in some situations the reaction may be such that the person cannot continue with their lives. Even if they cope in the short term, the problem may re-emerge later and influence their health – and their healthcare.

Case Study 8.5

Mrs G was the life and soul of the community and a great coper. But she had never talked to anybody about the terrible time when her mother had had an intracranial haemorrhage and she had to manage on her own. Now every headache she or any one of her extended family got was treated as an emergency. When the doctor asked her: 'What exactly are you afraid of?' it all came out, and she and the practice were able to deal with issues more rationally.

Dean quote

You GP tutors would love hearing about the case I've just been asked to see on the surgical ward. A young woman had presented with abdominal pain, and all the tests that the surgeons could think of doing were normal. When I sat down beside the patent's bed I asked her 'When did this pain start?' She answered 'When my husband took my son back to Nigeria.'

Psychological symptoms may equally be the sign of a physical crisis or brain disease. Changes in the internal milieu may be expressed psychologically: for instance, alterations in calcium levels may change a person's perception of pain, and the side effects of medication may also cause changes in behaviour.

Case Study 8.6

A 35-year-old man presents to casualty with hypomania. On a careful history from his mother it transpires that he is on high doses of steroids for ocular myositis. When the prednisolone is slowly reduced his hypomania abates.

If the patient is a parent or in a family, emotional responses can alter children's health or damage the family or social group in wider and more longterm ways. A child's whole life may be altered.

Case Study 8.7

A young family of husband, wife, toddler and new baby daughter came to emergency evening surgery. 'The problem is him,' said the mother pointing to the toddler. 'He is pissing everywhere. And tonight he pissed on the baby.' The doctor could not help himself laughing. 'You laugh, doctor? But she is the most important person in the world.' Pause. 'Oh my God, doctor, what have I just said?' And she hugged the toddler and at follow-up the problem had resolved.

Studies show that the main or most important diagnosis in general practice is a psychological one (anxiety, depression, etc.) in a large number of cases that present to the professionals (see section on 'Symptoms and circumstances' below). What patients choose to offer to their doctors is influenced by many things – the social conditions locally, the availability of other forms of help, whether they think the doctor can help – but perhaps most particularly by how they expect to be received by the doctor when they introduce this topic. Many people still feel shy of discussing their feelings with doctors, because they think they will be seen as 'not really ill', 'making a fuss', or perhaps that the doctor will make a mistake and by thinking they are upset will miss a serious condition. Cultures vary, but in many groups there is still a stigma attached to mental illness of all kinds.

Practical Exercise

Make a note of the main issues relevant to each patient you see with your GP, especially:

❏ Why the patient came to the doctor, and what they wanted
❏ The main diagnosis or diagnoses made by you and the GP
❏ How the patient behaved in the consultation
❏ Whether you felt, or the patient exhibited, any obvious emotions during that time, and what they were.

Do you note any difference between these four headings when you use them? Do you think using these ideas expands the importance of psychological issues in general practice?

Student quote

'We've been taught about the iceberg of disease, and I guess that everyone is anxious in some way about themselves, or they wouldn't come to the doctor! When I went to my doctor and he was offhand about my symptoms, it only made things worse.'

Case Study 8.8

It was the second time that the medical student had been to the doctor with chest pain. He had been told he was as 'fit as a fiddle' but that had not reassured him. 'What was he worried about? Had he seen something which upset him?' He told the doctor about the post mortem on a lung cancer patient he had seen, and how he could not get out of his mind how like his Dad the patient had looked.

Practical Exercise

Think about the times you or your family went to the doctor. How were you received? Does this influence how you would like to practise in any way?

Madness

At the other end of the illness spectrum, the serious distress of madness (which is classed in medicine as 'psychosis', but described by some patients after recovery as 'being crazy') makes some people reluctant to come to doctors, either because they are suspicious that they will come to harm or because their pattern of thinking makes doctors irrelevant. Family or friends who might otherwise bring them to the surgery may not be perceived by the distressed individual as being 'on my side' either. However, although specialist psychiatry is particularly concerned with these problems, there are many reasons why hospital is not the best environment for people who are seriously distressed, so primary care staff have a significant role in detecting and helping to manage serious distress.

Thinking and Discussion Point

▢ Does this category (madness/psychosis/serious distress) make sense to you? How is it helpful and how unhelpful?
▢ What do you think the main needs of people who are going through such an experience are? Who might answer these needs? (You might like to read some more – see the Further reading list at the end of this chapter.)
▢ If you have met someone who seems to you to be in this category, what did you feel about the situation, for yourself, for the ill person, and for the professional? Did you understand anything of what the patient was going through? Did you feel safe?

Practical Exercise

If your answer to the last question is positive, or if you meet someone who was seriously distressed but now seems 'better' and your GP thinks it is all right for you to do so, see if you can find time and a suitable place to ask the patient if he or she would help you to understand the background by telling you about the experience and what it felt like, as far as both the illness and the treatment were concerned. Make it very clear that the patient is absolutely free to refuse and that this is only for your education.

Doctors' responses

It is common to hear people complain that when they were upset the doctor didn't seem to take any notice, or if they did they seemed just embarrassed or made some very unhelpful suggestions. Everyone is different in how they respond to distress – some people naturally find it easy and something they like to do, others want to run a mile. If you are in, or nearly in, the latter category you might think that is ok or that GP work is not for you. But this wouldn't be the answer if, say you didn't (as most people don't) want to see dead bodies or do a rectal examination. These things are part of professional medical work: we need to learn how to do them, how to do them well and how to cope with the distress it causes us. It is just the same with psychological work. We need to learn how to approach the subject, the questions to ask, how to feel confident we are doing the right thing and how to cope with our own feelings.

Patient comment

'Have I ever had any psychiatric help over the years? Well, I suppose I have, rather in the sense that someone adrift at sea might shout "Help!" to a passing supertanker, be thrown a lifebelt, and the tanker go on its way.'

Thinking and Discussion Point

How do you feel about dealing with psychological distress? For instance, do you feel comfortable, overwhelmed, or don't you feel it's your job? What support would you like to have, now and later in your professional life, to cope with this work?

Red flag symptoms

- 'I want to kill myself.'
- 'I can hear people talking about me all the time in my head.'
- 'I feel so bad I want to harm someone.'
- 'I am going crazy and I need help.'

Assessing mental state

One of the ways a doctor may feel more secure in the presence of someone who is behaving strangely is to check their mental state.

Practical Exercise

How do we assess someone's mental state? Think back to your teaching in psychiatry and look out your old notes. Consider a patient that you are currently working with. As well as taking a history, doing a physical examination and seeing all this in the context of their life and social situation carefully observe their appearance, behaviour, speech, mood, thoughts, perception and cognitive function. What are the predisposing and precipitating factors that brought them to this place and what perpetuating factors might you need to think about in helping them through? Write up your findings for this patient and discuss them with your tutor.

Adjusting to life changes

In between the 'normal' anxiety of every patient who comes to a doctor and the deep distress of a suicidal or psychotic patient, most thoughtful doctors detect a group of people who seem particularly drawn to seeking help about a medical condition when they are also going through a difficult or turbulent phase in their lives.

Thinking and Discussion Point

- Have you noted people coming in with this sort of background problem to your GP?
- Do you have experience in your own life, or the lives of your family or friends, when circumstance seemed to make you ill or drive you to see a doctor?

There are many different words to describe this interaction between social circumstances and health. 'Life events' are the experiences which people have that seem particularly associated with increased illness or increased attendance at doctors. Clear associations are found with moving house or losing someone who was loved. 'Life transitions' or 'adjustment reactions' are other names for a similar phenomenon, and this suggests that, rather than things happening to us, there are phases which everyone experiences as they go through life, and there are times of particular vulnerability, such as adolescence or retirement. Particular 'crisis points' are now widely recognized, for instance the 'mid-life crisis' of late middle age. We shall return to these ideas when we look at 'depression'.

Case Study 8.9

Julie was 11, and had been brought by her mother to see the doctor four times in six weeks with minor complaints. 'Are you having a difficult time at the moment Julie? You look as if life at the moment is a bit tough.' In the silence that followed, she looked at her mother: 'Doctor, I think you're quite right. Julie's just gone to big school, and is finding it quite hard as all her friends are at the other one. We do talk about it, but it is affecting her.'

Psychosomatic is the name given to those illnesses or diseases for which there seems to be a clear connection, even a causal one, between stress and physical illness. The conditions that used to be quoted classically were ulcerative colitis, asthma and rheumatoid arthritis. The idea that there is a particular group is now questioned: most physical conditions are influenced by state of mind and reactions to circumstances, and many patients now ask 'Could this be stress-related?'

Mad, bad or sad? The debate about mental health

Case Study 8.10

A GP was talking about one of his patients, a 65-year-old woman. The patient was very distressed with symptoms of a psychotic depression and yet the symptoms kept changing. Everyone involved, including the woman's family, had their own opinions and even these varied over time. Various medications produced side effects and did not appear to help very much. The GP had become perplexed and worried by the woman's (and family's) plight and questioned 'Is she mad, bad, or sad?'

You may have noticed that this chapter often refers to different or changing ways of looking at things. This may be uncomfortable or unsettling, but it is to help you recognize that the area of psychological issues/psychiatry/mental health is a 'contested' field. There are different ways not just of describing what we all observe, but also of thinking about and explaining these observations ('discourses'), and these ideas are themselves still changing or developing. In this respect it is probably no different from the rest of your medical studies, but the arguments seem sharper in mental health in general. There are debates about the use of drugs, diagnoses, ways of managing distress or compulsory treatment that start from completely different points of view.

Thinking and Discussion Point

- Do you agree with what has just been said about different discourses? If so, what do you think creates these differences of opinion?
- What are the important things you need to be aware of when practising as a doctor in the wider community?

Some of these changes may be due to the way in which society in general seems to think. For instance, in the lifetime of the authors of this chapter, consensual homosexual acts between adult men have ceased to be considered as crimes in the UK, and being gay has stopped being a recognized condition in psychiatry, for which people are 'treated'. (We are still not at the point at which everybody agrees that adults are free to express their sexuality as they wish, provided they do not harm other people, so some forms of sexual desire or behaviour still cause distress, and people will come to doctors to be helped.)

Some of the issues that seem particularly important in mental health debates at the moment are:

- power, control and respect for autonomy,
- danger and safety,
- depersonalization, stigma and being a case rather than a person,
- dependency and relationships.

Case Study 8.11

The old man had always been eccentric, and the doctor regularly had to deal with neighbours who did not like his singing or the plastic flowers planted in his front garden. The doctor secretly admired odd behaviour, but it was when the rubbish began to accumulate outside, and the old man shouted abuse through the letterbox at anyone who called, that he realized he had to take a new view of what was going on. In the words of the immediate neighbour, 'something must be done'.

Practical Exercise

- ❑ As you see patients in your current attachment, listen to what other members of the team or relatives and neighbours have got to say, and to how the patient describes his or her own condition.
- ❑ Do these suggest different ways of looking at the problem and, if so, do these differences help you to see different solutions, or do they make things even more difficult?
- ❑ If people disagree on what approach should be used, and there is conflict, whose ideas should win?

Classification and assessment: how do we make sense of it all?

Different people approach even this problem in different ways. Classical medical teaching is that diagnosis must precede treatment, but this is not always possible. When physical specialists are often perplexed by the lack of physical signs in psychiatry, psychiatrists, by using questionnaire 'instruments' of various sorts, claim that their classifications are as clear and objective as any. But even within that branch of the profession, opinions differ. The psychodynamic school might look at what has to be worked with, the behavioural at what life problems need to be worked on, and so on. There is a radical mode of thought that rejects all labelling as stigmatic: labels are seen as traps for overworked or under-involved people, who just follow someone else's thinking and do not listen carefully to what the patient is really saying. A helpful way of combining different approaches in general practice is through the concept of narrative – the story a person is trying to tell. We shall come back to that concept later in this chapter. One thing we can be sure about: distressed people often get physically ill, and people with a physical illness often find this very distressing. We are dealing not with 'either/or', but with 'both/and'. Our classifications must be inclusive, not exclusive, and allow us to keep open minds.

Case Study 8.12

The new young GP had a special interest in depression. His patient, aged 55, had just lost his mother, and was tired and listless. At the third session, when there seemed no improvement, the patient muttered, 'I don't know, everything seems to be psychological these days – but I feel ill.' The doctor quickly remembered that he had not done a physical assessment. The erythrocyte sedimentation rate (ESR) was raised and the patient had multiple myeloma, as well as a difficult bereavement reaction.

Practical questions in classification

Some people say that questions are more useful than answers. In the area of mental health classification in primary care, you might think some of the following questions were useful.

- Is the condition *dangerous*, in the sense of a threat to life or offering the possibility of serious harm to self or others?
- Does the condition seem to be triggered mainly by *outside events*?
- Is there something that can be *usefully done* and, if so, is it to be done by the health service or by other agencies?
- Does addressing the problem mainly depend on what the patient does for *himself or herself*?
- Is it an *acute condition, a long-term condition*, or has there been a recent change?
- Does it seem mostly related to a *physical illness*, which needs treatment too?
- Is there a *pattern* in the person's behaviour that seems to cause much of the difficulty or offer important clues?
- Does the person seem to be thinking in a way we understand, or is their *thought in some form of disorder*?
- Is the person's *age, culture or gender* crucial?
- Does the condition seem to have been initiated, or made worse, by some *psychoactive substance*?
- Even if we understand the distress and the reaction seems normal, do we need to help because of the *degree of distress*?

Your other readings in psychiatric classification may look quite different: consult your recommended reading in this field, as there is not scope to cover it all here. You will notice that most of these classifications are also a mixture, and that in the individual case people often recommend looking at a psychiatric assessment from several different points of view – a 'multi-axial' approach (Tylee *et al.*, 1995) which also underlies the International Classification of Diseases (ICD) (World Health Organization, 2010). Grouping might depend on:

- symptoms,
- behaviour,
- a recognized pattern or syndrome,
- probable cause,
- society's judgement of what is acceptable,
- what the patient will agree to,
- what treatment is available.

As you read down this list, some of the headings may have become uncomfortable to use and may raise questions for you that must be faced and may need to be revisited. Certainly, outcome will depend on resources for treatment, for instance, but diagnostic assessment also might do so.

Thinking and Discussion Point

Try looking at some of the people you have met, or cases you have come across, who might be in the following jumbled categories in relation to the questions at the start of the 'Practical questions in classification' section:

- learning difficulties
- child abuse
- suicidal threat
- phobias
- alcoholism
- bereavement
- anorexia nervosa
- Alzheimer's disease
- panic disorder
- postnatal depression
- retirement crisis
- psychopathy
- hypochondriasis
- school refusal
- delirium
- post-traumatic stress disorder
- mania
- obsessive–compulsive behaviour
- schizophrenia
- divorce.

Whatever groupings seem to be most helpful (and it is likely that, like other areas in medicine, there will continue to be changes), medicine is a subject for which practical skill is needed, and you might like to match some of these conditions with the practical questions in classification above, and with your own. You will notice that sometimes this necessitates putting together two conditions that do not have a common or similar cause. You might also like to write down the words which ordinary people would use to describe them in your particular community.

Dangerousness

In doing the exercise on the previous page (in the section on 'Practical questions in classification') you might find something odd. For instance, when dealing with the first question (about dangerousness), you may pick out suicidal depression, anorexia nervosa, delirium, drunkenness, acute schizophrenia, child abuse and psychopathic behaviour. But the way of approaching it will have to depend on some of the same sort of questions, such as the following:

- What sort of threat is there, and to whom?
- Is it acute, in the sense of needing immediate action, or will it wait for a different sort of assessment?
- What are my duties, and how far will the law allow me to go?
- Should other people be informed?
- What sort of resources can we muster to cope?
- Do I need help and, if so, of what sort?

Case Study 8.13

At the end of a Saturday morning surgery, the doctor received a message that one of his male patients 'was not very well – would he call round?' The receptionist had been unable to find anything else out, and said that the wife had seemed very 'cagey' on the phone. Irritated, but in a hurry to get to his son's football match, the doctor decided just to call in quickly on his way home. He left his main bag in the surgery and just took a stethoscope and a prescription pad. When he arrived, he found the husband was in an acute and violent paranoid state. Trapped in the bedroom, with no emergency drugs and no mobile phone, the doctor took over an hour to fight his way to the home phone to ring the police. When six officers arrived, the patient was clearly overwhelmed and immediately settled down; he was admitted to an acute psychiatric ward, and recovered in three weeks without a final diagnosis being made. The doctor missed the football match.

This case, a rare occurrence it needs to be said, illustrates some issues that are obvious but worth emphasizing:

- the doctor was himself one of the people at most risk;

- asking for help is not a sign of weakness but . . .
- thoughtless rushing about is not likely to be helpful so . . .
- think ahead and consider safety issues as well;
- most acutely psychotic people will give in to a show of numbers;
- doctors' irritation is one of the major causes of poor management.

> ## Thinking and Discussion Point
>
> - So what might have improved the outcome?
> - What problems does the doctor face in his future care of this couple?

Symptoms and circumstances

If dangerous, mad behaviour is (fortunately) rare and containable (and in many cases, as above, just one episode in a life which afterwards may well return to normal), the usual presentations of distress in our society are very different, and often much less easy to typify or describe. One of the reasons, as we have seen, is that unhappiness and illness go hand in hand. Being ill makes us anxious; worrying can make us ill. So it is much more difficult to sift out from all those with symptoms which concern them enough to bring them to a doctor, the particular individuals whose main issue is psychological distress. Community surveys have suggested that psychiatric morbidity rates from as little as 3.7 per cent to 65 per cent. It all depends how it is defined. What is clear is that at least one in ten consultations are overtly about psychological problems in most practices, and that the more a professional looks, the more is likely to be found.

We can say with certainty what sort of symptoms should alert the doctor to psychological distress, but we cannot ever say that certain symptoms are always excluded. In other words, we could be sure that in some cases a person is distressed, but it is hard to be sure that they are not, given all the ways in which most cultures try to inhibit open expression of distress in general.

Symptoms have usually arisen from feelings, emotional states of one sort or another. Two common psychological diagnoses are *anxiety* and *depression*. Although these could be seen as increased or reduced arousal, in practice these states are often mixed and one may progress to the other: acute worries may produce long-term tension, which looks more and more like depression as the days pass and the feelings or circumstances persist (Figure 8.1).

Anxiety

Anxiety may be easier to detect than depression. Anxiety is usually episodic, and we are all aware of the likelihood of tension headaches (as in Case Study 8.3) being possible signs, as are the symptoms of panic: a pounding heart, dry mouth, breathlessness, waves of nausea, sleeplessness or diarrhoea. Management of the symptoms is half of the battle here, as their very presence is part of a vicious cycle which makes the person even more anxious because of secondary concerns – the dry mouth which makes public speaking impossible, the disgrace of public sickness or dashing to the lavatory, and so on. These help to persuade sufferers that there is something seriously amiss, adding further to anxiety levels. The second half of the battle is to get to the root of the anxiety.

Case Study 8.14

A young woman presented with recurrent chest pain and wheezing which she insisted were due to a physical illness undetected by the doctors. Negative tests were initially of no avail in unravelling the problem, until she began to talk about her mother's illness from breast cancer, and she and the doctor were able to make the connection between her physical feelings and the unresolved grief she felt after having lost the person she had seen as both her greatest challenger and her greatest supporter. Once she was prepared to make the link and work on it, she abandoned her demands for further specialist referrals and agreed to work with a counsellor.

Thinking and Discussion Point

The challenge in Case Study 8.14 was the patient's own decision that anxiety and grief were not 'real' symptoms, and that because she did have real symptoms the doctors must be missing something.

In observing other health professionals at work, note how they re-educate as well as diagnose. You should collect phrases and approaches that seem to you to help doctor and patient to reach an understanding. In dysfunctional or difficult consultations, what seems to make things go wrong?

The long-term management of people who tend to become anxious, are constitutionally 'highly strung' or who worry constantly about their health is perhaps less easy now than two or three decades ago, because of the current understanding of the hazards of most long-term anxiolytic treatment. The psychopharmacology and physiology of anxiety make it very unlikely that a medication will be developed in the near future that reduces anxiety without in the long term running the risk of dependency, and of seriously disabling symptoms on withdrawal. This is one of the areas in which the prescriber runs great risk of doing more harm than good: it is not uncommon to find that the symptoms of an anxious person who has become dependent on tranquillizers and then withdraws remain permanently worse than the original symptoms.

Practical Exercise

Think of the patients you saw in your last session. Could their symptoms arise from an emotion that you detected that went unnoticed?

Symptom peaks

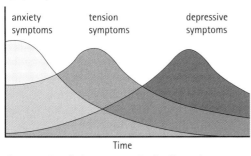

Figure 8.1 A typical symptom series for distress in primary care.

Dependency is the link between the relief obtained by socially accepted and available drugs, such as nicotine or alcohol, and medical or 'dangerous' street drugs, such as barbiturates, tranquillizers and heroin. Although each may have a particular pattern, the withdrawal syndrome is often much the worst feature for the patient, and (as with barbiturates, for which tolerance levels are all-important) is potentially lethal.

The message for those treating anxiety is not to be pressed into unwise prescribing, even in the short term, and to look wherever possible towards behavioural or lifestyle management methods which empower patients to deal with their own anxiety. Examples include relaxation tapes, yoga classes, behavioural treatment of phobias, exercise regimes, etc.

Practical Exercise

Discover what treatment methods are available in your current clinical attachments, how they are administered and by whom. What can you learn from the patients you meet?

Depression

Depression is more difficult to detect than anxiety but has more clear-cut treatment schedules, even if the best methods are disputed and outcomes still open to question. Like anxiety, headache and appetite loss may be pointers, but sleeplessness is classically described as waking early (whereas people who are anxious often have difficulty getting to sleep). Overwhelmingly the best way of making the diagnosis initially is simply to think of it. Doctors differ in their abilities to detect it, but this can be changed, at least in the short term, by training (Tylee *et al.*, 1995). It seems that a lot of patients meet doctors who prefer to turn a blind eye, or are too busy, or who in some way cannot cope with what they see as being a painful or difficult assessment. This is perhaps excusable if the doctor is overworked, or even depressed: it is difficult to deal with a problem in someone else that one cannot cope with oneself. But much of this points to the failures in detection being due to failures in the detection instrument – the clinician.

Once the diagnosis has been made and accepted, the attitudes and aims of patient and clinician may determine how the illness is seen and treated: as a disease to be eradicated, at one extreme, or as an opportunity for reflection and change, at the other. Perhaps best results combine different approaches.

Case Study 8.15

A young music publisher presented to a doctor about heavy drinking, but in assessment revealed that the drinking was happening to cover increasingly bleak moods and feelings of disappointment and disgust. After a programme of abstinence, he began on high levels of antidepressant treatment with weekly counselling, and was able to confront the experiences of a bleak and intellectual childhood, and the way in which he 'set up relationships to fail'.

A different model for the causes and management of depression derives from the work of Professor George Brown and colleagues (Brown and Harris, 1978), examining the social origins of depression in women. A pattern emerges of a model in which a potentially vulnerable person, faced with a current crisis and losing or failing to gain a proper support system, may be unable to cope. The characteristics of the urban women in Brown's original studies that seemed associated with depression were:

- poverty,
- no job or outside interest,
- low self-esteem,
- no extended family,
- no close confidante,
- poor communication with spouse,
- more than three young children at home,
- death of mother in childhood,
- death of a close relative or friend in the previous few months.

The interplay of personality, experience and relationships with lack of support or recent crisis has not been explored in every context but rings true with clinical experience in primary care. Many patients describe a 'last straw' that makes life apparently intolerable or distress overwhelming, and such experiences, although important, often seem too minor to create the disturbance that has resulted unless attention is paid to the other issues that affect the patient. The aspect of current support at home or being in control of one's work in the working environment is insufficiently emphasized in some approaches. What the social model does is to reveal the interplay of factors, and this may be helpful to the observer in general practice when the patient appears more disturbed by a physical symptom than is appropriate or understandable. Figure 8.2 illustrates typical components that lead to major symptoms.

Who can help provide help and how?

These different models suggest ways in which psychological disturbance can be managed in primary

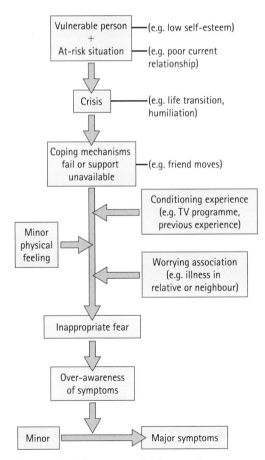

Figure 8.2 Typical components leading to major symptoms.

care. Prescribing issues are dealt with in detail elsewhere, but, particularly in depression, there is now agreement as to what constitutes good and safe prescribing, and this does not mean the use of medication without other approaches to reinforce positive and neutralize negative aspects of the situation. It also opens up the area for the work of those members of the team who have little or no ability to prescribe, but who nevertheless can be vital in management. A health visitor with a young family, a district nurse with an elderly couple, counsellors, groups and even reception staff all have a part to play, whether formal or informal.

The activities which may help the patient within the frameworks set out above include being able to explain and talk about the problem (ventilation), being given time to identify and clarify the main issues, being given 'permission' to express the distress (by crying, being angry, etc.), and then being provided with a frame of reference, in terms of support or interpretation, to show the patient a new way of coping with apparently insurmountable problems or distress. There is dispute about the best forms of intervention here, and their effectiveness; but what can never be in dispute is that a human response as well as a pharmacological one is a moral and therapeutic necessity.

Transitions have been noted as points of particular vulnerability, and this seems easiest to understand because such change involves a life event or loss. The loss may be obvious, such as when a bereavement has occurred, or when a person becomes redundant, retires or gets divorced. However, even apparently happy events, such as the birth of the first baby or moving to a new home, may contain loss of freedom or intimacy between a couple in the first situation, and of familiar patterns, environment and friendships in the second. In addition, humiliation or a feeling of defeat or being trapped adds strongly to the experience of loss if the event or loss is severe.

Fears (anticipation of loss) may underlie and underline such losses. Everyone at some time has to confront fears of isolation or annihilation, but illness or depression can swiftly strip away the barriers people put up against such thoughts, even if the condition itself may be apparently minor. The simple question 'What are you most afraid of now?' may be what is needed to allow people the chance to express (and so confront and gain support in facing) a fear that is causing symptoms.

Stepped care model

A stepped care model for treating patients with mild to moderate levels of psychological distress or such conditions as adjustment reactions, anxiety and depression has the following steps (NICE, 2010):

- Step 1: Recognition and diagnosis
- Step 2: Treatment in primary care
- Step 3: Review and consideration of alternative treatments
- Step 4: Review and referral to specialist mental health services
- Step 5: Care in specialist mental health services.

With mild mood symptoms, watchful waiting with follow-up within two weeks is sensible. A focus on lifestyle factors such as drugs and alcohol intake, social interventions and exercise and sleep hygiene are helpful. If the symptoms persist, brief psychological interventions may be provided by the GP, practice counsellor, primary care mental health worker or through workplaces and colleges. Guided self-help and computerized cognitive behavioral therapy (cCBT) are other options available in primary care. If the symptoms require more intervention, CBT or medication such as selective serotonin reuptake inhibitors (SSRIs) may be prescribed by a GP. Where symptoms are worsening, a discussion with and referral to specialist services is in order, and where there is a risk to self or others a crisis team referral may be made.

Systems and frameworks

A way of thinking about personal development and its pitfalls that takes account of the way in which people interact with each other and their environment as part of normal human life may seem a long way from the idea of depression as a disease. But in this model apparent breakdown, or intense distress, may be a breakthrough to a new understanding. Certain patterns of thought or behaviour may be signposts within a family group or a culture. Systemic thinking sees the way in which individuals are part of a structured group with particular ways of doing things or thinking,

and suggests that these ways, usually supportive, can on occasions be unhelpful, or may help the doctor and patient to see why something is so much of a problem to an individual. Questions such as 'What would your mother have made of this?', 'What would your father have wanted you to do?', 'How would your relationship with X change if you got better?' may help someone to see the framework of their emotional life and begin to help them to challenge the destructive parts and be supported by the aspects which will enable them to make progress.

The narrative approach

All doctors in training are taught how to take a history from patients (see Chapter 3 on the consultation and Chapter 5 on diagnosis and management), but this may differ from the story a patient may want to tell. What has happened to patients, what they have done, thought about, wanted or planned, and how they react to the crises, excitements or disappointments in their lives so far may all be crucially important to their own mental or emotional state. It may be difficult for the doctor to make sense of the patient's presentation (and so even harder to provide an adequate response) without an understanding of some of these parts of a patient's story. Yet in all healthcare encounters time is short, so with the best will in the world doctors often find themselves firing questions at a patient when it is not clear what is going on. This may be because the doctor is afraid of losing control of the consultation if the patient heads off on a personal track, but in reality what the resort to closed questions often loses is just these details and insights that will help that doctor make sense of the presentation, and so help the patient to make sense of the problems in the context of his or her individual life. If the patient is frightened, confused or chaotic, a measure of control of the discussion may be vital, if offered in a sensitive and kind way, but getting the balance right is a key skill for professional practice. In most situations outside medicine when we are not sure what is going on, we keep quiet until we are, and that may be a more helpful way forward in primary care too. We have two obvious choices if we wish to do that: to give the patient the time he or she needs right now and accept the problems of running late, or to arrange a suitable time (and possibly longer) in the near future. There are advantages and disadvantages of each, but either way this work must to be done properly. Access and continuity in primary care are key issues. As stories unfold, it may become clear that others (such as partners or family members) may have another side to tell. The assessment and management of mental healthcare in general practice are often provisional, iterative and on the move – more like driving a car through a big city than painting a picture. Also, we may not be the only drivers available. If it is clear that there is a long, deep and significant story that has to be told, it may be appropriate to refer to someone else in the primary care team – a counsellor, psychiatric nurse or other mental health specialist – or to the relevant agency in secondary care.

Learning about possible narratives will require us to think more broadly than just about medicine. In training, it will usually be very helpful to give yourself time to make a full assessment of some people. In our own lives, it will mean, too, that the things we enjoy in our spare time – soap operas, novels, plays, films or reading newspapers – will not only be a source of pleasure (although that's important enough) but also of insight into how people 'tick', and what sorts of things can cause distress or can help people to move on. In the process, it is crucial we understand our own selves better.

Effects on the professions: the way forward

So, in sum, several things can undeniably be said about clinical practice in primary care. One is that it is hard to limit demand, and to work to time, so that there may be few opportunities for a doctor to work as much at length or at depth with a patient as either would wish. The clinician has to develop ways of working at speed, of making assessments rapidly and taking imaginative shortcuts. The available resources to be expanded are the patient's own enthusiasm, skill and time (so that helping people to help themselves is a key aim of this type of medical practice), and the clinician's own intuitive understanding.

Most medical work turns a blind eye to the emotional aspects of the condition or its treatment. Primary care is largely where such feelings demand to be expressed, and where people will often bring distress or dread. A practitioner can either try to avoid recognizing the feeling that is being brought, or can help to give it expression and shape. Either way, the emotion is there, and will affect the doctor as well. Every practitioner working in this field must develop ways of being able to deal with the effect of distressing emotions on himself or herself, within the doctor–patient relationship immediately, with colleagues, or outside the surgery (Higgs, 1994).

Finally, few things point as clearly to the moral position we take, or values we hold, as our own and our profession's approach to psychological issues. We can reduce the people we meet to biomechanics, or defend ourselves from involvement with real life by prescribing medicines at every turn. But if we sincerely intend to do the best for our patients, to minimize harm to them, to increase their autonomy and their own control over their minds, bodies and lives, to help them become whole again, then we need to become skilled in detecting and managing distress in a way that expresses human values and recognizes potential as well as pathology in the people we meet.

SUMMARY POINTS

To conclude, the most important messages of this chapter are as follows:

- In sorting and responding to psychological distress in primary care, account must be taken of all the issues that may influence the situation, relating to physical conditions, social circumstances, relationships, goals and values of both the patient and the system in which he or she lives and works.
- Appropriate management of patients and of their presentation should include an understanding of what the professional brings, as well as what the patient brings.
- Medication is only one aspect of management, and team care and self-care are vital to progress, recovery and prevention of future distress.
- Listen to the story the patient may be trying to tell.

References

Brown, G. and Harris, T. 1978: *Social origins of depression*. London: Tavistock.

Higgs, R. 1994: Doctors in crisis: creating a strategy for mental health in health care work. *Journal of the Royal College of Physicians* 28(6), 538–40.

Matthews, K., Milne, S. and Ashcroft, G.W. 1994: Role of doctors in the prevention of suicide: the final consultation. *British Journal of General Practice* 44(385), 345–8.

NICE (National Institute for Health and Clinical Excellence) 2010: *NICE guidelines*. www.nice.org.uk/usingguidance/commissioningguides/cognitivebehaviouraltherapyservice/steppedcaremodels.jsp (accessed 3 October 2010).

Tylee, A., Freeling, P., Kerry, S. and Burns, T. 1995: How does the content of consultations affect recognition by general practitioners of major depression in women? *British Journal of General Practice* 45(400), 575–8.

World Health Organization 2010: *International Classification of Diseases (ICD), 10th revision*, version 2007. http://apps.who.int/classifications/apps/icd/icd10online/ (accessed 17 October 2010).

Further reading

Primary care

Dowrick C. 2009: *Beyond depression*. Oxford: Oxford University Press.

Elder, A. and Holmes, J. 2002: *Mental health in primary care – a new approach*. Oxford: Oxford University Press.

Kendrick, T., Tylee, A. and Freeling, P. 1996: *The prevention of mental illness in primary care*. Cambridge: Cambridge University Press.

What it's like to be mentally ill

Barker, P., Campbell, P. and Davidson, B. (eds) 1999: *From the ashes of experience: reflections on madness, survival and growth*. London: Whurr Publishers.

Dunn, S., Morrison, B. and Roberts, M. 1996: *Mind reading: writer's journey through mental states*. London: Minerva.

Read, J. and Reynolds, J. (eds) 1996: *Speaking our minds: an anthology of personal experiences of mental distress and its consequences*. London: Open University/Macmillan.

Rogers, A., Pilgrim, D. and Lacey, R. 1993: *Experiencing psychiatry*. Basingstoke: Macmillan/MIND.

Different ways of looking at mental health

The Open University has produced books under the heading 'Mental health and distress: perspectives and practice'.

Psychiatry

American Psychiatric Association 1994: *Diagnostic and statistical manual of mental disorders*, 4th edn (DSM-IV). Washington DC: American Psychiatric Association.

Gelder, M., Harrison, P. and Cowen, P. 2006: *Shorter Oxford textbook of psychiatry*. Oxford: Oxford University Press.

Gelder, M., Andreasen, N., Lopez-Ibor, J. and Geddes, J. (eds) 2011: *New Oxford textbook of psychiatry*. Oxford: Oxford University Press.

Oxford University Press publish both a shorter textbook and the longer New Oxford textbook.

Goldberg, D., Benjamin, S. and Creed, F. 1997: *Psychiatry in medical practice*. London: Routledge.

Communicating

Corney, R. 1991: *Developing communication and counselling skills in medicine*. London: Routledge.

Narrative medicine

Brody, H. 2002: *Stories of sickness*. New Haven: Yale University Press.

Greenberg, M., Shergill, S.S., Szmukler, G. and Tantam, D. 2003: *Narratives in psychiatry*. London: Jessica Kingsley Publishers.

Narrative in a secondary care case format

Greenhalgh, T. and Hurwitz, B. (eds) 1998: *Narrative-based medicine: dialogue and discourse in clinical practice*. London: BMJ Books.

An interesting series of essays, but see particularly the contributions of Launer, Elwyn and Gwyn, and Holmes.

Launer, J. 2002: *Narrative-based primary care*. Abingdon: Radcliffe Medical Press.

SINGLE BEST ANSWER QUESTIONS

8.1 James had a high pressure job in finance, so important that, as he told himself and anyone else who enquired, he was too busy to bother with friends of either sex. He lived alone. In fact he was desperately lonely and hardly spoke to anyone outside work. To cope with the pressures, he began to drink heavily and was finally sacked. He came to see his doctor with headaches and sleeplessness and it was not long into the interview before his depression and overuse of alcohol was clear to the GP, though James did not appear to want to accept these diagnoses.

a) The doctor should admit him to hospital at once under section if necessary, as his depression is serious

b) It's no business of the doctor what James does in his private life and the GP should concentrate on the headaches

c) The doctor is his only lifeline to help him out of this mess

d) He is very much more at risk of suicide as a drinker than a non-drinker in this situation

e) Seeing him every day is the best way to help him.

8.2 Joanne has just gone to senior school, but not the one of her choice. She is a shy child, all her friends are now at another school nearer her home but this new school is a long and complicated journey from home and in what her very dominating father, who has brought her in,

SINGLE BEST ANSWER QUESTIONS CONTINUED

describes as 'a rough area'. Shortly after starting term Joanne, who was enuretic as a 5 year old, begins to wet the bed again. Which of the following is *not* a diagnostic possibility requiring investigation?

a) Diabetes mellitus
b) Anxiety from being bullied at school
c) Early sexual experience, including rape
d) Urinary infection
e) Developmental delay.

8.3 A practice counsellor:

a) Can only see a patient six times
b) Is now usually employed by the local council
c) Would be the first point of referral for someone who is drinking heavily
d) Usually works with the patient's goals in mind
e) Will keep the doctor informed about what the patient talks about.

8.4 A teacher is depressed following a crisis at the school. Her GP should:

a) Encourage her to think positively and pull herself together as teaching is such a rewarding and important profession

b) Put her on antidepressant therapy immediately
c) Refer her to a counsellor even though she doesn't want to go
d) Telephone her head teacher to warn the head of the vulnerability of his member of staff and possible danger to children
e) Give her some time off work and see her again near the end of the week.

8.5 We are all alarmed when someone appears to be talking to themselves (in the absence of a mobile phone). Schizophrenic 'front rank' symptoms (Schneider) include:

a) Talking to himself about how no one cares for him
b) Hearing two people talking to each other about him in his head falsely accusing him of being a homosexual
c) Hearing his mother's voice calling to him, though she has been dead for several years
d) Hearing a hated tune going round and round in his head repeatedly
e) Hearing a voice in his head warning him about unpaid bills.

CHAPTER

CHRONIC ILLNESS AND ITS MANAGEMENT IN GENERAL PRACTICE

- Tripartite approach to chronic illness care
- The patient
- The population
- The disease

- Summary points
- References
- Further reading
- Single best answer questions

Most chronic illnesses present the patient with a tough challenge. Usually the challenge can be lived with; less often can it be overcome. The task that faces the doctor is also challenging. It requires technical expertise, a personal partnership with the patient, and more recently acknowledgement of the need to deliver a service to the whole population. For the modern general practitioner this implies a responsibility to all registered patients. The treatment of chronic illness is helped by a keen grasp of the complex effects the illness has on the individual. It also requires a clear structure within which effective and predictable long-term care can be provided.

LEARNING OBJECTIVES

By the end of this chapter you will be able to:

- understand different chronic illnesses by type;
- understand the impact of chronic illness;
- describe five different illness models;
- know the prevalence and workload associated with the common chronic illnesses in primary care;
- understand the role of screening for chronic illness;
- construct a programme for the long-term management of common chronic illnesses.

Tripartite approach to chronic illness care

The commonest cause of the deaths of most people alive today will be a chronic illness. In most cases this illness could have been postponed, at least, if not prevented. Most chronic illnesses should be better managed. The key to improving chronic illness management lies in systematic structured care or what has been proposed as the Chronic Care Model (Wagner *et al.*, 2001). The risk of ill-health or death from chronic illness varies amongst different groups in a population. The risk is often greater amongst those who are more socio-economically deprived. It makes sense, therefore, to target efforts to improve the care of diseases such as ischaemic heart disease, diabetes mellitus and chronic obstructive pulmonary disease as closely as possible to those at greatest risk.

Chronic illness care presents a dilemma for general practitioners (GPs) and primary care teams. Can the ethos of personal care, which has been at the core of general practice throughout the twentieth century, be maintained in an environment that also demands precise disease management skills and the delivery of national strategies to local populations (van Lieshout *et al.*, 2011)? A tripartite approach to the care of chronic illness

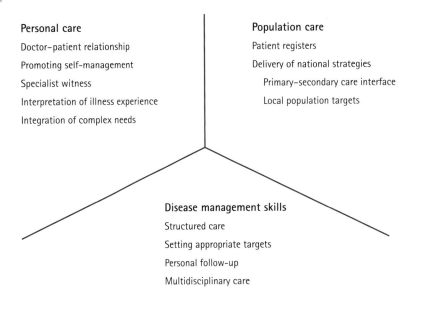

Personal care

Doctor–patient relationship

Promoting self-management

Specialist witness

Interpretation of illness experience

Integration of complex needs

Population care

Patient registers

Delivery of national strategies

Primary–secondary care interface

Local population targets

Disease management skills

Structured care

Setting appropriate targets

Personal follow-up

Multidisciplinary care

Figure 9.1 A tripartite model of chronic illness management in primary care.

is now essential in primary care (Figure 9.1). Personal care must be integrated with a population strategy. In both of these the achievement of high-quality chronic illness management depends on excellent disease management skills.

In this chapter, the management of chronic illness is considered first from the point of view of the person with the disease. The population statistics of the major chronic illnesses and their impact are then examined. The chapter ends with a detailed presentation of structured care and the strategies available to GPs in delivering high-quality chronic illness care to all the patients registered with them.

The patient

When chronic illness presents

When a chronic illness is diagnosed, the possible consequences of the illness and of its treatment will be apparent to the doctor. The patient may have little sense of what lies ahead. Although chronic illnesses become chronic with time, they often start out as 'chronic' to the doctor. Asthma, diabetes and hypertension are good examples. For patients, on the other hand, most illnesses generally start as acute illnesses, and are expected to be limited in time. So the realization that the illness might be here to stay or might come and go is one of the first hurdles to address in coming to terms with chronic illness. 'Surely, with the right treatment this illness can be cured?' the rheumatoid arthritis patient might reasonably ask. Such reasoning might continue: 'After all, if you doctors can transplant hearts, and diagnose disease in babies in the womb, you must be able to treat my arthritis.'

The advances of modern medicine have done more to help us understand chronic illnesses than to relieve or cure them. This may be bewildering to patients who develop a chronic illness. They may have to compare the relative impotence of modern medicine in the face of their illness with the dramatic improvements achieved in such fields as microsurgery or the relative control of the great killers of the past such as tuberculosis and other major infections. They have to face the fact that chronic illnesses remain a common burden in our society. Doctors can help them to understand chronic illness, and can help to limit its intrusion into their lives, but for the most part chronic illnesses cannot be cured, and it is one of the duties of doctors to help patients to come to terms with their illnesses, rather than to reject or deny them.

Chronic illness by type

One of the defining features of many common chronic illnesses is that they are diseases of process or processes rather than disorders of structure. Typical examples of this type of chronic illness include asthma, hypertension, rheumatoid arthritis, inflammatory bowel disease and schizophrenia. A shared aspect of these diseases is the diffuseness of the disordered process in the tissue or system. In asthma there is a complex inflammatory response in the airways that may continue long after symptoms appear to have resolved. In hypertension there is a generalized over-pressurizing of the arterial system that may be chemically or humorally mediated through the central barometer of arterial pressure or through the peripheral baroreceptors. In rheumatoid arthritis there is an over-reaction of the immune system in which the synovium of the joint is confused with foreign matter and is attacked. In inflammatory bowel disease the immune system again reacts inappropriately and attacks the bowel endothelium in similar fashion. In schizophrenia there appears to be a diffuse deficiency or imbalance in one or more neurotransmitters in the brain, with resulting disorganization of intellect and emotion.

In each of these diseases, the process whose failure is causing the signs and symptoms of the disease is spread throughout the tissue or system. It cannot be removed surgically, and cannot easily be overridden through a chemical or humoral switch. In all of them the underlying disorder is complex and usually beyond the reach of the drugs at our disposal. But in all of them we can exert some influence on how the disease is expressed in most patients.

These illnesses contrast with another group of illnesses which are also chronic either in their development or in their impact but which are more amenable to one-off treatments offering long-term relief. These more 'amenable' diseases are distinguished by either the relative simplicity of the disease process or their limited extent within the body. Examples include atheroma of the coronary arteries, benign hypertrophy of the prostate, cataracts of the eyes, osteoarthritis of the hips and peptic ulceration. The approaches outlined in this chapter may be suitable for these diseases also. However, where there is a realistic and reasonable hope of cure or sustained remission following a course of treatment, the approach and attitude of the doctor and the patient are likely to be influenced by this expectation.

Between these two poles of chronic illness lie a number of illnesses for which there are effective treatments but whose treatments need to be taken continuously. Examples of these are Addison's disease, hypothyroidism, idiopathic atrial fibrillation, myasthenia gravis and pernicious anaemia. The treatment of these diseases is more predictably effective. The diseases mentioned in this group are specific deficiency or function disorders that can be treated either by replacing the deficiency or by correcting the disordered function. By comparison with the first group of diseases, they are simple diseases.

Three categories of chronic illness have been identified here, according to responsiveness to treatment. The three categories are used in Table 9.1 to classify some of the more common chronic illnesses seen in Western Europe.

The impact of chronic illness

The development of a chronic illness may have a profound effect on the patient's life through morbidity (symptoms and interference with the activities of daily living), disability, handicap, impairment, interference with personal relationships, loss of confidence, loss of earnings, loss of self-image, and stigma. In order to be able to respond appropriately to the needs of the patient, the doctor has to understand how the illness is affecting the particular patient and how the patient sees the problem. Mrs B's situation is a good example.

Case Study 9.1

Mrs B is the head teacher of a primary school in Central London. She is 52 years old and has smoked all her adult life. Last year she came to see her GP, Dr A, with a bad attack of bronchitis. She was told by her doctor that it was likely she had asthma in addition to her bronchitis. Dr A prescribed an antibiotic for the bronchitis and an inhaler for the asthma. Mrs B disagreed with the diagnosis of asthma and took the antibiotics only. Within about two weeks, she was much bet-

Table 9.1 Common chronic illnesses categorized by responsiveness to treatment

Difficult to treat	Treatable – one stop	Treatable – continuous
Asthma	Coronary atheroma	Addison's disease
Chronic obstructive pulmonary disease	Hypothyroidism	Cataract of eye
Diabetes mellitus	Osteoarthritis of hips/knees	Depression
Hypertension	Peptic ulceration	Epilepsy
Inflammatory bowel disease		Prostate hypertrophy (benign)
Multiple sclerosis		Idiopathic atrial fibrillation
Osteoarthritis		Manic–depressive psychosis
Parkinson's disease		Myasthenia gravis
Rheumatoid arthritis		Pernicious anaemia
Schizophrenia		

ter and felt vindicated in her opinion about the asthma. She continued to have difficulty climbing the stairs to the third floor at the top of the school but put it down to the ravages of age and cigarettes. Her peak flow when Dr A measured it in her surgery was 240 L/min. It should have been 480 L/min.

When Dr A saw Mrs B six months later with osteoarthritis in her knee, Dr A took the opportunity to repeat her peak flow test. This time it was 375 L/min. With a 56 per cent improvement, reversibility was demonstrated and Dr A knew that the diagnosis of asthma was correct.

Thinking and Discussion Point

What do you think Dr A should do now? Should she tell Mrs B that she has asthma? How would Mrs B best be helped in her current situation?

If we are ever in doubt as to how we should approach a tricky situation with a patient, it is useful to ask ourselves what we would want if we were in the patient's shoes. Sometimes the answer to that question is that the doctor should take over and simply tell the patient what to do. In acute appendicitis, for example, the patient does not usually want to get into much discussion about what should be done. More often than not, however, patients would like to have the opportunity to express their own views and to have those views

taken into account in the doctor's decision making. This is especially true in chronic illness.

Case Study 9.1 (continued)

Dr A told Mrs B that she was very pleased that the peak flow test was now much better and asked Mrs B how the inhaler had worked. Mrs B blushed and said that she had not used the inhaler but that the antibiotics had made her chest much better in a matter of 10 days. Dr A then asked Mrs B if her chest caused her any difficulty now. Mrs B said, 'None at all except that I get short of breath climbing the stairs at school.' Dr A said she thought that might be due to her asthma. Mrs B frowned and said that she didn't have asthma. She said she knew what asthma was from her own daughter's experience of asthma and she certainly did not have that.

Thinking and Discussion Point

Dr A has a dilemma. Should she pursue the issue of the asthma now or wait until the problem recurs and deal with it then? Dr A decided to leave the asthma for now and get on with the management of the arthritis in Mrs B's knee.

When there appears to be a conflict between the view of the patient and the view of the doctor, it is sometimes because each is approaching the problem from a different perspective. Patients' priorities are often different from those of doctors. The patient may accept different degrees of illness or disability depending on what has to be gained or sacrificed in undertaking a particular treatment. For example, a doctor's desire to control hypertension by prescribing drugs to be taken every day may be unacceptable to a man for whom illness represents moral frailty and for whom medication represents capitulation to that frailty.

Patients sometimes feel isolated by their illnesses. They may feel isolated because family and friends do not or cannot understand what it is like to have the illness, or they may feel stigmatized by their disability or appearance. The doctor may be in a special position with the patient with a chronic illness, acting as what Heath (1996) has called a 'specialist witness' and also as a specialist 'interpreter' of the illness experience. The experience of chronic illness provokes complex reactions. The feelings and ideas generated sometimes have to be worked through carefully in order that emotional blocks to effective treatment can be overcome and that action to avoid secondary complications can be taken.

The population

The sensitivity that Dr A showed in her management of her patient should be matched in modern practice by a strategy that addresses the needs of the population as a whole. With the electronic patient record it is relatively easy to list all the asthmatics on Dr A's register and to identify those whose treatment needs to be reviewed. A review may be needed because asthma control is inadequate, seen for example from evidence of admissions to hospital. Or a review may be

needed because a patient is requesting frequent repeat prescriptions of short-acting beta-agonist inhalers without using any 'preventer' inhaled steroid inhalers.

In considering the approach that a medical practice might take to serving its registered population, it is useful to think of the models of illness that might underpin the thinking behind such a strategy. This is in turn could help a practice to design the approach it wanted to use and the structure of the service it developed.

Models of illness

Five different illness models have been proposed by Memel (1996) to explore the experience of chronic illness and the role and function of doctors who work with people who have chronic diseases. These models demonstrate how the perception of chronic illness can vary, and how the patient and the doctor may often approach the problem of chronic illness very differently (Table 9.2).

Thinking and Discussion Point

As you read the short summaries of each model, reflect on your own viewpoint. Is there anything new here? Are you thinking on more than one level at any time? What is the patient's angle, and is it reflected in the model?

The *medical model* is the traditional starting point of doctors. This model assumes that the main variable in a chronic illness is the disease itself and that all patients are much the same when it comes to considering the disease. The medical

Table 9.2 Attributes of the five illness models

	Models of illness				
	Medical	Functional	Social	Sociological	Biopsychosocial
Doctor-centred					
Patient-centred					
Multi-dimensional					
Technical					
Professional					

model has been essential to the development of medical science. It encourages the recognition of patterns of disease and patterns of response to treatment. If there are differences between patients, then, according to the medical model, the differences that count are more likely to be aspects of the disease than aspects of the patient or his or her environment. The chief concerns within this model of seeing illness are medical and technical. The patient's presentation and experience are interpreted in terms of disease patterns. In medical practice, the effect of this model can make patients feel like outsiders to the management of their own illnesses.

The *functional model* of illness is concerned with how the patient copes with his or her everyday life. This model contrasts with the medical model in being person-orientated rather than disease-orientated. Its aim is to look at functional ability such as mobility, self-care, social integration and independence, and to consider the impact of symptoms. However, it is similar to the medical model in being centred on the concerns of the professionals, because the assumption inherent in this model is that the definition of functional ability is a technical one. Nonetheless, functional scales provide an assessment of the illness that is patient-centred in its orientation, and that assessment may be more accessible to the patient than one based purely on the medical model.

The *social model* considers the disease from the viewpoint of social organization and the society in which the individual resides. It is concerned with the influences of society on the individual. It interprets the illness and its consequences in terms of the limitations which society imposes on the individual. Thus the social model addresses the effects of chronic illness in terms of social disadvantage. The dimensions of the social impact of chronic illness are broad and include financial penalties for individuals and their families, access to employment, access to education and training, and access to recreation and the arts. A particular advantage of this model is the emphasis it places on the patient's viewpoint. In most areas of public and social service, and increasingly in the commercial world as well, there is an awareness of the needs of people with disabilities. Customers and clients with disabilities are not only catered

for, but their needs and opinions are sought out. One problem associated with the social model of chronic illness is the tendency to adopt a global view of disability and impairment and handicap. The effect of such simplification is to emphasize the visible elements of disability such as paralysis, blindness or deafness, and to underestimate the less visible aspects of chronic diseases such as chronic schizophrenia and learning disorders.

The *sociological model* of chronic illness contrasts with the first three models described here in being concerned with observing and describing the experience of people with chronic illness rather than defining a specialized framework within which to categorize chronic illness. Medical sociologists have explored both the meaning and themes evident in the life experience of people with chronic illness and the perspectives of the professionals who work with sufferers. Bury (1982) has proposed the idea of 'biographical disruption', which follows the onset of chronic illness. The patient has to review his or her identity that has been so altered by becoming someone with a disease or disability. The concept of biographical disruption is a powerful aid to doctors, who are usually the ones who have to label the onset of the chronic illness. By being sensitive to the potential disturbance and disorientation that can follow the diagnosis of a chronic illness, the doctor can promote the acknowledgement and resolution of some of the conflicts that the onset of the illness will inevitably provoke. It was the sociological model that encouraged the exploration of the ways in which the doctor–patient relationship can promote or hinder effective diagnosis and treatment. The sociological model is a model for understanding chronic illness, not for managing or controlling it.

The *biopsychosocial model* was developed to explain how the impact of chronic illness can operate at several levels at once. It embodies an holistic approach that encourages the doctor and the patient to look at the process of the disease and its physical, psychological and social effects simultaneously. In the General Medical Council's document *Tomorrow's doctors*, published first in 1993 and most recently updated in 2009, every medical school in the UK has been charged with ensuring that the holism of the biopsychosocial model is demonstrable throughout undergraduate medical training. As this is achieved, the medical, functional and social models of illness will become less conspicuous in the teaching and practice of medicine.

These models of illness provide a key to analysing how patients, doctors and society might respond to chronic illness. In Mrs B's case, there was a clear difference between the patient's and the doctor's views.

Case Study 9.1 (continued)

Six months later, Mrs B developed another attack of bronchitis and came to see Dr A again. This time her peak flow was 200 L/min and she was having considerable difficulty climbing the stairs at school. Even before the infection, she had been scheduling her visits to the classrooms on the top floor so that she could get up there in stages. Dr A prescribed the antibiotics again and once more raised the question of asthma. Mrs B was adamant that it was not asthma. She did agree to try to stop smoking. Dr A persuaded her to use a steroid inhaler for her chest. 'I don't mind what I take so long as you don't call it asthma,' Mrs B declared. Dr A never found out why Mrs B was so adamant to avoid the diagnosis of asthma. She was prepared to work on Mrs B's terms so long as she could get Mrs B to try the asthma treatment. Mrs B found the inhaler a great help.

There are several advantages to the position adopted by Dr A. She has made it clear to Mrs B that she was on her side and prepared to compromise in tackling the illness. It may be that the prospect of the diagnosis of asthma was unacceptable to Mrs B for what it meant to her self-image as a headmistress or for its implications about her future health. Whatever the reason, Dr A succeeded in prescribing the treatment and engaging Mrs B in a dialogue about her breathlessness. In the longer term, this approach will have given Mrs B confidence in raising other difficult health issues. The disadvantage of not naming asthma is that it may lead to delay in obtaining the right treatment if attacks of asthma were to occur in the future. Failure to agree the diagnosis of asthma may make subsequent discussion of Mrs B's breathlessness unduly complex. It is sometimes difficult to be sure about the diagnosis of asthma in older people and in children. Having the label of asthma can get patients onto the fast track to treatment. Achieving a compromise with the patient may ultimately ensure that the relationship between the doctor and the patient is one that promotes the best disease management.

Chronic illness facts and figures

Chronic illnesses are relatively common and comprise a substantial part of the work of GPs (see Chapter 7 on common illnesses). They are also major components of the work of specialists in internal medicine. In some areas, such as rheumatology, they are the backbone of the discipline.

There are three main sources of our knowledge of the prevalence and impact of chronic illnesses in the UK. The first is the *General Lifestyle Survey* (GLS, formerly known as the General Household Survey), which is conducted by the Office for National Statistics (formerly the Office of Population Censuses and Surveys) and is reported annually (Office for National Statistics, 2010). The second source is the *NHS Information Centre* which presents annually the results of the Quality and Outcomes Framework element of the General Practitioners' Contract (www.ic.nhs. uk/). This latter instrument reports on the prevalence and process of care of a limited number of chronic illnesses, including coronary heart disease, hypertension, diabetes mellitus, asthma, chronic obstructive pulmonary disease and epilepsy. A more detailed analysis of morbidity statistics used to be carried out jointly at the time of the national census by the Office for National Statistics and the Royal College of General Practitioners. The last time this was produced was in 1995 (McCormick et al., 1995) and the figures are now out of date. They do provide the most detailed analysis of morbidity data in general practice ever collected, and remain an important reference point.

The final and most accurate source of epidemiological data on chronic illness comes from *specific epidemiological studies*. These are carried out in distinct populations among people whose names are drawn from the electoral register or from complete population lists such as GPs' patient lists. In the UK more than 99 per cent of the population is registered with a GP so GPs' registers are likely to be good sources of epidemiological statistics. In epidemiological studies specific diagnostic definitions and tests are used to identify 'cases' and to determine prevalence and severity. There are likely to be significant differences between prevalences on GPs' lists and prevalences in epidemiological studies, not only because definitions used in practice are likely to differ from epidemiological studies but also because patients may only present to their GP when a disease becomes symptomatic even when they have had the disease for some time according to agreed definitions (Nacul *et al.*, 2011).

The answers obtained in the General Lifestyle Survey help to paint the picture of chronic illness as a common significant problem experienced throughout the population in all ages and social groups.

The following questions were asked in the General Lifestyle Survey in 2009 (Office for National Statistics, 2010). About 15000 people aged 16 years and over in 8206 households took part (response rate 73 per cent).

- 'Do you have any longstanding illness or disability or infirmity? (By longstanding I mean anything that has troubled you over a period of time or that is likely to affect you over a period of time.)' Yes: 31 per cent.
- 'Does this illness or disability (these illnesses or disabilities) limit your activities in any way?' Yes: 19 per cent.

In Table 9.3 we have compared the 'prevalence' figures derived from the Quality and Outcomes Framework of the contract for General Practitioners in England in 2009–2010 with prevalence figures derived from a variety of recent epidemiological studies (Ashworth and Krodowicz, 2010). These studies reported the prevalence of the diseases referred to in different areas of England and Wales and in different population groups.

Thinking and Discussion Point

- Do these figures contain any surprises? Did you think ischaemic heart disease was more common?
- Did you expect hypertension to be the commonest of the chronic diseases?

It is clear from the Table 9.3 that in the diseases for which there is a general practice diagnostic

Table 9.3 Chronic disease prevalences identified in epidemiological studies, current diagnostic prevalences (where available) from data collected for the Quality and Outcomes Framework (QOF) of the GP contract, and estimated number of cases in each category seen by a GP per year

Disease	Epidemiological prevalence (%)	Diagnostic or consultation prevalence QOF (%)	Cases/GP per year
Asthma	6.5	5.8	86
Hypertension	35	11.4	200
Backache	4.0	–	80
Osteoarthritis	3.0	–	60
Ischaemic heart disease	3	3.7	34
Chronic obstructive pulmonary disease	3.5	1.65	24
Diabetes mellitus	3.0	2.1	22
Cerebrovascular disease	1.0	1.5	20
Epilepsy	0.5	0.6	8
Alcohol-related disorders	0.2	–	4
Schizophrenia	0.150	–	5
Multiple sclerosis	0.09	–	2

Number of cases likely to be registered with a GP in one year have been computed from epidemiological studies where available or from the United Kingdom NHS Quality and Outcomes Framework (QOF).

prevalence the true prevalence is higher than the prevalence estimated from reported consultations. It appears that a number of patients in these categories of disease do not consult their GP at all, or do not have their disease recorded by their GP. What explanations could there be for this discrepancy?

Practical Exercise

If you are currently attached to a primary care team, you may wish to discuss with your tutor the following exercise. This exercise is best carried out within the practice. It requires you to investigate the practice disease register which is likely to be a computer list based on the electronic patient register. You should also investigate a prescription listing from the computer to identify patients whose names have been missed from the disease register.

Questions to consider:

❑ How many patients are listed in your practice with asthma?

❑ How many patients are listed in your practice with epilepsy?

If your practice is computerized, ask the practice manager or computer manager if lists can be generated based on these two diagnoses. Ask also for a list of all patients for whom an asthma drug has been prescribed and a list of all patients for whom an anticonvulsant has been prescribed. Use the two lists of drugs for asthma and epilepsy below. Your tutor will tell you which drugs are never prescribed for the practice's patients and which can be ignored. Don't forget to add to the list the brand names for these drugs if they are supported by your computer. Check in your local formulary (e.g. *British National Formulary* – BNF) and branded product list (e.g. *Monthly Index of Medical Specialties* – MIMS) for new medications not included in these lists.

❑ *Asthma*: aminophylline, bambuterol, beclomethasone, budesonide, cromoglycate, eformoterol, formoterol, fenoterol, fluticasone, ipratropium, ketotifen, montelukast, nedocromil, salbutamol, salmeterol, terbutaline, theophylline, tiotropium, zafirlukast.

Make sure you include combination inhalers such as salmeterol + fluticasone, formoterol + budesonide, formoterol + beclometasone.

❑ *Epilepsy*: carbamazepine, clobazam, clonazepam, eslicarbazepine, ethosuximide, gabapentin, kufinamide, lacosamide, lamotrigine, oxcarbazepine, phenobarbitone, phenytoin, pregabalin, primidone, tiagabine, topiramate, (sodium) valproate, vigabatrin, zonisamide.

When you have obtained the lists of patients with asthma and of patients on an asthma drug, and the lists of patients with epilepsy and patients on an anticonvulsant, compare the total numbers in each. Why are these numbers different? What percentages of the total practice patient list are patients with asthma and patients with epilepsy? How do they compare to the percentages in Table 9.3? What explanation can you offer for the differences?

Undetected and unseen chronic disease

A reasonable interpretation of the discrepancy between the diagnostic or consultation prevalence figures (i.e. based on the GP contract reporting) and the epidemiological prevalence figures in Table 9.3 is that some people with chronic illnesses either do not attend their GPs at all in the course of a year or have never had their disease detected. In the cases of diabetes and epilepsy, this discrepancy can be nearly 50 per cent (Jacoby *et al.*, 1996; Holman *et al.*, 2011). What does this mean? There are a number of possible explanations. Some patients attend hospital clinics, rarely if ever see their GP, and do not have their names entered in the GP's register. Some patients have diseases that are asymptomatic. Some patients would rather have symptoms than have any contact with doctors and their devices! And some patients think that nothing can be done about their symptoms so why attend the GP anyway?

A GP in the UK is likely to see more than 75 per cent of the patients registered on his or her list in one year, according to the General Lifestyle Survey. This means that about 25 per cent of patients will not attend in any one year. Because patients with diagnosed diseases are more likely to attend than those without, the proportion of people who do not attend is probably much less than 25 per cent in the case of most people with known chronic illness. However, some patients with chronic illness who do attend their GP may not attend to discuss the chronic disease in question, and therefore the disease may not appear in the consultation statistics.

There is a problem in addition with the detection of certain chronic illnesses. Some chronic diseases are symptomless throughout their course until complications occur. Two examples of this problem are hypertension and non-insulin-dependent diabetes mellitus. Almost all published studies of hypertension prevalence have shown that hypertension is detected in only 50 per cent of those people who actually have hypertension for which treatment is indicated. Recently, there has been a marked increase in the recording of blood pressure in primary care in the UK, due to the linking of GPs' incomes with specific chronic disease service targets. So the detection of raised blood pressure may have increased. In the meantime, the low detection rates up to now of diseases for which there are effective interventions serve to show that it cannot be left entirely to the individual to request screening tests for symptomless diseases if we want to reduce the morbidity which these diseases cause.

To complicate matters further, there is now concern that hypertension is over-diagnosed by physicians because of isolated elevations of blood pressure in their consulting rooms, called 'white coat hypertension'. It is not yet clear if white coat hypertension (where 24-hour ambulatory blood pressure is normal) carries added cardiovascular risk, but the diagnosis of hypertension does require surveillance of asymptomatic adults using explicit guidelines (see British Hypertension Society at www.hyp.ac.uk/bhs/). Diabetes is another disease that is asymptomatic in the early stages and in which early treatment can forestall the onset of complications. In both of these diseases, the rewards of effective detection are tangible. This is the argument for screening in chronic illness and it is why the UK National Health Service (NHS) has made part of the GPs' income dependent on them achieving certain minimum targets in the care of ischaemic heart disease, hypertension,

diabetes, asthma, epilepsy and chronic obstructive pulmonary disease.

Epilepsy is a little different. Epilepsy is not asymptomatic, yet it is easy to ignore for both patients and doctors. Take the case of Mr O, a fourth-year medical student.

Case Study 9.2

Mr O, a 24-year-old medical student, had had epilepsy since he was 18 years old. On the night he had his first fit he had just finished his 'A' level exams and had driven two of his friends to an end-of-year party. He had had his driving licence for four months. It was an all-night party, but because Mr O was driving, he didn't drink any alcohol. At about 5 in the morning, Mr O was dancing when he had a grand mal fit that lasted for about 2 minutes. Following assessment at an accident and emergency department that night, he attended the neurology outpatients. Six months later, he had two further fits and was started on phenytoin capsules. No cause was found for the fits and Mr O was in every other way in good health.

Mr O attended the neurology clinic regularly for the first 2 years, but he continued to have a fit once every six months or so and got fed up seeing the doctors. He simply obtained his prescription from his GP and kept taking the tablets regularly. At this stage he had finished his first 2 years in medical school. His GP assumed he was still attending the neurologists and he assumed the GP knew he was not.

There is good evidence that both patients and doctors have low expectations for epilepsy, even though research has shown that it can be completely controlled in more than 80 per cent of patients by taking only one drug (Shorvon *et al.*, 1978). It may be an aspect of the stigma associated with epilepsy that sufferers do not attend doctors, for they do not attend neurologists any more than they attend their GPs.

Case Study 9.2 (continued)

It came as something of a surprise to Mr O, when he was placed finally in the neurology department of his medical school, to learn that amongst people with epilepsy his epilepsy treatment was poor. To be taught by the consultant whose clinic he attended as a patient that the great majority of epileptics should be controlled free of fits was galling. On the one hand, he was his own worst enemy by not attending the clinic, but he could not recall hearing that his epilepsy should be completely controlled. Mr O was effectively treated eventually, his convulsions were completely controlled, and he regained his driving licence. Without a driving licence, he would have had difficulty practising as a GP, which is the career in medicine he had chosen.

Thinking and Discussion Point

As a GP, how could Mr O go about ensuring that other sufferers from epilepsy had a better deal than him?

Screening and surveillance of chronic disease

Screening

It is apparent from the unsatisfactory detection of hypertension and non-insulin-dependent diabetes mellitus that screening of these diseases is needed. But how should this be carried out? Two principles are paramount (Hart, 1975; Sackett and Holland, 1975):

- The screening test should be specific enough to ensure that the number of false positives (positive test but no disease) is manageable, and sensitive enough to give confidence that most actual cases are detected.
- The disease or risk factor detected should be amenable to prevention or treatment.

There are two approaches to screening in general practice: population screening and opportunistic screening.

- In *population screening*, the screening test is offered to the whole population being screened (e.g. letters of invitation for cervical smear to all women aged 25–64 years).
- In *opportunistic screening*, the test is offered to members of the group to be screened who happen to present at the surgery (e.g. cholesterol testing of all adults with a family history of

ischaemic heart disease who happen to attend for whatever reason).

In most chronic illnesses, population screening is not carried out because the resources to do it are simply not available. Furthermore, it is not clear that the rewards to patients and society would justify the inconvenience and costs. In a disease such as hypertension, in which up to 50 per cent of cases go undetected, a more acceptable approach is to screen once a year all adults over the age of 30 who attend the surgery. Since, in the UK, about 75 per cent of people attend their GP once a year and 97 per cent attend every 5 years, opportunistic screening seems to most GPs a more suitable way of screening for hypertension.

Most chronic illnesses cannot be detected by screening because there is not a screening test for the disease which is specific and sensitive enough. Chronic diseases or chronic disease risk factors for which effective screening can be carried out include diabetes mellitus, hypertension, hyperlipidaemia and chronic renal failure.

Thinking and Discussion Point

Asthma is a common disease, affecting more than 25 per cent of the population in the course of their lives and more than 6.5 per cent of the population at any point in time. Can you think of a screening test for asthma? This test, if it is to be used, has to be sensitive enough to detect most cases of asthma (e.g. at least 75 per cent) and specific enough not to have too many false positives (e.g. 25 per cent or more). (See the end of the chapter for a discussion of this question.)

Surveillance

Having detected hypertension, what should the GP or practice nurse do?

Practical Exercise

If you are currently attached to a primary care team, you might discuss the following exercise with your GP tutor. Compare your findings with the advice given by the British Hypertension

Practical Exercise continued

Society in their guidelines for the management of hypertension (www.hyp.ac.uk/bhs/).

Ask your tutor to identify for you five patients with established hypertension. Obtain the medical records for these patients and record for each of them the following information:

❏ date of detection of hypertension,
❏ reason for recording of blood pressure at time of detection,
❏ date of commencement of treatment,
❏ number of blood pressure recordings between first detection and start of treatment,
❏ number of changes of treatment since first detection,
❏ number of blood pressure recordings per year since detection,
❏ investigations carried out since first detection.

Discuss the findings with your tutor and ask his or her opinion on the representativeness of your findings of blood pressure management in the practice.

In addition to the 50 per cent of people with hypertension who are undetected, only about 50 per cent of those with detected hypertension for which treatment is indicated are actually on treatment. Furthermore, only 50 per cent of those on treatment are on adequate treatment. These three observations make up what has become known as the rule of halves in hypertension. Their significance lies in showing that not only is it necessary to detect hypertension, but also that its ongoing treatment demands careful surveillance by the primary care team. It is hard to decide whether this performance in hypertension care is simply the best that can be achieved in a symptomless condition in which patient motivation is low, or whether it reflects poor management by the primary care team. It is up to primary care teams to ensure that they provide the highest possible quality of care. Often patient attendance and uptake of the service will remain low despite the best efforts of the primary care team.

The disease

Agreeing the management plan

How far doctors and nurses should go in ensuring patients attend for treatment and comply with the treatment advised is a matter for debate. At the beginning, the patient with a chronic illness should be asked what he or she expects from the primary care team and the patient should be told what the primary care team expects from him or her. There should follow a degree of negotiation in which a plan is agreed between the patient and the primary care team and, if possible, this should be written down. If the primary care team has a structure for managing chronic illness, the patient should be informed about it. Without a structure, the management of chronic illness is very much a hit-and-miss affair. How would you approach Mrs G, whose story follows?

Case Study 9.3

Mrs G is 71 and has had insulin-dependent diabetes mellitus for the last 10 years. She lives alone in sheltered accommodation in London, all the rest of her family having moved to the USA. She has recently developed a neuropathic ulcer in her right foot and is unable to come to the surgery. She has macular degeneration of the retina and her visual acuity is limited to 6/12 on both sides. Her diabetes is poorly controlled and her last glycosylated haemoglobin (HbA1c) was 12.2 per cent (desirable <7 per cent).

Thinking and Discussion Point

How would you organize Mrs G's care? What services should be provided at home and what should be provided in hospital or other health service centres?

The main challenge in Mrs G's case is to provide effective care at home. She has advanced diabetes, with probable involvement of the vasa nervorum of her foot causing her neuropathy. Her diabetes is out of control and she is entering a rapid downward spiral. It is likely that in becoming housebound she has lost contact with the services for her diabetes and is now at risk of a major infection or acute ischaemia of her feet or vital organs.

Does she need to see a diabetologist to give advice on her insulin? Is the chiropodist attending her at home? Should she have the advice of a neurologist about her peripheral neuropathy? What about her eyes? Will active surveillance of her eyes prevent the additional insult of diabetic retinopathy to add to her senile macular degeneration? Is she able to draw up her own insulin? Who is dressing her ulcer? What aids would help at home? When was the last time her renal function was checked? Is she getting meals on wheels? Could she attend a day centre for elderly people?

Mrs G's situation is not unusual. The role of the primary care team is to coordinate her care, and one member should take the lead. A case conference with other members of the community health and social services, if not also the diabetic team, may be especially useful. Many hospital diabetic teams have the capacity for nursing outreach and community-based diabetic teams are an increasing feature of NHS care. Support in the community of people like Mrs G is probably the ideal to be sought, but there is no reason why she should not attend the diabetic clinic in the first instance if she is not already doing so.

Mrs G needs an explicit plan of care in which the roles of the various healthcare professionals are stated and she knows what to expect from whom. The primary care team should be able to assess their own performance in delivering services to people like Mrs G to ensure that patients do not fall through the net of services. What is required is structured care of her illness.

In major psychiatric illness, formal care in the community occurs under the title of The Care Programme Approach (CPA; Department of Health and Social Security, 1990). The CPA was introduced in the UK in 1991 in response to growing concern about the care of mentally ill people in the community. It promotes inter-professional collaboration and ensures that both psychiatric and social needs are addressed. A key worker is appointed who may or may not have a role in the treatment of the patient. This person is responsible both to ensure decisions made within the CPA

are carried out and to act as the main point of contact of the patient with the care team. The CPA is now enshrined in UK Government Statute. There is much about the CPA which is reflected in formal, structured care of chronic illness in general practice, but the principle behind both is simple: people with chronic illness need clear objectives, clear leadership and a clearly identified key worker in the management of their illness.

Structured care of chronic illness

In the section that follows, the various elements of the structured care of chronic illness are outlined. It is not necessary for all elements of this programme to be included in every case of chronic illness care. It would be wise to ask: 'If they are not included, would the care be better with them than without?'

The goal of providing high-quality care to a population of patients should not conflict with the GP's primary aim of serving patients within a personal relationship that extends over time and across consultations. In a now celebrated clinical trial in diabetes care, Kinmonth and colleagues (1998) found specific disease-related outcomes were worse among GPs who had undertaken training in a more person-centred approach than among those who continued with routine care. They pointed out the need for those who are committed to more person-centred consulting also to keep their focus on disease management. Structured care of chronic illness is designed to ensure that disease management goals are kept to the fore.

The idea behind structured care is that of a safety net which operates at a number of different levels. It begins at a population level, promoting a systematic approach to the population or disease group under consideration. It should define the goals of management, who is responsible for carrying it out and what the management approach will consist of. It should address the resources that are required, the impact on other aspects of the service, and the systems that will be used to serve the programme. Finally, it should include a process for reviewing the effectiveness of the programme and for making changes in response to that review.

What population?

- *What disease?* This could be set by diagnostic criteria such as level of blood pressure or by specific prescription such as anticonvulsant.
- *What target population?* Identify all those known with the disease criterion.
- *Are the patients at risk being identified?* Compare the number known with the disease with the number predicted from national figures for the practice population size.

What goals are set?

- *Individual*: What should each patient expect from the treatment? For example, a hypertensive might expect to have blood pressure controlled according to the guidelines of the British Hypertension Society, or according to a practice-agreed derivative of those guidelines.
- *Group*: What should be achieved with all known members of that disease group? For example, the aim might be to review all asthma patients on inhaled steroids at least once a year.
- *Practice*: What should the practice achieve in its administration and management programme for the disease? In epilepsy, the aim might be to conduct a practice audit of epilepsy once a year, to review the epilepsy guidelines and protocol every 3 years, and to establish effective liaison with the local neurologist.

How will the programme be delivered?

- *Advertisement within the surgery*: How will patients be informed of the service?
- *Organization*: Whether to run a service as part of normal surgery consulting or to provide special disease-oriented sessions such as a diabetic clinic.
- *Clinical leadership*: Should this service be led by one of the doctors or one of the nurses or the manager or another team member?
- *Clinical care*: Should the service be provided by all doctors and nurses (probably essential in asthma due to the numbers of asthmatics in the population) or by one or two interested clinical staff (a more practical requirement for a less common disease such as epilepsy)?
- *Administration*: Who will be responsible for

maintenance of the disease and prescription registers, and the recall system?
- *What clinical disciplines should be involved?* A dietician and chiropodist might be essential for diabetes mellitus.

What resources are needed?

- *Personnel*: doctor and nursing time, administrative support.
- *Time*: impact on existing general medical services.
- *Accommodation*: e.g. room for nurses to run special clinics.
- *Equipment*: e.g. blood glucose monitoring equipment, placebo devices in asthma, choice of cuff sizes for sphygmomanometry.
- *Finance*: cost of providing special equipment, carrying out audit (potentially very expensive, depending on the extensiveness of data collection and the existence of computerized clinical records).

What information will be kept?

- *Computer systems*: a modern prerequisite for structured care of chronic illness. The manual recording of disease and prescription registers is almost unbearably tedious.
- *Manual systems*: it can be done, but it is essential in establishing any programme of clinical care to ensure that the administrative system serves the clinical objectives. If the system is manual, it has to be kept as simple as possible so that accurate and complete recording can be achieved.

How will the patients be reviewed?

- *Establish a disease register*: cross-check against prescription register.
- *Establish a prescription register*: cross-check against disease register.
- *Formal annual review*: this may not be possible for all patients, so prioritize patients.
- *Recall systems*: either from set recall mechanisms within a computerized record or from a manual card index or from repeat prescriptions. Computerized repeat prescriptions may provide the easiest and most efficient access to patients who need recall. Most NHS practices operate a repeat prescription system in which

patients are given access to a limited supply of repeat medication. The amount is determined by the prescribing doctor during a clinical consultation. Requests for repeat prescriptions that have not been authorized bring to the attention of the practice staff patients who should have attended but who have not. Reluctant patients can be encouraged by the issuing of limited supplies of their drugs!

Summarize into a protocol

■ *Team meetings*: Structured care is best provided by a team in which each discipline can play to its strengths – doctors concentrate on medical care, nurses on nursing, managers on managing, and clerical staff on appointment systems, records and filing. If structured care is to work, all the desired action points have to be agreed by the relevant team members.

■ *Written protocols*: Plans that are written down are likely to be clearer and more realistic. Agreements that are recorded can be challenged and developed. Audit is made considerably easier if the basis of what is being assessed has been recorded. New members of the team will find it easier to take part in an enterprise which requires collaboration if the purpose and method of the work have been written down.

Ensure standards

■ *Audit*: Self-review by the practice team of its performance in the structured care of chronic illness is the best way of ensuring that change and development take place. Audit requires adequate resources to be carried out effectively. Under-resourced, it becomes a source of irritation. Properly prepared, it is encouraging and promotes high quality.

SUMMARY POINTS

The most important messages of this chapter are as follows:
■ Chronic illness is a major element of most areas of clinical medicine.
■ Chronic illness is often detected or diagnosed late and then often under-treated.
■ The impact of chronic illness is complex, and understanding chronic illness requires a model of illness that takes into account the medical, functional, social and sociological aspects of the disease.
■ Screening is essential in chronic illnesses such as diabetes and hypertension, but does not have a place in the detection of most chronic illnesses.
■ The proper long-term management of all chronic illnesses requires a programme of formal structured care involving multidisciplinary members of primary and secondary care teams.

Screening in asthma, yes or no? The answer!

The diagnostic criterion for asthma is variability (or reversibility after administration of a bronchodilator) in peak expiratory flow rate (PEFR) or in forced expiratory volume in the first second (FEV_1) of at least 20 per cent. Asthma cannot be diagnosed on a single test. A screening test would therefore have to be applied either on two separate occasions or before and after the administration of a bronchodilator. While it is unlikely that all symptomatic asthmatics are currently taking treatment, the first two principles of screening would nonetheless have to be met. And since there is as yet no evidence that screening for asthma would detect disease for which treatment would be worth prescribing, there could be no justification for screening for asthma.

References

Ashworth, M. and Krodowicz, M. 2010: Quality and outcomes framework: time to take stock. *British Journal of General Practice* 60(578), 637–8.

Bury, M. 1982: Chronic illness as biographical disruption. *Sociology of Health and Illness* 4.2, 167–82.

Department of Health and Social Security 1990: The care programme approach for people with a mental illness referred to the specialist psychiatric services. HC(90)23/LASSL(90)11. London: HMSO.

Hart, J.T. 1975: Screening in primary care. In: Hart, C.R. (ed.) *Screening in general practice.* Edinburgh: Churchill Livingstone, 17–29.

Heath, I. 1996: *The mystery of general practice.* Oxford: Nuffield Provincial Hospitals Trust.

Holman, N.F., Farouhi, N.G., Goyder, E. and Wild, S.H. 2011: The Association of Public Health Observatories (APHO) diabetes prevalence model: estimates of total diabetes prevalence for England, 2010–2030. *Diabetes in Medicine* 28(5), 525–82.

Jacoby, A., Baker, G.A., Steen, N., Potts, P. and Chadwick, D.W. 1996: The clinical course of epilepsy and its psychosocial correlates: findings from a UK community study. *Epilepsia* 37(2), 148–61.

Kinmonth, A.L., Woodcock, A., Griffin, S., Spiegal, N. and Campbell, M.J. 1998: Randomised controlled trial of patient centred care of diabetes in general practice: impact on current wellbeing and future disease risk. *British Medical Journal* 17(7167), 1202–8.

McCormick, A., Fleming, D. and Charlton, J., Royal College of General Practitioners, Office of Population Censuses and Surveys, and Department of Health 1995: *Morbidity Statistics from General Practice. Fourth National Survey 1991–1992.* London: HMSO.

Memel, D. 1996: Chronic disease or physical disability? The role of the general practitioner. *British Journal of General Practice* 46, 109–13.

Nacul, L., Soljak, M., Samarasundera, E., Hopkinson, N.S., Lacerda, E., Indulkar, T., Flowers, J., Walford, H. and Majeed, A. 2011: COPD in England: a comparison of expected, model-based prevalence and observed prevalence from general practice data. *Journal of Public Health (Oxford)* 33(1), 108–16.

Office for National Statistics (2010): *General Lifestyle Survey.* London: HMSO. Also available online at: www.statistics.gov.uk/downloads/theme_compendia/GLF09/GLFoverview2009.pdf (accessed October 2010).

Sackett, D. and Holland, W.W. 1975: Controversy in the detection of disease. *Lancet* ii, 357–9.

Shorvon, S., Chadwick, D., Galbraith, A. and Reynolds, E. 1978: One drug for epilepsy. *British Medical Journal* 1, 474–6.

van Lieshout, J., Goldfracht, M., Campbell, S., Ludt, S. and Wensing, M. 2011: Primary care characteristics and population-orientated health care across Europe: an observational study. *British Journal of General Practice* 61(582), 22–30.

Wagner, E.H., Austin, B.T., Davis, C., Hindmarsh, M., Schaefer, J. and Bonomi, A. 2001: Improving chronic illness care: translating evidence into action. *Health Affairs* 20(6), 64–77.

Further reading

Anderson, R. and Bury, M. (eds) 1988: *Living with chronic illness, the experience of patients and their families.* London: Unwin.
This is an authoritative and highly informative account of the meaning of chronic illness from the perspective of the sufferer.

General Medical Council 2009: *Tomorrow's doctors. Outcomes and standards for undergraduate medical education.* London: GMC.

Littlejohns, P. and Victor, C. (eds) 1996: *Making sense of a primary care-led health service.* Abingdon: Radcliffe Medical Press.

Littlejohns and Victor have gathered together a group of authors who have a good grasp of the main issues facing GPs as purchasers of health care. The book is relevant to this subject in describing how GPs might respond to rising demand, because rising demand is the central issue now in chronic illness care.

Wagner, E.H., Austin, B.T., Davis, C., Hindmarsh, M., Schaefer, J. and Bonomi, A. 2001: Improving chronic illness care: translating evidence into action. *Health Affairs* 20(6), 64–77.

This paper summarizes the challenges of delivering care for chronic illness in healthcare systems that remain predominantly orientated towards acute illness care.

SINGLE BEST ANSWER QUESTIONS

9.1 The clinical responsibility of a GP in modern healthcare can best be described as follows:

a) The GP's responsibility is solely for the patient with whom he or she is consulting
b) The GP's responsibility is for the clinical care of the patient who has consulted with him or her for as long as that patient is registered
c) The GP has responsibility for the clinical care of all the patients registered with him or her whether or not they have consulted recently
d) The GP only has clinical responsibility for patients who have sought his or her advice
e) The GP's clinical responsibility relates only to clinical conditions about which the patient has consulted.

9.2 In communicating the diagnosis of a chronic illness the GP should:

a) Ensure that the patient knows the precise diagnosis before the consultation concludes
b) Be careful not to allow the patient to misinterpret the nature of the illness by being vague
c) Avoid euphemisms (e.g. 'a bit of wheeze in the chest' when the diagnosis is asthma) that fail to tell the full story
d) Base the information that he or she chooses to give on the knowledge and understanding of the patient
e) Be direct and straightforward to avoid confusion.

9.3 A 45-year-old woman is taking levothyroxine for hypothyroidism which she has had since she was 28 years old. She asks for a repeat prescription. Her thyroid stimulating hormone (TSH) is usually normal at 0.13 mmol/L. It was last done 2 years ago. The most appropriate action is:

a) You should give her three months of levothyroxine authorized three monthly for the next year
b) You should invite her for a TSH blood test and not give her any medications until she attends for the blood test
c) You should invite her for a TSH blood test and give her enough levothyroxine for a month
d) You should give her the usual three-monthly prescription and invite her for a TSH blood test at her convenience
e) You should give her the usual three-monthly prescription and remind her to have the TSH blood test in a year.

9.4 In your general practice you find that you have a much lower prevalence of diagnosed hypertension than would be expected for your practice list characteristics. Your practice decides that it is going to make a big push to identify more people with hypertension. What should the practice do?

a) Invite by letter annually to attend for a blood pressure review all patients aged 35 years and over who have not had a blood pressure recording in the previous three years
b) Invite by letter annually to attend for a blood pressure review all high-risk patients (family history of cardiovascular disease, diagnosis of ischaemic heart disease, or diabetes mellitus, or chronic kidney disease, or cerebrovascular disease, or hypercholesterolaemia)
c) Take the blood pressure of all adults aged 35 years and over who attend the surgery who have not had a normal blood pressure recording in the previous year

SINGLE BEST ANSWER QUESTIONS CONTINUED

d) Take the blood pressure of all patients in high risk groups (same as in B above) who attend the surgery

e) Write to all patients aged 35 years and over on the practice list advising them of the value of hypertension surveillance and recommending that they have their blood pressure checked at their next healthcare consultation.

9.5 A 45-year-old housebound paraplegic patient is found to have raised blood pressure when he attends the accident and emergency department with a laceration on his hand. His GP is informed. What should be done?

a) The patient should be referred to the district nurses for assessment of his blood pressure

b) The patient should be referred to the local cardiology department for management of his blood pressure and ambulance transport should be arranged

c) A domiciliary assessment by a cardiologist should be requested

d) The patient's GP should assess the patient at home, arrange for serial recording of the patient's blood pressure and carry out screening tests for underlying causes and associated conditions

e) The patient should be invited to attend the GP's surgery and to arrange his own transport.

CHAPTER

10

TREATING PEOPLE AT HOME

- ■ Home care by GPs
- ■ Deciding when to visit
- ■ Home visits – facts and figures
- ■ Out of hours
- ■ Reason for visits
- ■ Treating at home can cause problems!
- ■ Services for housebound patients

- ■ Managing housebound patients with teamwork
- ■ Services delivered at home
- ■ Summary points
- ■ References
- ■ Further reading
- ■ Single best answer questions

Treating people in their own homes provides general practitioners (GPs) with a fascinating and privileged insight into their lives. It often reveals important elements of their medical problems. It is also time consuming. Doctors have to consider carefully who needs to be seen at home and who can actually get to the surgery, in order to use the doctor's time most effectively. People who are housebound are often treated at home by a variety of health professionals. New approaches to the management of illness, including so-called 'hospital at home', can enable people to be discharged early from hospital and can allow highly dependent patients to be managed at home with a mixture of high-tech medicine and intensive social care.

LEARNING OBJECTIVES

By the end of this chapter you will be able to:
- ■ understand the reasons for treating patients in their homes;
- ■ understand the role of home visiting in the work of a GP;
- ■ describe the workload related to treating people at home;
- ■ discuss the variety of arrangements for treating patients out of hours;
- ■ list the services available for housebound patients.

Home care by GPs

In the British Isles, the GP is often identified as the doctor who comes to the house when a member of the family is ill. This view is surprisingly common, even though home visits make up only a small fraction of the work of the GP. It is confirmed in popular television and stage drama and in literature, where many of the emotion-laden encounters between GPs and their patients occur in the setting of the patients' homes. In most other parts of the world, home visiting by doctors is even less common, although whichever the country, consulting with a patient in his or her own home is a highly significant event for both the patient and the doctor, and is likely to be remembered by both.

Home visits afford the GP a privileged insight into the personal life of the patient, and they give the patient exceptional access to the GP. Moreover, information obtained at home may be crucial to the management of the illness. Consider the case of Mr F.

Case Study 10.1

Mr F, a 63-year-old unemployed widower, had chronic venous ulceration of both lower legs that required twice-weekly compression dressing by the practice nurse in the surgery. Despite this intensive treatment, the ulcers would not heal. Dr S had to see Mr F at home when he developed pneumonia. He was shocked to discover the poverty of Mr F's circumstances: he had no bed and slept every night in his armchair. He suffered terrible body odour that was not helped by his being unable to bathe, because of his dressings, and he was clearly depressed. By involving social services, Dr S enabled Mr F to get financial support to purchase a bed and bed coverings and sort out his social security benefits so that he could improve his circumstances at home. Within four weeks of him starting to sleep every night in bed, his ulcers, which were due to venous incompetence and had been made worse by his legs always being dependent, healed and he was able to bathe. His mood improved considerably and he renewed contact with his son, whom he had not seen for more than 2 years.

Deciding when to visit

Home visits are likely to take more than twice the time required for a surgery consultation (current average in the National Health Service (NHS) is approximately 10 minutes) when one takes into account the time for the journey there and back. Who should be visited, when and by whom are key issues for every GP who wants to manage his or her time effectively. How would you respond to the next case, in which the mother of a 3-year-old boy requests a visit for her son who has a sore throat?

Case Study 10.2

Mrs M phones Dr S's surgery at 8.30 a.m. to request a home visit for her son, Jason, aged 3, who has been disturbed through the night with a sore throat.

> ### Thinking and Discussion Point
>
> Before reading the next part of the case study, think what questions you would ask Mrs M before deciding whether or not to visit her son at home.

Case Study 10.2 (continued)

Mrs M says she does not want to bring Jason to the surgery because he has been awake all night and has a high temperature. She is worried it might develop into pneumonia if she takes him out.
Dr S explains to Mrs M that there is no risk to Jason of developing pneumonia by going outside and that his fever might even be helped by taking him out of doors.

There is a clash of beliefs here, with little research evidence to support the position of either Dr S or Mrs M. Dr S's belief is supported by his experience and his rationale that there is no pathological basis on which to suggest that short-term changes in ambient temperature might influence the progress of infection. Mrs M's belief is based on the authoritative opinion of her own mother and family that pneumonia is due to the cold temperature entering the body and allowing the infection to become deep seated. When she was a child, the doctor always visited the children when they were ill.

Case Study 10.2 (continued)

Dr S tries to resolve the impasse by offering to see Jason as soon as he arrives in the surgery so that his mother can take him straight home without delay. Mrs M accepts the offer with great reluctance.

From the GP's viewpoint, there is the risk of setting a precedent here by visiting at home a child who in his view could come to the surgery safely. If he did visit the child at home, it could be seen to undermine the position of his receptionists. He had instructed them to discourage any home visiting except in an emergency. Home visiting is an aspect of general practice that affects the whole team and for which there should be a clear policy.

The situation in relatively minor self-limiting illness is made complex by differences between the expectations of doctors and those of patients. Nonetheless, it is more a matter of convention and etiquette than life and death. However, major life-threatening illness can also present difficult dilemmas, as the experience of Mr J demonstrates.

Case Study 10.3

Mr J is a 52-year-old taxi driver who had a myocardial infarction a year ago. He made a good recovery and was able to resume his work after about six months. One weekday morning, he woke up feeling tired and weak. By 10.45 a.m., he was short of breath and called the surgery asking for a doctor to visit straight away. Dr S had attended Mr J during his heart attack the previous year and had come to know him very well since. He knew Mr J was an anxious man and that he had a deep fear that another heart attack would not be far off. Dr S recognized that this fear was quite reasonable in someone who had already had a heart attack at the relatively young age of 51. Dr S was himself in the middle of a busy morning surgery and was running about half an hour late. He still had eight more patients to see. Should he simply call the ambulance or should he visit Mr J at home himself?

Thinking and Discussion Point

What are the arguments for and against Dr S visiting Mr J at home immediately as against calling the emergency ambulance? Give this scenario to your GP tutor and find out how he or she would want to deal with it?

Mr J could be having another myocardial infarction with associated left ventricular decompensation. He might be suffering from one of a number of other causes of breathlessness completely unrelated to his heart. Could he be suffering acute anxiety with air hunger?

The dilemma facing Dr S is hard to resolve. He knows Mr J had an uncomplicated myocardial infarction with minor damage to the myocardium. He had streptokinase at the time and a subsequent angiogram was remarkably free of coronary disease, with the exception of the affected blood vessel. The doctor thinks a further myocardial infarction is unlikely. If he sends Mr J off to hospital in an ambulance, he will be reinforcing Mr J's belief that he is a man with precarious health which needs a dramatic response every time. If there is some other cause to his breathlessness, he may need to attend hospital anyway and Dr S will have added unnecessarily to the burden of his own morning's work. On the other hand, if the problem is simply an acute anxiety attack, it is in Mr J's and Dr S's interests to manage it at home. If the problem is respiratory rather than cardiac, it could perhaps be managed in an organized fashion from Mr J's home rather than by 'blue light' emergency, with all the stress and disruption that would ensue in the emergency department of the local hospital.

Case Study 10.3 (continued)

Dr S decided to see Mr J at home straight away. Mr J was quite distressed by his breathlessness, with a respiratory rate of 32 breaths/min. He had slight pleuritic pain in his right lung base, and he had a tachycardia of 102 beats/min. His blood pressure was normal at 146/84 mmHg. Having ruled out a pneumothorax, Dr S thought he either had pleurisy or a pulmonary embolus. Mr J had just returned from holiday in Kenya and the journey had involved a 5-hour flight. He had swelling and redness in his left lower leg. Dr S decided a deep vein thrombosis (DVT) with pulmonary embolus was the most likely diagnosis and immediately sent Mr J by ambulance to see the medical registrar of the local hospital. Mr J was admitted to hospital, had a D-dimer test and ultrasound scan that confirmed the DVT, and a lung scan that confirmed the pulmonary embolus. He was started on heparin intravenously and warfarin by mouth. He was discharged after 5 days with elastic compression hose on both legs, and a certificate to stay off work for at least a month.

Thinking and Discussion Point

Now that you know the outcome, has it influenced the way you see this case? Do you think Dr S was kicking himself when he got back to the surgery for not calling the ambulance in the first place? Or do you think he saw some value in the home visit?

The element of confidence and control which might have been imparted by the visit by Dr S is hard to measure. However, the overall experience of an arranged emergency referral to hospital with a tentative diagnosis is likely to be more constructive and acceptable than an emergency arrival at the accident and emergency department. The cost to Dr S is considerable in terms of both the personal stress and the impact of the event on his other patients. Was it worth it? This judgement is influenced by the doctor's feelings towards the patient and the relationship they have together. It is affected also by the support the doctor receives from his or her colleagues and staff on return to the surgery. Some GPs feel such home visits are not justified and resent colleagues who embark on what they themselves see as futile mercy errands leading to unacceptable stresses back in the surgery while the on-call GP is out on the emergency. This is a good reason to have protocols for the conduct of home visits, both in an emergency and otherwise.

The basic principles governing home visits by GPs in the UK have come under increasing scrutiny in the UK over the last 15 years with the development of out-of-hours GP cooperatives. The new contract for UK GPs in 2004 in which GPs could opt out of the 24-hour commitment, which had previously been an essential element of their work, profoundly affected the way out-of-hours services were seen and had an important knock-on effect on attitudes to home visiting. At their height, GP cooperatives in the UK formed the National Association of GP Co-operatives (NAGPC) which developed policy and guidance statements for its members. Among other policies, the NAGPC stated that 'general practice has never been and can never be an emergency service along the lines of the police or ambulance'.

While it recognized that there may be occasions when the GP would attend an acute emergency, it stressed that it was unlikely to be in the interests either of the acutely ill patient or of those patients being treated in the surgery for the GP to attempt routinely to augment the care provided by the emergency services. There was a notable exception to this principle. In some locations, patients lived very far from the emergency services and it was essential for their GP to be able to provide a relatively immediate response to most medical emergencies. However, most ambulance services in the UK now include highly trained paramedics who can assess and treat life-threatening arrhythmias, cardiovascular and respiratory emergencies and major haemorrhages. This statement has not been superseded and it retains widespread support among GPs.

Some of the problems that might lead to a more easily defined rationale for home visiting are listed in Table 10.1.

Sometimes, patients who request a home visit by the GP will happily travel to hospital by car or taxi if an urgent hospital assessment has to be made as a result of the visit. This willingness to travel to the hospital by car yet unwillingness to attend the GP's office may simply reflect a difference between the patient's view of the role of the GP and their view of the role of the hospital doctor. It may represent the patient's acceptance of the need to travel on learning that he or she is a 'hospital case', or it may represent the patient's horror of travelling in an ambulance.

Within the NHS, GPs are not obliged to attend patients in their home provided in 'the doctor's

Table 10.1 Reasons for visiting or for not visiting patients in their homes

Reasons to visit patients in the home	Patients who should be able to attend the surgery
Some acute emergencies, e.g. acute left ventricular failure, acute abdomen	Almost all children
	All ambulant patients
Patient too ill to travel, e.g. severe vertigo, advanced chronic obstructive pulmonary disease, terminal illness	Most adults with viral illnesses
Patient unable to travel, e.g. paraparesis, motor neuron disease, severe agoraphobia	

reasonable opinion' the patient's 'condition is such' that the patient should attend a doctor's premises. In the USA, Medicare, the national health insurance system, will support physician visits to the home if the services are reasonable and necessary and if a plan of care is established and reviewed. What is reasonable and necessary is defined in terms of observation and assessment, teaching and training of the patient, and therapy, management and evaluation of the illness (Oldenquist *et al.*, 2001). Also, there is good evidence, for example, that home-based assessments improve the likelihood that elderly patients will remain at home. The demands of home visiting on GPs' time have led to the introduction of home visiting by practice assistants in Germany, a scheme that has been associated with a reduction in home visiting (van den Berg *et al.*, 2010).

There is information for medical students on how to do a home visit in Chapter 4 on skills.

Home visits – facts and figures

The average home visiting rate in England and Wales in 1991/92 was 299 per 1000 patient-years, according to the Fourth National Survey of Morbidity in General Practice (Table 10.2; McCormick *et al.*, 1995). This amounted to around 600 visits per GP per year, or about three visits per working day. About one in nine of these visits took place between 10 p.m. and 8 a.m. More recent data on home visiting in the UK are not available. According to anecdotal reports by UK GPs, the number of home visits during office hours has continued to fall, although there is no reliable information about true home visiting rates.

Under the new contract for UK GPs, GPs can opt out of providing out-of-hours services between 6.30 p.m. and 8.30 a.m. This change has had a significant impact on GPs' working conditions and that is evident in changes in out-of-hours home visiting. Out-of-hours visiting will be discussed in the next section. Changes in rates of daytime visiting were already happening since the early 1990s and were not the result of the new contract. In 1996 Aylin *et al.* showed that people over the age of 85 had a home visiting rate of 3009/1000 patient-years in comparison with a rate of 103/1000 patient-years in people aged 16–24 years and a rate of 477/1000 patient-years in people under the age of 5 years. People in social class V had higher rates of home visiting than those in social class I. However, home visiting rates can vary greatly between practices, even allowing for age and sex differences, so that in the study which recorded these figures, some practices had home visiting rates as low as 100 visits per GP per year (Aylin *et al.*, 1996). This compared with practices at the other extreme, with a visiting rate of 1110 visits per GP per year. These differences could not be explained solely by the ethnic or social structure of the practice populations. At least some of the variation was determined by practice characteristics. These could be as diverse as the structure of the appointment system (Was there a facility for fitting in urgent consultations? Could advice be obtained over the phone?), the willingness or otherwise of the doctors to do home visits (Did the doctors accept all requests for home visits without question? Did receptionists try to avoid home visits by fitting patients in as an emergency during surgery consultations, or by getting the doctors to speak to patients

Table 10.2 Home visit rates in England and Wales, 1991–92

	Home visits per 1000 patient-years	Number on average list	Average GP visits/ year
All patients	299	2000	600
Patients under 5 years	477	138	66
Patients 16–24 years	103	256	26
Patients over 84 years	3009	28	84

The denominator '1000 patient-years' allows for patients who have moved away or died and is more accurate than '1000 patients'. Data from McCormick *et al.*, 1995. More up-to-date figures are not currently available.

requesting home visits on the phone?) or the advertising of practice arrangements (Was it clear to patients what constituted the need for a home visit in the eyes of the doctors?). In Australia, there has been a reduction of 50 per cent in home visits in the 10 years up to 2007 (Joyce and Piterman, 2008).

If you are currently attached to a primary care team, you might discuss the following exercise with your GP tutor. Having carried out the exercise, are there any other members of the team who could give you an opinion about the result? It might help to let them see the national figures compared to those of the practice.

Thinking and Discussion Point

How many home visits have been done in office hours in your tutor's practice in the past three months? Count the number of home visits in the period in question from the visit book, or its equivalent if computerized. Multiply that number by four. Divide the resulting number by the number of patients on the practice list and multiply by 1000. This is your tutor's practice's daytime visiting rate per thousand patients per year. How does it differ from national figures above reported in 1996? Can you offer any explanation for similarities or differences compared with the national figures given above?

Out of hours

Reliable data on the proportion of home visits made out of office hours are not available. There was a fall of 27 per cent in home visiting rates in the UK between 1981/2 and 1991/2. This was matched by a substantial rise in night visits during the same period. Changes in the organization of out-of-hours care in Britain, beginning with GP out-of-hours cooperatives in the 1990s and culminating in the new GP contract in 2004 with the introduction of the new option to end 24-hour responsibility for patient care, have changed the workload of GPs considerably, but the needs and demands of patients are unlikely to have changed much in that time (Jessop *et*

al., 1997; Department of Health, 2002). Among the innovations that have taken place, there have been dramatic increases both in the number of GP out-of-hours cooperatives and in the number of out-of-hours primary care centres. A GP out-of-hours cooperative is a formal business arrangement amongst GPs within a particular area. The aim of the cooperative is to share in the provision of out-of-hours general medical services to patients registered with participating GPs so as to achieve maximum efficiency of service and minimum costs in manpower, time and expense. Out-of-hours primary care centres are local centres manned by primary care professionals providing out-of-hours services on behalf of local primary care teams. This service is usually an emergency service, but in some examples routine care is also provided in these centres. Within the NHS, a new plan for out-of-hours care called the 'Out of Hours Review' was implemented in 2004 alongside the new contract for GPs (Department of Health, 2002). It was intended to introduce a fully integrated out-of-hours service in which all telephone calls out of hours would be received by NHS Direct, the patient telephone advice line. Where clinical care was required, it would be provided by existing GP services (e.g. out-of-hours cooperatives), but also by walk-in centres, primary care centres and accident and emergency centres. These services would be integrated with or have close liaison with minor injury units, social services, community nursing, the ambulance service and mental health and palliative care units. NHS Direct has continued to operate since then, and it remains the intention of the NHS to centralize all out-of-hours telephone contacts.

At present, services vary greatly from area to area, with many GP cooperatives still in operation. Patients use NHS Direct to a varying extent, with many still having direct access to GP cooperatives and other services.

A notable change in the pattern of out-of-hours provision is the increasing number of contacts that were being dealt with by telephone advice (Studdiford *et al.*, 1996). Salisbury (1997) reported that almost 60 per cent of contacts out of hours with one GP cooperative were conducted by telephone alone. The rate with which contacts were managed by telephone varied amongst out-of-hours cooperatives from 10 per cent to 65 per cent, according to Jessop and colleagues (1997). This differs strikingly from the rate of 1 per cent reported for GP deputizing services in 1994/5 by Cragg *et al.* (1997).

The whole issue of telephone consulting is now receiving more attention in the UK, with special training programmes and research projects being developed in a number of different centres. By contrast, there has been a long tradition of telephone consulting in the USA, where up to a quarter of primary care contacts have been by telephone (Studdiford *et al.*, 1996). Telephone consulting allows assessments to be made and advice given to patients who are either unwilling or unable to come to the surgery. In many surgeries it is only when the doctor gets to the patient's home that he or she learns about the reason for the home visit request. My own experience suggests that it is not uncommon for the doctor to discover to his or her dismay that the home visit was not justified purely on clinical grounds. So the development of formal telephone consulting may well prove to be an advance in limiting the current expansion in demand for general medical services. It may also improve access to GP services and reduce the time and travelling costs for consumers. Telephone consulting has been used for chronic disease surveillance for which the patient carries out home monitoring. This can be useful in the care of hypertension or diabetes mellitus, for which the results of home tests done by the patient can be discussed with a doctor or nurse and appropriate advice given.

One fear that accompanied the introduction of the new system in the UK was that patients would be more readily referred to accident and emergency departments which would in turn become swamped with primary care problems with which they were ill equipped to deal. So far this appears not to have happened, according to a recent study by Ingram *et al.* (2009).

Reason for visits

Diseases of the respiratory system are the commonest diagnoses made during home visits (Aylin *et al.*, 1996). These include upper respiratory tract infections, pneumonia, asthma and chronic bron-

chitis. Diseases of the respiratory tract account for 40 per cent of home visits for children and 20 per cent for adults. In 11 per cent of home visits, the category of diagnosis (drawn from the International Classification of Diseases – Version 9) was 'symptoms, signs, and ill defined conditions'. In people aged 65 years and over, respiratory diseases account for 17 per cent of home visits and diseases of the circulatory system account for 16 per cent.

Treating at home can cause problems!

In contrast with Mrs M's experience of Jason's sore throat is that of Mr V.

Case Study 10.4

Mr V is 45 years old and has acquired immune deficiency syndrome (AIDS). He is now receiving terminal care at home and is being looked after by his partner and the local district nurses supported by the Macmillan team. Requests for a visit to Mr V are put in the home visit book by the receptionists without question.

But Mr V's situation led to other difficulties for Dr S.

Case Study 10.4 (continued)

Mr V had a necrotic bedsore on his buttocks that was discharging heavily. Dr S visited him on Friday morning. Mr V's pain was poorly controlled and the doctor decided to start him on morphine. Dr S is part of an out-of-hours cooperative, so between 6.30 p.m. on Friday and 8.00 a.m. on Monday morning, emergency visits would have to be done by other local GPs in the cooperative. Dr S wanted to warn any doctors who might come to see Mr V about his condition so that they could be informed about how best to relieve his pain and also to ensure that they would protect themselves against contamination. Could Dr S tell the answering service that Mr V had AIDS (and tell the answering service to warn any doctors who might visit) without asking the patient's consent?

Thinking and Discussion Point

- What arrangements does your GP tutor use for out-of-hours cover?
- What are the arguments for and against disclosure of the information about Mr V?
- To whom can a doctor disclose confidential patient information?

Patients who require treatment at home may not always be able to see the doctor they usually see at the surgery. They should nonetheless expect the same degree of confidentiality from the attending doctor. They should assume that their doctor will share information about them with other doctors either directly or through the medical record. However, just as a patient can rightly expect the doctor to hold medical information in confidence from other members of the primary care team, such as receptionists, so it should be assumed that such confidentiality is observed with the telephonists and administrators of an out-of-hours service.

What are the issues in Mr V's case? Dr S may be concerned that a colleague in the cooperative who visits Mr V may take inadequate precautions on coming into contact with Mr V's body fluids. He may worry that Mr V or his carers will fail to communicate the nature of his disease, either because of embarrassment or because he is too ill or they are too distressed to do so. Dr S's anxiety for the safety of his colleagues is not adequate cause to disclose Mr V's diagnosis beyond his medical or nursing attendants without his informed consent. There are other actions that Dr S could take. He could discuss his dilemma with Mr V or Mr V's carer. He could leave a message in the home to be given to a visiting doctor on his or her arrival. The principal issue here is the patient's right to confidentiality and the doctor's duty to observe that right. This right is paramount, except where the risk of injury to others is such that breaching the confidence is the only way in which that risk can be avoided. The onus will then be on the doctor to prove that breaching the confidentiality of the doctor–patient relationship was justified. Because it is not ever possible to be certain that patients are free from infection, doctors are warned to assume that all body fluids are contaminated until proven otherwise and to take appropriate precautions. By the same token, the risk of infection from contact with body fluids is not in itself adequate reason to breach patient confidentiality. However, doctors should always aim to reduce such risks by making information about infectivity as accessible as possible to patients, their carers and fellow professionals.

Home visiting often brings to the fore medico-legal and ethical issues that seem less pressing in the surgery office.

Services for housebound patients

Some people become housebound in the course of their illness, so that they are unable to attend their GP or other health professionals in their offices. If they have carers who can look after their daily needs such as shopping, banking and cleaning, they may only require particular health services on an intermittent basis. If, on the other hand, they need daily nursing care, they are likely to require carefully coordinated services from district nurses, and may in addition need physiotherapy, chiropody and occupational therapy at home. The GP will have a key role in assessing the needs of housebound patients and obtaining the assessment of other professionals at the appropriate stage of the illness.

The cost of hospital admissions and the higher risk of accidents and infections for people in hospital have led to earlier discharge of patients from hospital and the development of 'hospital at home' services. 'Hospital at home' is defined as a service that provides treatment by healthcare professionals in the patient's home of illnesses that would otherwise require acute treatment in hospital. In a systematic review of randomized trials of 'hospital at home', Shepperd and Iliffe (2001) could not support its development as a cheaper alternative to inpatient care. However, more recent studies give cause for optimism and it is likely that attempts to reduce the length of hospital stay by providing high-tech medical services at home supported by intensive social services home care will continue.

A particular problem arises when the housebound patient has a chronic illness that requires on-going surveillance. The elements of structured care that are described in the section on chronic illness apply equally here. However, account needs to be taken of the patient's ability to demand visits when they are required. Mrs W provides a good example of the problem.

Case Study 10.5

Mrs W was 74 years old when she developed insulin-dependent diabetes mellitus. She had been admitted to hospital for a left knee replacement, as she had severe osteoarthritis in both knees and could not walk more than 10 metres without severe pain. She had hypertension, for which she took enalapril 10 mg daily, and she was hypothyroid, for which she took levothyroxine 0.1 mg daily. She was partially blind and could not draw up her own insulin, although she did inject the insulin herself. The district nurse visited her every 3 days to draw up her insulin. Dr S would call about every three months to take her blood pressure. A year after the diagnosis, the practice nurse was carrying out a diabetic audit and noticed that Mrs W was on insulin but did not appear to attend either the hospital or the practice. It became obvious that no surveillance of her diabetes was taking place.

Thinking and Discussion Point

What should be done? Who should do it?

Managing housebound patients with teamwork

It may prove embarrassing for patients such as Mrs W to ask the doctor or nurse to visit to take their blood pressure or to demand checks for their diabetes. Anyway, most patients will not have a detailed concept about what is required in chronic illness management. It seems reasonable to convene a meeting about Mrs W with all the team members involved in order to decide who should have responsibility for what element of her care. Such a meeting is likely to raise other issues such as the need for chiropody, which would be a key service for a diabetic of Mrs W's age. If the meeting is held with Mrs W, she will have the opportunity to say what way she would like her care to be organized. It is wise to determine who has the main overall responsibility to ensure the service is delivered effectively. The best person to do this may well be the district nurse rather than the GP, since it is the district nurse who is seeing Mrs W most frequently.

Services delivered at home

In addition to the GP and district nurse, there is a wide variety of home services that are provided for housebound patients. These are listed in Table 10.3 in two categories – health services and social services.

Table 10.3 Health and social services provided in the home

Health services for the housebound	Social services for the housebound
General practitioner	Home care (personal care, meals, shopping, banking, laundry)
District nurse	Occupational therapist
Health visitor	Bathing attendant (some districts only)
Chiropodist	Meals on wheels
Nurse specialists (paediatric, diabetic, etc.)	Social worker
Early discharge teams	

SUMMARY POINTS

To conclude, the most important messages in this chapter are as follows:

■ Home visiting offers a privileged insight into the lives of patients, but is time consuming and should be justified by the severity or urgency of the illness or by the immobility of the patient.

■ Within the NHS, each GP does 600 home visits on average each year, of which about 65 are done between 10 p.m. and 8 a.m.; the rate of home visiting for people aged 85 years or more is 30 times that for people between the ages of 16 and 35.

■ Rates of home visiting in the NHS vary from 100 per GP per year to 1100 per GP per year, a difference that cannot be explained solely by patient need.

■ Respiratory diseases are the commonest diagnoses recorded on home visits, accounting for more than 20 per cent of diagnoses on visits to adults and for more than 40 per cent of diagnoses on visits to children.

■ Housebound patients are sometimes under-treated through their own unwillingness to demand appropriate treatment at home; a structured approach to their care such as that described in Chapter 9 ('Chronic illness and its management in general practice') may help to ensure effective continuing care of people who are confined to their homes through illness or disability.

References

Aylin, P., Majeed, F.A. and Cook, D.G. 1996: Home visiting by general practitioners in England and Wales. *British Medical Journal* 313, 207–10.

Cragg, D.K., McKinley, R.K., Roland, M.O. *et al.* 1997: Comparison of out of hours care provided by patients' own general practitioners and commercial deputising services: a randomised controlled trial. I: The process of care. *British Medical Journal* 314, 187–9.

Department of Health 2002: *Raising standards for patients. New partnerships in out of hours care.* London: Department of Health. Also available online at: http://www.doh.gov.uk/pricare/implementoohplan-guide.pdf

Ingram, J.C., Calnan, M.W., Greenwood, R.J., Kemple, T., Payne, S. and Rossdale, M. 2009: Risk taking in general practice: GP out-of-hours referrals to hospital. *British Journal of General Practice* 59(558), e16–e24.

Jessop, L., Beck, I., Hollins, L., Shipman, C., Reynolds, M. and Dale, J. 1997: Changing the pattern of out of hours: a survey of general practice co-operatives. *British Medical Journal* 314, 199–200.

Joyce, C. and Piterman, L. 2008: Trends in GP home visits. *Australian Family Physician* 37(12), 1039–42.

McCormick, A., Fleming, D., Charlton, J., Royal College of General Practitioners, Office of Population Censuses and Surveys, and Department of Health 1995: *Morbidity Statistics from General Practice. Fourth National Survey 1991–1992.* London: HMSO.

Oldenquist, G.W., Scott, L. and Finucane, T.E. 2001: Home care: what a physician needs to know. *Cleveland Clinic Journal of Medicine* 68(5), 433–40.

Salisbury, C. 1997: Observational study of a general practice out of hours co-operative: measures of activity. *British Medical Journal* 314, 182–6.

Shepperd, S. and Iliffe, S. 2001: Hospital at home versus in-patient hospital care. *Cochrane Review*, Issue 2. Oxford: Cochrane Library.

Studdiford III, J.S., Panitch, K.M., Snyderman, D.A. and Pharr, M.E. 1996: Telephone in primary care. *Primary Care* 23(1), 83–97.

van den Berg, N., Meinke, C., Matzke, M., Heymann, R., Flessa, S. and Hoffmann, W. 2010: Delegation of GP-home visits to qualified practice assistants: assessment of economic effects in an ambulatory healthcare centre. *BMC Health Services Research* 10, 155.

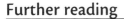

Further reading

Aylin, P., Majeed, F.A. and Cook, D.G. 1996: Home visiting by general practitioners in England and Wales. *British Medical Journal* 313, 207–10.

Hallam, L. 1994: Primary medical care outside of normal working hours: review of published work. *British Medical Journal* 308, 249–53.

Hallam, L. 1997: Out of hours primary care. *British Medical Journal* 314, 157–8.

SINGLE BEST ANSWER QUESTIONS

10.1 A 54-year-old man with no previous medical history of note phones the GP's surgery at 10.15 a.m. requesting a home visit by the doctor. He tells the receptionist that he has had crushing central chest pain for 20 minutes, he is sweating profusely and he feels faint. The receptionist should:

a) Arrange for an urgent home visit by a GP within 2 hours
b) Arrange for the duty doctor to call the patient back as part of his duty doctor calls
c) Offer the patient a same day appointment
d) Arrange an emergency home visit by the duty doctor
e) Make a 999 call for an emergency ambulance.

10.2 A 39-year-old mother of five children aged 4–21 years suffers from recurrent menorrhagia. This month her period has been particularly heavy and she feels exhausted and weak. She asks for a home visit. By careful questioning the GP satisfies himself that she has not lost a dangerous amount of blood and suggests she attends the surgery. She goes into a rage and accuses the doctor of failing in his duty to attend to a patient who is unwell. What should the GP do?

a) The GP should advise the woman that this is not a reasonable request for a home visit and offer her a suitable appointment in the surgery
b) The GP should arrange to visit the woman at home and plan to deal later with what he sees as the inappropriateness of her attitude
c) The GP should offer her a suitable appointment in the surgery within the next 7 days and refuse to discuss the matter until he sees her then

d) The GP should advise the patient that her attitude is unacceptable and that if she wants treatment she should attend the accident and emergency department of the local hospital
e) The GP should advise the woman that her behaviour is unacceptable and she should seek to register with a different GP.

10.3 A 75-year-old man with terminal lung cancer is being looked after at home by his wife. He is receiving morphine slow release tablets 60 mg twice daily for back pain due to secondary spread of the cancer but has great difficulty swallowing the tablets and his pain is unbearable. His wife has been told by the palliative nurse specialist that in these circumstances he should have his morphine by continuous injection under his skin. The equipment is in the house. She phones his GP at 11 a.m. to ask her to do it. What should his GP do?

a) His GP should contact the palliative nurse specialist and request a same day home visit with a view to the palliative team starting morphine by syringe driver
b) The GP should visit the patient and set up the syringe driver herself
c) The GP should ask the district nurses to set up and commence the syringe driver
d) The GP should visit the patient, give an appropriate injection of morphine and arrange for repeated 4-hourly injections of morphine until the total required daily dose is known and the syringe driver can be set up
e) The GP should change the presentation of morphine to oral liquid.

SINGLE BEST ANSWER QUESTIONS CONTINUED

10.4 An elderly lady of 82 requests a visit for her husband who has a high fever and is breathless. When the GP visits he suspects the husband has pneumonia and admits him as an emergency to hospital. He notices that the flat, which is rented from the council, is squalid with filthy tissues all over the floor which is sticky with dirt. There are many plates and cutlery with half-finished meals, and the home smells foul. The wife, who is cognitively normal, explains that they have not been able to keep up the housework but that they are managing fine. What should the GP do about the wife?

a) Admit the wife to hospital as an emergency social admission until the flat can be cleaned
b) Suggest the wife arranges to employ a cleaner to help keep the flat clean
c) Refer the couple to social services and request an urgent home care assessment
d) Advise the wife that this is an unhealthy environment, especially for her husband, and she should sort it out before he returns home
e) Advise the wife that this is not a pleasant environment for her or her husband but that it is up to them as a couple as to how they live.

10.5 A mother phones at 9.30 a.m. about her four and a half-year-old boy who has had an upper respiratory tract infection over the past 3 days. He has had fever with rigors for nearly 2 days. He has vomited twice in the last 24 hours. He has a blanching maculo-papular rash on his neck, trunk, upper arms and upper thighs. There are no other complaints. His mother is very worried. She asks the GP to see him at home. What should the GP do?

a) The GP should arrange for the boy to be seen at home by a GP within 2 hours
b) The GP should ask his mother to bring the boy to the surgery at an agreed time later in the day
c) The GP should arrange for the boy to be seen at home during the same day after morning surgery which is scheduled to finish at 12.30
d) The GP should ask the mother to call an ambulance
e) The GP should give the mother advice about fever control, recommend paracetamol solution (120 mg/5 mL) 7.5 mL 6 hourly, and suggest she contacts the GP if the child's condition worsens.

CHAPTER

11

HEALTH PROMOTION IN GENERAL PRACTICE

- Background
- Health promotion and public health
- Health literacy
- Health inequalities
- Health promotion for 'healthy' patients
- Health promotion for patients with early signs and symptoms

- Health promotion for patients with non-communicable diseases
- Summary points
- References
- Further reading
- Single best answer questions

This chapter provides some background to the discipline of health promotion and the links with public health. Theory and rationale are to some extent discussed but the emphasis is on practice within the context of general practice. There has been considerable growth and interest in this field during the last 5 years and evidence-based practice has been enhanced by the range of publications now available from the National Institute for Health and Clinical Excellence (NICE), Cochrane Reviews and the Royal Colleges together with the requirements of the General Medical Council and Department of Health directives. Population health priorities influence health promotion practice with a growing understanding of the need to facilitate behaviour modification as an integral aspect of clinical practice. Behaviour modification is linked to social context and hence health promotion in general practice potentially contributes to the process of reducing health inequalities.

LEARNING OBJECTIVES

By the end of this chapter you should be aware of:
- definitions, parameters and opportunities for health promotion in general practice;
- theories and models that inform health promotion practice;
- terms such as social and modifiable determinants of health, disease prevention, health literacy, health inequalities;
- skills for brief intervention, motivational interviewing and supporting behavioural change;
- NICE guidance and sources of evidence related to health promotion practice.

Background

Since the last edition of this book health promotion has become more prominent in the routine work of general practice, especially with regard to smoking cessation. Health promotion is a broad topic with links to public health, psychology, sociology, education and social marketing. What is health promotion and what are the research,

evidence and literature bases that inform practice? The scope of health promotion practice goes beyond the clinical arena, but for this chapter the focus is based on the application of health promotion within general practice.

The most frequently used definition of health promotion is from the World Health Organization (WHO) Ottawa Charter, 1986: 'Health promotion is a process of enabling people to increase control over and to improve their health' (World Health Organization, 1986). The Charter has been at the forefront of the discipline with its three principal approaches of *advocacy*, *enablement* and *mediation* within five domains:

- building healthy public policy;
- creating supportive environments;
- strengthening community action;
- developing personal skills;
- re-orienting health services.

Despite the apparent simplicity of the WHO definition, health promotion is contested, complex, eclectic, challenging, swathed in jargon, littered with acronyms, political in nature and prone to misinterpretation. For example, advice giving may be based on sound scientific evidence, such as smoking is harmful to health, but how that advice is presented (i.e. the intervention), and whether this is evidence-based best practice is sometimes questionable. There is the potential to raise anxiety, rather than facilitate behaviour change, if intervention evidence is not sought or is misunderstood.

A simple definition offered by Tones and Green (2004) is 'Health promotion is healthy public policy × health education', the argument being that the healthy choice is in essence the easy choice. Others have avoided definitions but offered models for practice such as Beattie (1993), supplemented with discussions on approaches by Ewles and Simnett (2003) and Prochaska and DiClemente's Stages of Change or Transtheoretical Behaviour Change model (1986). This model has become familiar, being the favoured approach for smoking cessation and other lifestyle modification and being based on psychological paradigms. This model is limited in effectiveness, however, if certain conditions are absent. The individual must be assessed and 'ready' for change and 'motivated' to change, with an enabling personal and social context (Wylie, 2004a).

The very term 'health promotion' is one that can have multiple meanings; it is not exclusive to any elitist group and can be part of everyday language. We also struggle with the term 'health' and what it means, accepting that this is variable for individuals and society (Duncan, 2007). There is a working definition of health promotion

used for medical education that may help: 'the study of the response to the modifiable determinants of health'. This definition focuses on two aspects: a *response* which equates to an intervention, whether something small scale and simple, such as giving a patient a leaflet, or a more strategic intervention, such as commissioning exercise referral programmes locally; and *modifiable determinants*, whereby there are sound arguments to support the case that the key determinants have been identified and are modifiable (Wylie and Thompson, 2007). For example, advising a person to stop smoking may be reasonable clinically but the patient may not be able to act on such advice if their circumstances are not favourable to what could be a major change in behaviour for them. Referral to an appropriate cessation service will be necessary when the patient demonstrates 'readiness to change'.

Most activity that is defined as *health promotion* or *health improvement* is funded from the public purse and as such is associated with political agendas and ideology, is of public interest and can provoke public debate and hostility. An example of a current concern for the public is around the prevalence of obesity, with questions such as: How much investment should be focused on prevention? Should we treat obesity without trying to reduce the prevalence? Should obese people pay for their healthcare? Such questions are of interest to society not only because the obese patient will present with chronic conditions and comorbidities, generally managed in general practice, but also because such a person will become less economically active within society. This chapter has limited space to discuss moral and ethical issues but nevertheless it is important to be aware that health promotion practice is not value-free practice.

Health promotion for some, especially those in academia, is seen as a post-modernist discipline and a synergy of philosophies that can be applied in a variety of arenas. It is a young and emerging discipline, applied mainly outside the medical context, but it can and does have a place within the healthcare sector (Wylie, 2004b). In fact, within the context of general practice and primary care, health promotion has become an integral part of provision, and the growth of the discipline has been nurtured there (Boyce *et al.*, 2010).

The other branch of medicine that is closely linked to health promotion is that of public health. Health promotion differs from public health in three important ways:

- It explores the question 'What causes health?' rather than 'What causes disease and what are the patterns/trends of disease?'
- Its evidence base relates to intervention efficacy, which is multifactorial and often complex, using both qualitative and quantitative methodologies.
- It can have both an individual focus and a population focus.

Improving the evidence base is an ongoing challenge, especially for medical practitioners, but increasingly NICE guidance and Cochrane Reviews cover public health-related work, offering the clinical health promoters evidence-based approaches that potentially improve the health of patients.

Health promotion and public health

The health promotion movement and public health have had some shared history. The famous cholera outbreak in London in the early nineteenth century was a classic public health issue. First, by plotting the details of the outbreak, it was clear that there was a location issue and some link or association was made with a specific water pump. Although at this stage it could not be fully explained, an intervention could be implemented, which was to close access to the contaminated water pump, inform the public and arrange alternatives. The epidemiological data identified the noxious agent (i.e. the water pump); it was closed and people were given safe alternatives. But was this *health promotion*? If health promotion is defined as 'the study of, and the study of the response to, the modifiable determinants of health', this historical episode was both public health work and health promotion (Wylie, 2002). The public's health was at risk and, by an intervention or response, this risk was reduced (Naidoo and Wills, 2000).

Both fields have expanded as more complex data and research have become accessible and reliable. The social determinants of health are now incorporated into public health reports and local information easily accessible on the internet, from public health observatory sites, census information and the Office of National Statistics (ONS). These data include housing, income, educational attainment, obesity, smoking behaviour, alcohol consumption and dental health, crime and breast feeding rates. Such is the importance of these data that from these general practices can gain insights into the probable health needs of the community they serve. The correlation between poor health outcome and social determinants of health has led to the recognition of the existence of health inequalities and these can potentially be addressed by well-planned and resourced interventions. If you are in a London general practice, depending on how west or east you are affects the life expectancy of your patients. Based on analysis by the London Health Observatory (2011) using Office for National Statistics data, if one travels east on the Jubilee line past the eight stops between Westminster and Canning Town, two stops, on average, mark nearly a year of shortened lifespan.

Such phenomena are experienced elsewhere such as affluent and non-affluent areas of Glasgow, across cities in Europe and further afield where there is great disparity between the minority indigenous population and affluent majority. These disparities are to some extent explained not by medical sciences but by the social sciences and the social determinants of health. Social disadvantage, be it related to health literacy, income or living in a violent environment, for example, put people at greater risk of poor health and lead to a greater tendency to engage in activities deleterious to their health. The higher prevalence of smoking, drug and alcohol abuse, obesity, domestic and traffic accidents as well as poor sexual health and experiences of violence are all factors that influence primary healthcare provision in more deprived areas (Marmot *et al.*, 2008; Marmot, 2010). Marmot has researched this extensively. His 2008 article, 'Closing the gap', was followed by the Royal College of Physicians policy statement, *How doctors can close the gap* (Royal College of Physicians, 2010), giving credence to the notion that doctors, especially in primary care and general practice, have a role in acknowledging and addressing health inequalities.

Thinking and Discussion Point

Health promotion, public health and general practice share common ground. How could they differ practically in the general practice setting and how could 'successes' be defined? For example consider childhood immunization provision:

- What are the priorities for health promotion?
- What are the priorities for public health?
- What are the priorities for general practice?

It is these variable priorities that can influence how success or efficacy is defined. Health promotion may be concerned with proximal changes that are measurable or observable, such as parent engagement and inquiry, suggesting the process of informed decision making is being facilitated. Public health may look at distal data and uptake within a defined population, able to identify needs. Figure 11.1 suggests a number of stages as part of a continuum that can contribute to evaluation of interventions, be they health promotion or public health.

Types of indicators:

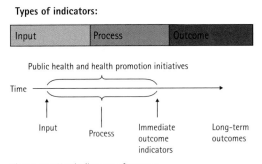

Figure 11.1 Key indicators of success.

Practical Exercise

Using practice data, assess the numbers of patients who are recorded as smokers, how many have been referred to smoking cessation services and how many are now recorded as non-smokers. If possible, do some demographic analysis.

Before we can gauge 'success' or 'failure' a number of variables could be considered. Public health data can indicate the smoking prevalence in an area or population group, for example young men 17–24 years of age:

- How likely are they to engage with the general practice?
- What information is available at the practice?
- How skilled are the practice team to engage with the patient about smoking behaviour?
- What social issues are influencing behaviour or could influence behaviour change?
- What cessation referral systems are available and suitable (e.g. evening, local)?

These are key factors that can contribute to 'success' with regards to input and intermediate outcomes. When planning interventions, the Ewles and Simmett flowchart provides guidance (Figure 11.2, Ewles and Simnett, 2003).

The public health concern about smoking in young men in a specific area will inform the need and approach to designing an intervention, where multiple factors and resources inform the process. Public health 'success' may be concerned with measureable improvement long term with regard to a reduction in smoking prevalence in a specific group, whereas health promotion 'success', especially within general practice, may relate to the number of opportunistic encounters, assessment of readiness to change and engagement with a local cessation service. NICE guidance offers further information (NICE, 2006).

The two fields – health promotion and public health – are mutually beneficial to each other and this is particularly evident within general practice (Boyce *et al.*, 2010).

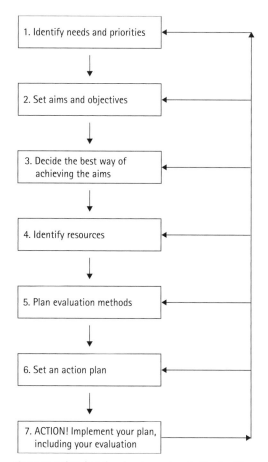

Figure 11.2 Flowchart for planning and evaluating health promotion (Ewles and Simnett, 2003).

The boxes in the flowchart read:

1. Identify needs and priorities
2. Set aims and objectives
3. Decide the best way of achieving the aims
4. Identify resources
5. Plan evaluation methods
6. Set an action plan
7. ACTION! Implement your plan, including your evaluation

Health literacy

Since we have universal compulsory education in the UK it may seem difficult to appreciate that literacy and numeracy levels still cause concern. Only 9 per cent of the population in England can fully engage with modern information technology and 56 per cent of the population have sub-optimal skills to achieve their full potential (Protheroe *et al.*, 2009). Interventions associated with shared decision making and informed consent are relevant for those with high enough literacy and numeracy skills and there could be inherent risks if such factors are not considered. Problems can arise with taking medication, understanding instructions and care of self or others where communication is a challenge and in these situations there may be limited options to challenge, modify or access appropriate services. While tools

have been developed in the USA to rapidly assess literacy levels in the healthcare context, these have yet to be implemented in the UK, although trials are underway. Hence health inequalities can be exacerbated when patients' low literacy levels are not considered or addressed. Poor health literacy is likely to impact overall on patient health.

Consider encounters in general practice where poor health literacy could influence practice:

- English not first language;
- poor or inadequate education experience;
- limited abilities;
- hearing, visual or speech impairments;
- low or non-existent literacy levels in first language or mother tongue;
- sub-optimal quality of translation and interpreter arrangements;
- lacking basic knowledge about health and self-care;
- limited understanding of symptoms and significance.

There are more factors but just a few of the above together can impact on an already distressing health situation with information overload adding to the confusion. A leaflet translated into Bangladeshi, for example, may be of limited use if the intended recipient, a Bangladeshi speaker from a rural community, has limited or no reading skills. If the information is also complex it will have been written well above a reading age of 12, which is considered the reading age for most public information in people's first language. Information, giving medication directives and self-care guides may be less than useful if health literacy has not been considered and some adaptation made. For example when explaining prenatal haemoglobinopathies screening to patients it should be remembered that there are risks related to the screening, there is no 'cure' and one option would be termination if the fetus is affected. But to date, how adversely a baby will be affected cannot be determined. Other day-to-day issues may be related to accessing smoking cessation services, whereby support for non-English speakers or those with limited English is poorly resourced or non-existent.

Even those with high levels of education attainment can be confused by medical information. Writing in the *New England Journal of Medicine* in November 2009, Parker *et al.* present a dilemma experienced by parents who were themselves doctors and were prescribed Tamiflu for their child. They experienced further distress and confusion because the prescribed dose was 3 or 4 teaspoons, but the package came with a syringe marked with milligrams (Parker *et al.*, 2009). Were the parents to give teaspoons of medication or use a syringe and be precise? Providing information, in distressing circumstances, calls for clarity, accuracy, as well as an awareness of decision complexities, thereby enabling informed choices. It frequently requires additional time, especially for those who have limited literacy skills.

Thinking and Discussion Point

Explaining how to use asthma inhalers correctly and why this is necessary can be time consuming. What potential problems may arise when the patient is from an East European country, without an interpreter, and given he speaks limited English? Consider a similar situation with a Spanish-speaking patient where you consider yourself able to speak Spanish. Finally, imagine this as a three-way consultation with an interpreter present. Discuss how interpreter services in your area or practice are used, and the strengths and limitations of such a service

Practical Exercise

Select two or three leaflets from www.patient. co.uk on sexual health and/or cancer prevention. Try to access the same leaflets in another language but one you have some competency in. Translate the leaflets back into English and compare with the English version. Identify what has been lost, embellished, misunderstood or incorrect.

If our skills are limited to word-by-word translation the essence will most certainly be limited and any nuances or caveats missed. Equally, if our skills are good we may discover the leaflets have been:

- poorly written in the first instance in English;
- well written but poorly translated;
- a combination of the above;
- well written and translated but for a sophisticated level of literacy;

- well written and translated to an acceptable standard.

The complexity of the information can also add to difficulties. People with comorbidities (or caring for those with comorbidities) and multiple social issues can miss out on opportunities as well as be at greater risk from mismanagement of medication. If you intend to provide a patient with written information you should consider readability and decide on its suitability for the specific patient and the situation.

The formula adapted by the Plain English Campaign is the FOG (Frequency of Gobbledegook). The test considers the number of sentences in a 100-word sample, the number of words in a sentence and other factors such as number of words with more than one syllable. Common comparisons about reading ability suggest that most of the literate general public can understand tabloid newspapers but fewer can understand broadsheet newspapers (Ewles and Simnett, 1999). If leaflets and other written material are given to patients, there should be consideration as to how complex and accurate the information is and if the patient can benefit from it at this time.

Thinking and Discussion Point

A woman has arrived in the UK from South Africa. Her UK employer has taken her passport and told her that UK doctors charge fees so best to avoid visiting a doctor. The woman had left school at 11 years of age with low level literacy and was ill-equipped to find out about healthcare for herself. She was also fearful of her immigration status. Meanwhile, her diabetes was not being controlled and her eyesight was deteriorating. By the time she sought help from a GP, irreversible damage had occurred. She struggled with all aspects of her diabetic care, such as managing a good diet with the income and facilities she had, getting help and using public transport, attending social events as well as healthcare appointments. She may appear to have English language skills but may need help with written information. What additional support may be available via the general practice?

Health literacy is not just about translation but encompasses similar issues to health promotion: being able to make informed decisions, knowing how and when to access healthcare, to self-care and to safely medicate. According to Protheroe, low literacy and numeracy levels are factors in health inequalities and increase the risk of adverse events. For those with good literacy skills and health knowledge, there is still a need to explore patient understanding, especially when dealing with complex and emotional issues (Protheroe *et al.*, 2009).

Health inequalities

Over the 30 years since the publication of the *Black Report* in 1980 and the *Health Divide* in 1987, health inequalities have been increasingly recognized as a public health priority within public health circles (Townsend *et al.*, 1988). However, it was not until 1998 that the issue truly arrived on the political agenda, when the Acheson Report was published (Acheson, 1998). Since the publication of the White Paper *Tackling Health Inequalities* (Department of Health, 2003), the need to address health inequalities has become part of contemporary healthcare practice. Within general practice these inequalities are encountered daily. Patients with multiple disadvantage experience greater levels of morbidity, comorbidity and complex social problems. Chronic illness, teenage pregnancy, poor postnatal outcomes, children on the 'at risk' registers, drug and alcohol abuse, intimate violence and premature death are some of the ways inequalities are experienced. Accidents are more common in areas of deprivation, both in the workplace and at home, and enduring mental health problems are more prevalent. The risk factors associated with poor health outcomes such as unsafe sexual behaviour, smoking and poor nutrition, for example, are encountered in communities with disadvantage. Although further research is still needed, Ashworth *et al.* have explored the quality markers for GP provision in areas of deprivation (Ashworth *et al.*, 2008).

As noted earlier, the most striking aspect of these inequalities is life expectancy. The role of general practice in addressing these inequalities may seem limited but, to reiterate, the Royal College of Physicians in their 2010 paper, *How*

Doctors can Close the Gap, state that addressing health inequalities is part of the role of all doctors, especially GPs (Royal College of Physicians, 2010). The social and physical environments, as well as the risk factors facing patients, become evident to local GPs. GPs can be advocates for change and can identify what additional support services may be needed and how healthcare needs to be adapted. For example, smoking cessation services may need to be in a local venue on a housing estate or may need to have more input and may need to be provided by local health trainers with appropriate language skills.

It is probable that ad hoc modifications to services and advocacy happen, but systematic and planned interventions offer more insight into addressing inequalities effectively. For example, Abdullahi *et al.* carried out a qualitative study to explore the low uptake of cervical screening in Camden, London by Somali women (Abdullahi *et al.*, 2009). They concluded that education, oral information and culturally appropriate services would improve uptake. In pluralist societies, translation and interpretation services can reduce inequalities but there is also a need to be aware of the limitations of such provision and the skills needed in consultations and information giving, given the subtleties of language.

Thinking and Discussion Point

A patient has an autistic child and is struggling to care. She was told by neighbours it was linked to the MMR and wants to know who is to blame. The already disadvantaged mother now has to negotiate with a number of agencies to get support and begins to feel it could have been avoided if she hadn't consented to the MMR. Take a leaflet about MMR vaccination or look at NHS booklets provided for parents of children under five and the sections on vaccination. Consider how this might be helpful in helping those with social disadvantages. What additional support should the practice provide to help parents give informed consent and what additional support could be given to this parent? What are the local data indicating about prevalence and trends of mumps, measles and rubella and do they reflect vaccination uptake?

As well as the written word, our colloquial speech can lead to misinterpretation and misunderstanding. Assumption about behaviours and attitudes may result in reduced opportunities. For example, Dormandy *et al.* (2008) found that GPs did not always offer antenatal sickle cell screening and Vogt *et al.* (2005) found evidence that older people with chronic obstructive respiratory disease were not necessarily offered smoking cessation referrals. While patient demand and expectation may guard against such shortcomings, those patients already disadvantaged may be unaware of their entitlement and/or the benefits.

In areas not noted for social deprivation, general practices should still be aware of health inequalities, with those patients who are disadvantaged experiencing greater levels of morbidity while being a minority within the wider community. Inadequate public transport services, for example, could be a barrier to healthcare services and a lack of social programmes for older vulnerable people may lead to isolation, depression and insufficient physical activity. 'Walking for Health' initiatives may favour the more affluent patients. Care provision may be limited for those with social disadvantage, especially where the workforce, whether voluntary or not for profit, perceive or experience anxiety about working with chaotic families or in adverse settings. Healthcare provision in rural areas or areas of deprivation may therefore be sub-optimal and may even further contribute to inequalities, being less attractive to the potential workforce.

The 'simple' lifestyle change advice offered to patients is often based on the biomedical model; for example, we know the link between smoking and cancer. Health promotion interventions, however, have to be skilfully designed and implemented to meet the need of the individual patient and appropriate to the context of the local community if they are to be of benefit.

Practical Exercise

In your practice and in the area covered by your practice do a mini audit of the patient encounters during a 7-day period. Note the patients' postcodes, their reasons for accessing healthcare, smoking status and, if possible, employment or income status. What proactive processes are in place that address the needs of these patients with regards to health inequalities, whether practice based or not?

In Bromley by Bow in Tower Hamlets, London, an area of deprivation with significant health inequalities, a range of culturally sensitive health and well-being activities have been set up, able to provide information about a variety of social issues such as housing and benefits. Such input is justified in this area but the challenge may be more difficult in areas with very mixed patient groups, where a minority have disadvantage. The health promotion domains of the Ottawa Charter were exemplified by Dr William Bird, a GP in an affluent semi-rural practice in the Thames Valley, when he set up the 'Health Walks' scheme in 1995 which is now a national programme in partnership with Natural England. The scheme promotes and implements regular local and safe walking for those most in need.

Reducing disadvantage, per se, starts with childhood and various government initiatives, including the Sure Start scheme, have been set up with the aim of giving children the best possible start in life. Evaluation of these schemes is complex but overall these established centres have been recognized as positive contributors to potentially reducing inequalities (Kane, 2008).

Practical Exercise

Explore the local Sure Start centres in your practice area. Find out about the management and performance indicators. How are they assessed and regulated? Do they address local health inequalities issues?

Health inequalities have also been part of the climate change and sustainable health agenda. The scope of this chapter and book is limited with regard to climate change debates but in brief it is clear that those who are most vulnerable and already disadvantaged are the first to become the 'victims' of environmental changes.

Data are still being generated and analysed from two European tragedies – the deaths in Paris in August 2003 during a heat wave and the ongoing psychological and social disruption to some of the Cumbrian residents caught up in the flooding of November 2009. Could family doctors and community health services have been more proactive, and what could they have done to reduce the impact of those extreme weather conditions?

The research is on-going, but some factors are already evident. In Cumbria, those who suffered most had existing health problems and social disadvantage, and lacked the resources and skills associated with resilience, prompt adaptation and response. As the situation deteriorated, so their problems escalated. After the immediate crisis subsided, those who survived were further disadvantaged and likely to have on-going health and social problems. In the longer term, lessons learnt are likely to suggest that primary healthcare providers need to be more proactive; and weather charts for mid- and short-term forecasts should be sent to health professionals with additional warnings and comments. For example, access to healthcare was seriously impeded in Cumbria yet patients needed supplies of medications, nursing services and some reassurance, as well as food, water and heat. The key questions are: How quickly can local and healthcare services coordinate emergency care? Can the vulnerable be identified and supported and by whom?

In France, the health system differs, as did the weather, but extreme heat, poor neighbourhoods and those weakened by existing morbidity were effectively abandoned. Without food, access to help, cooling systems such as fans and 'friendly' neighbours, their existing chronic illnesses quickly overwhelmed them. There may have been limited options but it is notable that while all of Paris was experiencing very high temperatures, the deaths occurred in the deprived areas.

Beyond the UK, primary care is also often at the forefront of the health inequalities associated with indigenous populations. Cunningham and others highlight the disparity in life expectancy, and the prevalence of smoking, alcohol and drug abuse and obesity in many minority indigenous populations. These higher levels of risk factors and 'modifiable' health determinants present the GP with

a number of challenges with regard to potential interventions (Cunningham, 2010). The Ottawa Charter may offer some direction, for example advocating on behalf of the local community, reorienting health services to meet local need, creating supportive environments for change and contributing to public policy initiatives.

The health inequalities agenda is no longer for those marginally interested or those with some special interest and skills, but has to be an integral part of medical practice and within general practice this translates to a close alliance with patients, local populations and public health.

Health inequalities are global issues. Poverty and conflict can displace millions, encourage mass migration, and people trafficking and various criminal activities seen as necessary for survival. In the UK many GPs will have patients who have disadvantages associated with global inequalities, some as a result of torture. The Medical Foundation for the Care of Victims of Torture (www.torturecare.org.uk/contact_us/34) can advise and take referrals. Other agencies and charities, such as 'Project: London' (www.doctorsoftheworld.org.uk/project-london/default.Asp) offer direct support to such vulnerable people.

Health promotion for 'healthy' patients

Since the start of the NHS general practice has had a role in promoting health, enabling patients to access preventative medicine, such as screening, advice, routine care during change such as antenatal and postnatal care, baby clinics and sexual health clinics. The skills associated with this type of health promotion need to be honed and practised.

Preventative medicine can include routine monitoring, new patient checks and assessments. Data about an individual are recorded from taking a history, biomedical tests such as urine analysis, blood pressure readings and BMI calculations. It may become evident that more physical activity is desirable, risk factors such as high alcohol consumption levels may be identified or it may emerge that the patient is at risk of social isolation or burn out. For the 'well' patient, the situation may result in breaking bad or unexpected and unwelcome news. One or more of the 'five As' may be helpful – ask, assess, advise, assist, arrange – and thus form an enabling consultation. The WHO Diabetes Action Online resource (www.who.int/diabetesactiononline/about/fiveAs/en/index.html) relates the five As to diabetic patient-centred care but they are, of course, transferable to other settings. Two key questions to explore in these situations are 'What changes are advisable and possible?' and 'Is the patient accepting change?'

At a population level, the Quality Outcomes Framework (QOF) and payments for recording such data have influenced practices in organizing systematic profiling of their patients, thus offering the potential for early intervention where indicated (Ashworth *et al.*, 2008). Vaccinations are also part of the preventative agenda, whether for children and young people, occupational need, travel or because of age-related risks, such as influenza vaccination for older patients.

Screening more deliberately looks for disease, at an early or even precursor stage. It is potentially harmful as it can result in false negative and false positive outcomes and relies on the compliance of a critical mass of a specific target group. Most UK screening programmes are organized through general practice and as a consequence patients may request advice before consenting, with an expectation that the GPs and practice nurses will explain the screening process and why it is advisable. The level of informed consent provided is certainly contentious. As health professionals, the role of 'editing' information or selective information giving is a challenge.

While screening overall has benefits to the public, it has to be balanced against the potential harm and anxiety to the individual (Raffle and Gray, 2007).

Thinking and Discussion Point

Take, for example, a woman in her 50s with poor or limited English. She is reluctant to take time off work for breast screening. She has no experience of family or friends with breast cancer, she breastfed her four children, all born during her twenties, and has never used hormonal contraception. She is embarrassed, and fearful of a positive outcome. She will also find it difficult to get to the screening centre. What are the options for addressing this patient's anxieties and queries? Can practice protocols help?

Other screening programmes have similar dilemmas but also present GPs with challenges as they respond to:

■ those at high risk but anxious about screening;
■ those at low risk and not taking advantage;
■ those who are non-attendees/not willing /complacent;
■ those with 'positive' results or who have been asked to repeat/recalled.

Public information may be inappropriate for some because of language barriers, literacy levels or access difficulties, and the invitation itself may feel irrelevant to the recipient.

Advice is sought by many patients in general practice and a good source of generic information for patients is www.patient.co.uk. It is perfectly acceptable to not know all the answers, to be aware of limitations and in some cases seek advice from colleagues or refer patients elsewhere as appropriate. Advice can, of course, be categorized and frequently patients without any known morbidity ask about travel issues, and preventative care such as malaria precautions, use of sun block and vaccinations. Some will ask about their fitness for extreme activities, high-altitude trekking and high-risk activities such as diving and may need a signature for insurance purposes. In many cases there is uncertainty, contraindications and contested advice (e.g. over the use of hormonal contraception when the patient is planning SCUBA diving).

The skills needed in such consultations are associated with the 'personal counselling' quadrant of Beattie's model (Figures 11.3 and 11.4), guiding the patient with regard to authoritative information sources and being able to critique information (Beattie *et al.*, 1993). Other types of advice are associated with complex social and personal circumstances such as domestic violence, tackling bullying at work, locally or in a child's school, relationship problems, benefits and carers' needs. Such concerns verge on the psychological distress continuum – a well person in an at-risk situation, vulnerable to mental and emotional morbidity. General practices sometimes have access to welfare and social advisors, but care again should be taken not to give inaccurate or inappropriate information. The role of the GP as a listener and counsellor in such instances is valued.

Antenatal and postnatal care and education juxtapose health promotion, preventative care and screening. Pregnancy is sometimes welcomed, sometimes a 'surprise', and sometimes unwanted. Lifestyle, general health and well-being and pre-conception health are all factors that could influence progress as well as social circumstances. Women may have sought advice about conceiving and pre-conception care, such as diet and folic acid intake, weight loss or gain, help with smoking cessation and advice about alcohol. Such information is readily available but some patients may need more support and explanation, and more guidance for and referral for behaviour modification. Once pregnancy is confirmed, opportunities present to promote healthy eating and other lifestyle issues, to offer screening and antenatal education.

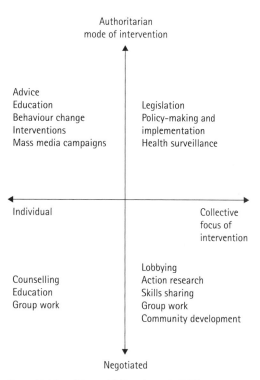

Figure 11.4 Beattie's model (Beattie et al., 1993).

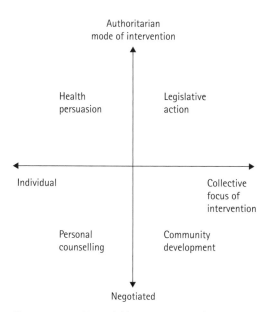

Figure 11.3 Beattie's model (Beattie et al., 1993).

As mentioned earlier, screening does carry risks and helping the woman make informed decisions is paramount but not always straightforward. Sickle cell screening, for example, can be a risk to the pregnancy, may cause emotional distress to the mother and may result in a dilemma about whether to continue with the pregnancy if the fetus is found to be sickle cell positive. Counselling services are available in high-prevalence areas and it is difficult to know how the child will be affected, what impact will having a child with sickle cell disease have on the family, and what would be the impact of a termination. Within a short space of time a woman, not necessarily unwell, has had a pregnancy confirmed, agreed to the screening and is now faced with an unwelcome situation.

In the setting of general practice these complex personal issues can be explored if they arise, but it is important to acknowledge that science does not have all the answers.

While pregnancy is a healthy situation for many, during the antenatal period a number of problems could arise that must be dealt with early to mini-mize harm. Smoking and obesity present serious health risks and early referral to behaviour modi-fication services is advisable but needs to be done with care. Motivational interviewing and support are indicated. Blood pressure and urine analysis may indicate preeclampsia and/or gestational dia-betes, conditions which need to be addressed with some urgency.

In areas of deprivation, health inequalities are especially evident in antenatal and postnatal out-comes, indicating the greater need for support. Higher stillbirths, low birthweight, complications and poor maternal health can be expected, as well as greater numbers of teenage pregnancies. Breastfeeding rates may be low, living conditions and income may be poor and higher prevalence of child and maternal morbidity experienced. Community midwives and health visitors pro-vide much of the routine care and support and will know what services are available locally and what interventions are in place. They will also have information about various health promo-tion campaigns at certain times of the year, such as child safety and breastfeeding awareness. They will have lists of local parent and child groups and will run baby clinics which offer routine advice on child development, manag-ing weaning and teething, nappy rash and other such concerns as well as the crying baby. While many parents source information from reliable websites and professionals as well as friends and family, and are able to discern good information, more vulnerable parents will need the support of professionals who are easily accessible. They may present more frequently at general practice. The Department of Health have published two books – *The Pregnancy Book* and *The Birth to Five Book* – for first time mothers and these are also available on-line (Department of Health, 2007a, 2007b). These books cover a wide range of issues and are a useful resource during clinics and consultations.

Sexual health is also an aspect of the health pro-motion role sometimes offered in general practice. While this can vary with local arrangements, such as whether there is a young persons' sexual health clinic provision, most general practices will be able to prescribe, advise or refer patients with regard to sexual health, whether related to con-traception, sub-fertility or infection prevention, screening and treatment.

In summary, the healthy patient is an infre-quent consulter in general practice, yet many opportunities exist to be proactive as a health promoter for that individual patient and for the local population. Good listening skills, awareness of reliable information and local referral options are essential, as well as demonstrating a willing-ness to be open to new knowledge, consult and use NICE guidance. Recording a summary in the patient's notes with regard to the essence of your intervention becomes an integral aspect of health promotion within the general practice.

Thinking and Discussion Point

A young woman, recently separated from her partner of 3 years, has resumed smoking. She has come because of an irritating and persistent cough. During the consultation she tells about her financial anxieties and her job being under threat. Would you raise the issue of her smok-ing? If so how and if not why?

Practical Exercise

In your practice review the cervical screening rates and identify the processes used to inves-tigate non-attendees. How does your practice compare with others locally for uptake of cervi-cal screening?

Health promotion for patients with early signs and symptoms

A patient may arrive at the practice with some concerns, or has been asked to see the GP or nurse following some routine investigations. The patient may be a 'well' patient needing a form signed for health insurance, requesting a 'sick note' because of a sports injury, or wanting the contraceptive pill. Another patient, recently made redundant, may be wondering what is best for an aged, frail and forgetful parent.

GPs have a role in understanding the medical, social and psychological issues that impact on patients and their well-being, but it can be difficult to prioritize and decide how best to proceed with what is presented. Preventative medicine links both population health and individual health. Rose *et al.* (2008) present complex arguments regarding large-scale programmes that prevent or identify disease in a small number of people and the caveats about such strategies. The alternative approach is targeting those at high risk. The continuum of disease has to be explored in the context of people's lives, with the GP often having to decide whether to intervene or not and to explain risks.

Moynihan (2010) discusses the challenges of identifying the 'pre-hypertensive' patient and whether they should or should not have drug treatment. Having blood pressure readings that are at the upper range of normal should, he argues, be 'treated' with lifestyle advice, but the pressure to prescribe is ever present and subsequently a well person becomes a 'patient with hypertension' yet no overall change is evident in population health and lives saved. Lifestyle advice may also be ignored by the patient given they feel well, changes may be difficult and they don't conceptualize the 'risks'. Blood pressure readings have come to represent this notion of when a patient is sick or well, at risk with the potential to reduce or manage risk, and when medication could make a difference but only to a few. Hypertension, on the other hand, is classed as the 'silent killer', with cardiovascular diseases still representing one of the major causes of morbidity and premature mortality and yet potentially it could be modified with lifestyle change.

Signs without symptoms are also identified by routine clinical encounters or through mass media alerts, and campaigns suggest that you see your GP if you notice signs such as a change in bowel habit, moles and lumps, or weight gain or loss. Mass screening such as cervical screening can also identify a 'change' that may justify further investigations.

Equally patients may present with concerns about symptoms that may be time-limited conditions or easily managed but some lifestyle advice may be appropriate.

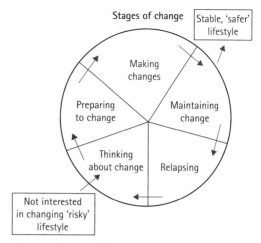

Figure 11.5 'Stages of Change' model (Health Education Authority, 1993).

Time invested, albeit 'brief intervention', in health promotion at these consultations is advised, given that the patients have themselves presented concerns. The Stages of Change Model (Figure 11.5) can guide the trajectory of the consultations, assessing where the patient is in terms of wanting to change and readiness to change as well as the opportunity to do motivational intervening (Health Education Authority, 1993).

Thinking and Discussion Point

Breast cancer awareness month is October. What are the pros and cons of such events for GP practices and for patients?

Practical Exercise

Review the patient information in the practice – posters and leaflets and website – and assess:
❑ Is it up to date and current?
❑ Is it likely to make a difference in prompting a patient to change/take action?
❑ Is it accessible to most patients? Who may be excluded?
❑ Does it link to local services/opportunities?

Health promotion for patients with non-communicable diseases

The growth in non-communicable diseases and complex comorbidities dominates the workload of general practice and although much of this work will be associated with clinical concerns, such as reviewing medication and regular monitoring of blood pressure and renal function, for example, improvements and/or maintenance of current health status can probably be enhanced with lifestyle intervention and modification.

The regular contact with these patients also provides regular opportunities to assess readiness to change and early detection of deterioration, whether physical, social or psychological.

Older smokers with chronic illness can benefit from referrals to smoking cessation programmes. Vogt and co-workers reported that some GPs have been reluctant to make these referrals (Vogt *et al.*, 2005, 2007). GPs are well placed to look at the wider social context of these patients, and to consider, if their partners and carers are also smokers, whether they should both be referred. Do they need motivational interviewing to assess readiness to change, and how easy are the cessation services for such patients to access? Patients need also to be aware of chance of relapse and that they will probably need to be referred to a cessation programme more than once.

Smoking is also associated with boredom and lack of social engagement, and withdrawal from former activities that may now seem unrealistic. Income and an increasing dependency on benefits may be influencing factors in patients with chronic illness who continue to smoke. As Tones and Green remind us, the healthy choice needs to be the easy choice (Tones and Green, 2004) so within general practice there is a need to consider whether benefits are being maximized and where to refer for further information and activities that may be beneficial, such as local Walking for Health groups.

Malnutrition, poor nutrition, dietary restriction and obesity have an important role in all stages of chronic illness. Patients with specialist needs – such as those with coeliac disease, raised cholesterol levels, kidney disease and obstructive problems such as oesophageal cancer – may need to be referred to the dietician. But many patients will benefit from becoming 'healthy eaters', reducing their BMI, and increasing intake of certain foods and vitamins, such as those with or at risk of osteoporosis. In general, eating habits have proved to be very difficult to modify. Within general practice an awareness of local context will help health professionals provide supportive information and advice.

Cultural habits, the availability of fresh fruit and vegetables at low cost, cooking skills and facilities, and local programmes to improve diets, sometimes with health trainers, all influence the options available.

For type 2 diabetic patients the DESMOND programme (Diabetes Education and Self Management for Ongoing and Newly Diagnosed) is now seen as an evidence-based option for referral, addressing not only dietary modification but also increasing patient understanding of the nature of the disease, other factors such as smoking and physical activity change and how to sustain change. It has been developed based on sound adult education principles (Davies *et al.*, 2008). For patients with type 1 diabetes DAFNE (Dose Adjusted for Normal Eating and Exercise) is in place and has also shown promising results with regards to helping people to modify behaviour and sustain change.

Alcohol consumption has become a greater cause of concern in recent years, not only because of social problems such as increased sexual risk associated with alcohol consumption (and drugs), but also trauma and an increase in chronic illness at younger ages. Liver diseases and chronic alcoholism remain major challenges for healthcare professionals, but within general practice the additional burdens, such as family breakdown, may also be obvious. Local social programmes for support may be variable and some will be based with not-for-profit agencies or charities. For those patients with access to the internet the 'Down your drink' website offers a pragmatic option for the GP and health professionals as well as the patient and their family (www.downyourdrink. org.uk/).

People may be defensive about their drinking and dietary habits but may freely offer details about their physical activity levels. People with chronic illness may have inadequate physical activity which exacerbates their condition, increasing the trajectory of the degenerative process. It may seem obvious that people tend to become less active with age and disease, especially where an individual has been sedentary for a number of years. However, being mobile and active is advisable for all, according to circumstances. Physical activity helps with general well-being. However patients may be uncertain about what is safe and possible and frequently will encounter directives such as 'check with your GP'.

Exercise on prescription has now become widely available as an option for GPs, with exercise specialists able to assess patients and devise programmes with high levels of supervision. Patient rehabilitation, for example following a stroke, can improve the outcome for patients. Often these programmes work in conjunction with clinical physiotherapists as a follow-on after the initial rehabilitation, with the overall aspiration being that patients will have the confidence to continue being active as best they can, using local facilities.

For older people with restricted options 'armchair aerobics' have been shown to be beneficial, especially when done within a social context.

Patients with chronic illness may benefit from lifestyle modification and this can be facilitated by accessing or referring to local services and provision, being aware of charities and not-for-profit organizations that can support social change and infrastructure, and engaging with the patient self-help groups often related to the disease, such as diabetes UK (www.diabetes.org.uk) and the British Heart Foundation (www.bhf.org.uk). Indeed, the growth of self-help groups has become beneficial to the wider healthcare workforce, enabling the public and patients to gain good reliable information as well as actively campaigning and advocating and fundraising for research and improved services.

Finally, carers, often registered at the same practice as their cared for, can be vulnerable and their needs should be addressed. Again, local provision varies but Crossroads schemes are widely available (www.crossroads.org.uk). For patients with cancer and their families, Macmillan Cancer Support offers a range of support to carers (www.macmillan.org.uk). Carers' needs vary, from first recognizing they are carers to adapting to a changing situation. Equally their own health, independent of the situation, may easily be neglected and subsequently they present late with serious or acute situations, which may precipitate a crisis with regard to care needs. It is in general practice that such situations can be anticipated and either alleviated or managed in such a way as to reduce potentially harmful and distressing outcomes.

Thinking and Discussion Point

Knee problems have been discussed at the practice team meeting and some feel surgery is justified while others argue that patients must have a successful weight reduction programme and the practice needs to design a protocol. Consider how this protocol could be designed and piloted.

Practical Exercise

Assess how many patients have been referred to exercise programmes, identify the chronic conditions they have and what follow-up is in place. For the same patients, assess their smoking status and their experiences of smoking cessation referral.

Everyday work in general practice will entail some aspect of health promotion but this is especially so with patients with chronic diseases. By glancing at any of the 100 cases in the book *100 Cases in General Practice* (Stephenson *et al.*, 2009) it becomes clear that GPs have an extensive role in health promotion and healthcare in their communities.

SUMMARY POINTS

To conclude, the most important messages of this chapter are as follows:

- Health promotion is an integral part of general practice work.
- Health promotion is difficult to define, is eclectic and contested, as well as political in nature.
- A number of theories and models are used to guide practice and identify relevant skills for practice.
- Within the context of general practice, health professionals can be health promoting in their practice and can engage specifically in planned health promotion interventions.
- The planning of health promotion activity facilitates evaluation, thereby contributing to the growing evidence base that is related to interventions rather than determinants.
- Evidence is from qualitative and quantitative paradigms.
- Ethical issues need to be identified and considered.
- Health promotion seeks to address health inequalities at local, national and international levels, through collaborative working, within and beyond the medical arena, endorsing WHO charters and declarations.

References

Abdullahi, A., Copping, J., Kessel, A., Luck, M. and Bonell, C. 2009: Cervical screening: perceptions and barriers to uptake among Somali women in Camden. *Public Health* 123, 680–5.

Acheson, D. 1998: *Independent inquiry into inequalities in health: a report*. London: The Stationery Office.

Ashworth, M., Medina, J. and Morgan, M. 2008: Effect of social deprivation on blood pressure monitoring and control in England: a survey of data from the quality and outcomes framework. *British Medical Journal* 337, a2030.

Beattie, A., Gott, M., Jones, L. and Sidell, M. 1993: *Health and wellbeing: a reader*. Basingstoke: Macmillan.

Boyce, T., Peckham, S., Hann, A. and Trenholm, S. 2010: *A pro-active approach. Health promotion and ill-health prevention. An inquiry into the quality of general practice in England*. London: The King's Fund.

Cunningham, C. 2010: Health of indigenous peoples. *British Medical Journal* 340, c1840.

Davies, M.J., Heller, S., Skinner, T.C., Campbell, M.J., Carey, M.E., Cradock, S., Dallosso, H.M., Daly, H., Doherty, Y., Eaton, S., Fox, C., Oliver, L., Rantell, K., Rayman, G., Khunti, K., on behalf of the Diabetes Education and Self Management for Ongoing and Newly Diagnosed (DESMOND) Programme 2008: Effectiveness of the Diabetes Education and Self Management for Ongoing and Newly Diagnosed (DESMOND) programme for people with newly diagnosed type 2 diabetes: cluster randomised controlled trial. *British Medical Journal* 336, 491.

Department of Health 2003: *Tackling health inequalities: a programme for action*. www.dh.gov.uk/en/Publicationsandstatistics/Publications/PublicationsPolicyAndGuidance/DH_4008268 (accessed May 2011).

Department of Health 2007a: *The birth to five book*. London: Department of Health.

Department of Health 2007b: *The pregnancy book*. London: Department of Health.

Dormandy, E., Gulliford Martin, C., Reid Erin, P., Brown, K. and Marteau, T.M. 2008: Delay between pregnancy confirmation and sickle cell and thalassaemia screening: a population based cohort study. *British Journal of General Practice* 58, 154–9.

Duncan, P. 2007: *Critical perspectives on health*. Basingstoke: Palgrave Macmillan.

Ewles, L. and Simnett, I. 1999: *Promoting health: a practical guide*. London: Baillière Tindall.

Ewles, L. and Simnett, I. 2003: *Promoting health: a practical guide*. Edinburgh: Baillière Tindall.

Health Education Authority 1993: *Helping people change: training course for primary care professionals. National Unit for Health Promotion in Primary Care*. Oxford: Health Education Authority.

Kane, P. 2008: Sure Start Local Programmes in England. *The Lancet*, 372, 1610–12.

London Health Observatory 2011: Health inequalities. www.lho.org.uk/LHO_Topics/National_Lead_Areas/HealthInequalitiesOverview.aspx (accessed May 2011).

Marmot, M. 2010: *Fair society, healthy lives – strategic review of health inequalities in England post 2010.* London: The Marmot Review.

Marmot, M., Friel, S., Bell, R., Houweling, T.A.J. and Taylor, S. 2008: Closing the gap in a generation: health equity through action on the social determinants of health. *The Lancet*, 372, 1661–9.

Moynihan, R. 2010: Who benefits from treating prehypertension? *British Medical Journal* 341, c4442.

NICE (National Institute for Health and Clinical Excellence) 2006: PH1 Brief interventions and referral for smoking cessation: guidance. http://guidance.nice.org.uk/PH1/Guidance/pdf/English (accessed May 2011).

Naidoo, J. and Wills, J. 2000: *Health promotion; foundations for practice.* London: Baillière Tindall.

Parker, R.M., Wolf, M.S., Jacobson, K.L. and Wood, A.J.J. 2009: Risk of confusion in dosing Tamiflu oral suspension in children. *New England Journal of Medicine* 361: 1912–13.

Prochaska, J.O. and Diclemente, C.O. 1986: Towards a comprehensive model of change. In: Millen, W.R. and Heathen, N. (eds) *Treating addictive behaviours: process and change.* New York: Plenum Press.

Protheroe, J., Nutbeam, D. and Rowlands, G. 2009: Health literacy: a necessity for increasing participation in health care. *British Journal of General Practitioners* 59, 721–3.

Raffle, A. and Gray, M. 2007: *Screening evidence and practice.* Oxford: Oxford University Press.

Rose, G., Khaw, K.-T. and Marmot, M. 2008: *Rose's strategy of preventive medicine.* Oxford: Oxford University Press.

Royal College of Physicians 2010: *How doctors can close the gap: tackling the social determinants of health through culture change, advocacy and education.* London: Royal College of Physicians.

Stephenson, A., Mueller, M. and Grabinar, J. 2009: *100 Cases in general practice.* London: Hodder Arnold.

Tones, K. and Green, J. 2004: *Health promotion: planning and strategies.* London: Sage.

Townsend, P., Whitehead, M. and Davidson, N. 1988: *Inequalities in health: the Black Report and the health divide.* London: Penguin.

Vogt, F., Hall, S. and Marteau, T.M. 2005: General practitioners' and family physicians' negative beliefs and attitudes towards discussing smoking cessation with patients: a systematic review. *Addiction* 100, 1423–31.

Vogt, F., Hall, S. and Marteau, T. 2007: General practitioners' beliefs about effectiveness and intentions to recommend smoking cessation services: qualitative and quantitative studies. *BMC Family Practice* 8, 39.

World Health Organization 1986: Discussion document on the concepts and principles of health promotion. *Health Promotion* 1.

Wylie, A. 2002: Health promotion in medical undergraduate curricula: a question of definition. Paper presented at the 10th Ottawa Conference on Medical Education, Ottawa.

Wylie, A. 2004a: Health promotion in general practice. In: Stephenson, A. (ed.) *A textbook of general practice.* London: Arnold.

Wylie, A. 2004b: Health promotion in medical undergraduate education; an exploration of the epistemology and the challenge. PhD, King's College, London.

Wylie, A. and Thompson, S. 2007: Establishing health promotion in the modern medical curriculum: a case study. *Medical Teacher* 29, 766–71.

Further reading

www.nice.org.uk
www.bhf.org.uk
www.plainenglish.co.uk/examples/gobbledygook-generator.html
www.heacademy.ac.uk/best

www.wfh.naturalengland.org.uk
www.nice.org.uk/usingguidance/commissioningguides/pulmonaryrehabilitationserviceforpatients
withcopd/specifying.jsp

SINGLE BEST ANSWER QUESTIONS

11.1 Mark, 29, has a football-related knee injury and needs a statement for fitness to work and some analgesic. He is a rare visitor and you take the opportunity to update his records. He tells you he smokes about 20 a day. How best should you respond to this information?

a) Provide information about the cessation service
b) Ignore the information and make no further reference
c) Explore his smoking history and ask him if he has any concerns
d) Give him a leaflet about the harm smoking does
e) Make him an appointment to see the nurse.

11.2 Mary agrees to the antenatal screening offer and wants to get a scan photo. She is 40, with BMI 32 and has been trying for this pregnancy for some time. Do you:

a) Make the arrangements without further discussion?
b) Explore her concerns, if any, about this pregnancy?
c) Tell her about the increased risk associated with her age and screening?
d) Tell her about the increased risks to her and baby with her BMI?
e) Ask what she knows about screening apart from the option to have a scan photo?

11.3 Jim, 56, has COPD and has come for his influenza vaccine. He is well known to the practice team and still smokes, although has cut down and rolls his own for economy as he is not working. On looking at his notes you realize he has never been referred to the cessation services in the practice.

a) Do you leave him alone with regards to his smoking?
b) Do you ask if he would like to have an appointment with the smoking cessation advisor?

c) Do you suggest a follow-up appointment at which time you will discuss his smoking?
d) Do you joke about his lifelong smoking – you can't teach old dog new tricks?
e) Do you give him a leaflet?

11.4 Khalid's blood pressure was raised when he went to the 'health check' bus at work and was told to see his GP. He is 49 and has BMI 29, otherwise well, with normal BP readings at the consultation and a non-smoker. His parents both died in their sixties with CVDs. Taking a history suggests his diet is calorie dense with saturated fats and refined carbohydrates. He exercises 'a little' but works long hours as a taxi driver. Do you:

a) Tell him not to worry – all is basically OK?
b) Decide to arrange fasting blood tests for cholesterol check and other tests for diabetes?
c) Advise him to lose weight and take more exercise?
d) Arrange for him to see the dietician?
e) Provide him with and discuss some information about healthy eating via the British Heart Foundation?

11.5 Paula's husband died six months ago after a stroke. She is lonely, eats out of boredom and fears the same could happen to her. She stopped smoking when he did 4 years ago but is often tempted. She noticed a poster about health walks which said 'check with your doctor' at some point. She wants to know more about these walks and if she can go on them.

a) You encourage her to join the scheme and explain more about it
b) You tell her to look into it
c) You take a history and consider depression
d) You suggest the exercise referral programme instead
e) You discourage it given she has not been very active in the past.

CHAPTER

12   HEALTHCARE ETHICS AND LAW

- Conflict and compromise
- Deciding for others: the question of capacity
- Moral and legal thinking in everyday clinical practice
- Sitting in: a suitable case for treatment
- The professional framework
- The law and professional regulation in practice
- Good practice and the moral stranger
- Moral antennae: paying attention to the issues
- Roles, rules and duties

- Duty
- An absolute duty?
- Four principles and scope
- Virtues and values
- Perspective and narrative
- Putting it all together
- Summary points
- References
- Further reading
- Single best answer questions

Broader questions about what is best for patients or staff, what it is right to do, or whether we are acting within the law commonly arise in practice for anyone who reflects on their work. This chapter suggests ways of approaching these issues and reaching conclusions that are satisfactory for all concerned.

LEARNING OBJECTIVES

By the end of the chapter, you will be able to:

- identify where moral and legal questions may arise in your work;
- understand how the law, professional regulation and medical ethics may ask different things of the practising doctor;
- confront the complexity of these requirements by using a framework to think though the issues;
- explore the different perspectives of all involved to create the best outcome possible in each situation.

Conflict and compromise

There may seem to be enough to do as a doctor, making clinical decisions at speed, without complicating things by asking 'whether something broadly accepted is really right', or 'what is really best' for this particular patient. Sometimes, however, those questions won't seem to go away, because the implications of the decision go beyond medicine, or because there is genuine conflict to be resolved. For instance, someone may ask the doctor to do something that the doctor thinks is wrong or cannot legally do. A diagnosis or a treatment may mean that someone can no longer do their job. Two patients may present at once with a shared complaint but different points of view about the best solution. Things that were hidden or unmentionable in families may suddenly need to be discussed, or members of that family may disagree about what should be done. The doctor may discover something that he or she feels should be reported to police or social services. All these problems may pile onto the doctor's desk in the same day.

Luckily these sorts of problems are not new to us. Negotiating life in a family or in the playground requires us to develop a sharp set of ideas about what is right or wrong, or what is best or most prudent to do in different circumstances. This is called a *moral sense*, and although we may each make slightly different decisions, the ability to detect and think about these sorts of things is as much part of human nature as wanting to eat nice food and making friends. As psychologists would say, the need for moral thinking and some of the skills are 'hardwired' into our brains.

So we have innate skills; but do we really need to do this extra work? Surely it is possible to bash on, ignoring the sort of problems outlined above? Our job as doctors is medicine, after all. Other things will somehow have to sort themselves out.

One of the flaws in this approach is that, whether we like it or not, the decisions we are making as doctors are not (or certainly not principally) for ourselves; they are for the welfare of other people.

There are lots of ways to look at ethical and legal cases, but try approaching the next case with the following ideas in mind:

- What are the main features of this case? (*summarize*)
- What moral and legal questions are we facing? (*focus*)
- Are we making any unwarranted *assumptions*? Should they be challenged?

Sometimes we need to think about the following:

- Can we analyse the dilemma in terms of our ethical *principles*?
- What are the possible *consequences* of different actions?
- Are there any *professional duties or guidelines*? Is there *law* about this situation?
- What are the *reasons* to accept or reject any possible solutions?
- What on balance should be done? (*conclude*)
- What are the *implications* of this for future practice?

Case Study 12.1

Tutor to patient: 'Good, you're well enough to go back to work now.'
Patient to tutor: 'But you don't understand what I have to deal with at work, doctor.'

Here are two people trying to reach a good decision. Each has special knowledge. There is conflict. Both have made assumptions. Behind those assumptions may be attitudes, and these may depend on cherished values or derive from bitter experience.

Thinking and Discussion Point

Take the above simple exchange and list as many different attitudes as you can think of (like 'Everyone should be at work unless they have a serious illness' or 'I've every right to take sick days off – everyone else does') that might be behind each statement. How might each affect the outcome and what compromises would have to be made to reach an agreement?
Try imagining the speakers swapping roles. What does this do to the ideas you have just had?

Have you heard a similar exchange while observing clinical work? If so, subject that exchange to the same processes.

Tutor quote

If you look carefully, you can detect legal or moral issues in almost every consultation. We don't necessarily need to address them, but we need to be aware what they are.

Deciding for others: the question of capacity

Making decisions with other people may not always be easy, but it may be even more complicated when we are being asked to make decisions for someone else; for instance, for someone who no longer seems to be able to make them for themselves. We need to think carefully how to approach complex decisions.

Case Study 12.2

A woman in her late forties presented to her GP with headaches. She was getting increasingly frantic about her mother's bizarre behaviour. Her mother had been diagnosed with early dementia and had been started on some medication. A carer had been arranged. Now the old lady was insisting on keeping mouldy food in the fridge and fiddling with the gas heating. She seemed withdrawn and did not even recognize her grandchildren or understand the surroundings of her own home. Neighbours had begun to insist something had to be done. The daughter thought her mother needed to live in a safer environment where there were trained staff, and wanted this organized quickly: she was worried there would be a crisis. However, when she had talked to her mother, the old lady, in spite of her apparent confusion, was very clear that she did not want to leave her own house. She had said she had always wanted to live out her days in her own home. 'There is no way I'm going to let them move me out of my house at my age. And remember whose side you are on.' The daughter wanted the doctor to intervene. He could raise the matter firmly with her mother, or make a referral to social services. She felt her mother was not in her right mind anymore and couldn't make rational decisions. 'After all, you have a duty to keep my mother safe, even if that means going against her wishes.'

In this case the doctor has a duty to both mother and daughter as his patients (and possibly to the wider society locally if things get worse), but it is also very clear there is no easy solution. Her patient is asking the doctor to consider acting against the wishes of her mother. Is this is a morally or legally acceptable thing to do? What does the doctor need to know? Has the old lady's judgement been called into question before? Do any others share the daughter's concern? Is there a real possibility something dangerous might happen?

When you are not sure what to do, there is a temptation to gather more and more information, to amass more details. Sometimes this seems to be just a way to avoid confronting a difficult moral issue. The bottom line in this case, however, is that the doctor has to make a judgement about whether the old lady knows what she is doing, whether she is capable of making proper decisions about herself, that is, about her mental 'capacity'. That is not something to be done lightly. There is extensive legislation governing those who lack capacity and the ways to go about making decisions for them about their health, home and finances. Each judgement is 'decision specific': there is no 'enduring declaration' of incapacity. Capacity is a flexible and relative status that may flux in the course of a patient's condition, and so a judgement will have to be made in reference to each new decision being considered.

Every doctor ought to be familiar with the outlines of the current law (see Box 12.1). However, the doctor must find a way of working so that proper concerns are not dismissed because of deference to a legal construct.

Student quote

'I know we are all looking for a black and white answer, but it seems to me that more often we are dealing with shades of grey.'

The Mental Capacity Act (Box 12.1)

The aim of the Act is to help those who care for others (over 16) who, through problems such as mental health problems, dementia or learning difficulties, may be considered unable to make decisions about not just their healthcare, but many aspects of their lives. It offers a framework for decision making in these situations.

Box 12.1 The Mental Capacity Act (England and Wales, 2005)

The Mental Capacity Act (England and Wales, 2005) is underpinned by five main general principles:

1) An individual must be assumed to have capacity to make judgements about themselves unless it is proven otherwise.
2) Individuals must be helped as much as possible to make their own decisions before they are considered to lack capacity.
3) If a decision seems unwise this in itself is not a measure of the individual's capacity to make that decision.
4) What is done must be done in the person's best interests.
5) The option chosen should be one that least restricts their basic rights and freedoms.

The Act provides for Independent Mental Capacity Advocates (IMCAs) who can be allocated to those judged to lack capacity to make certain decisions, but do not have friends or family who may be able to provide a view of what they may have wished for. IMCAs can also be involved where there is dispute amongst relatives or friends about what decision to take for someone who lacks capacity.

Thinking and Discussion Point

- What help or directions does the Mental Capacity Act give in this case?
- Do you think it still leaves the doctor uncertain as to what might or should be done? What other factors seem to you relevant to the decision?
- Do you think the way that things are done may be as important as what is done? If so, what should be aimed for and what avoided?

Student quote

'I think there's nothing medicine can't solve if you leave ethics and law out of it!'

Moral and legal thinking in everyday clinical practice

Ethics and law may seem quite separate from clinical medicine: after all, the thinking is not based on what scientists observe, but on reasoning about what is right or best, perhaps as outlined by 'experts'. On the other hand, both our cases above seem to suggest that ethical and legal thinking is intrinsic to the practice of medicine: in other words, we can't practise successfully as doctors without having an understanding of legal and moral thinking and how they might apply to the clinical problem in hand.

This latter idea seems to be backed up by the guidelines about various areas of practice published by statutory bodies, by the requirement before we practise to have some recognized medical insurance, and by what we see as the process in law when things appear to have gone wrong. But while the big issues that all these refer to feel like the exceptions to normal practice (and naturally none of us wants to fall foul of the law or the authorities), this chapter is just as concerned about the regular,

everyday, ordinary work that we do in general and community practice. New practitioners are often surprised by the way something apparently small can suddenly become of enormous consequence and, if it goes wrong, take a long time to sort out.

Tutor quote

I'm afraid I'm allergic to the idea that small concerns can be 'trivial'. Let's remember that the word 'trivial' comes from the Latin for 'crossroad' – where there is a decision to be made about which direction to take.

This chapter cannot cover every problem nor provide more than a sketch of moral and legal thinking, but it can offer frameworks and ways of approaching things: it can begin to provide the tools to help, pointing to the right approach in looking for answers when faced with confusing situations.

Ethics alert: some alarm 'symptoms' in consultations

- Feeling angry, or possibly any intense emotion
- Being tempted to tell a lie
- Trying to rush through something complex because you want to leave work
- Being very tired at the end of a long shift
- Using the phone when you should really see someone face to face
- Having to have a second consultation about the same problem (not as a follow-up)
- Two patients at once in the same consultation
- 'Better not write *that* down'
- Sitting in.

Sitting in: a suitable case for treatment

If you are a student or new GP about to sit in on a consultation with a teaching GP, there may be a series of obvious but important questions to ask. Is your focus on sorting out the patient's problems, or is it on helping you to learn medicine? Is the patient happy to have someone sitting in and hearing what is said? Has the patient been offered the option of the student leaving or of seeing another professional without a student?

Conventionally, these last questions bring together the two issues of *confidentiality* and *consent*. However, other issues may be lurking in the wings. You may be keen to learn, but have to get away to prepare for another class. The doctor may have to sort out an employment problem in the practice or squeeze other activities between the surgery and his or her afternoon visits. In the rush, you may find yourself watching or even being asked to do something that does not feel to you to be the best practice. Have you done all you could, or even the best you could in the circumstances? Have all the patient's concerns been properly addressed? Have you helped, or have you hindered, the primary clinical task?

Tutor quote

There are trade-offs to be made to get through a working day, and sometimes these leave us with lurking dissatisfaction or guilt – or even, perversely, a sense of pride in coping which our best selves know is only waiting for a fall.

The professional framework

Most medical schools these days do not ask qualifying doctors to swear an oath, but all who practise in the UK must work to the rules or guidelines laid down by the General Medical Council (GMC). Most other countries have similar arrangements, some directly following the lead of the GMC. Doctors could act completely within the law of the country they work in and still find themselves in trouble with their regulating authority. These rules, guidelines or statements act like a sort of evolving 'oath in progress'. We may not think about them all the time, and may not be able to quote them, but they exist to form and frame the world we work in. Some of this helps to make it clear when we might fall foul of the law, were we not doctors, and some of it helps to clarify legal requirements. Sometimes, however, it appears more complicated than that. So sometimes it feels like there is a never-ending stream of advice, demands and values to satisfy with every medical decision (Figure 12.1).

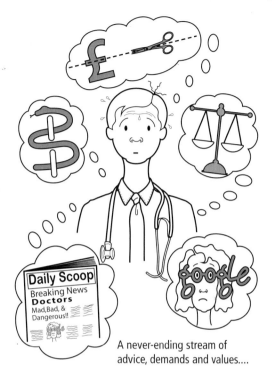

A never-ending stream of advice, demands and values....

Figure 12.1 Sometimes it feels like there is a never-ending stream of advice, demands and values to satisfy with every medical decision.

The law and professional regulation in practice

The frameworks of legal and professional regulation are both derived from what a society considers it right to do. As the emphasis or balance of thinking in any society may change, so may laws and professional regulations.

Tutor quote

Remember there might be important differences between what you can do in different countries. Any health professionals going to practise in another country would be foolish not to check out the approaches in that country.

Surprisingly the law often says little specific about things that matter a lot in medical practice. For example, until recently, the law in England and Wales on medical confidentiality was very sparse. But doctors are seen in law as having to do things that other people are usually not allowed to do, hence the need for examinations, regular appraisal and a special registration. The law expects doctors to get on with being doctors without the law having to intervene: it is only likely to become involved if something goes or is done wrong. What would constitute a crime may of course not be absolutely obvious; in the words of one English lawyer, 'the law doesn't tell you what to do, it only tells you after you've done it whether it was lawful or not.' But courts know all too well how difficult it is to make good judgements in the heat of the moment and so are reluctant to criticize doctors. What is more, they are likely to be cautious about making a legal decision that would have the consequence of depriving patients of medical care because doctors would be unable or too nervous to act. Most judgements will therefore follow rather than lead changes in public opinion; certainly in countries where the law is based on the English legal system, which relies to a great extent on cases and precedent.

'Being questioned' – a change for good?

Change in medical practice comes about for many reasons, but is sometimes spurred by the discovery that previous practices were dangerous, or allowed errors and even crimes to go unnoticed. In 2000, Harold Shipman, a single-handed GP, was convicted of murdering 15 elderly patients with overdoses of sedative or analgesic drugs. (It is suspected that he killed many more than that.) Shipman's activities were brought to light by another local GP who raised concerns about the high death rate in Shipman's practice. After an extensive enquiry, the case highlighted flaws in the systems used to manage the prescription and dispensing of controlled drugs. Several changes have been made to this process since then, based on the outcome of this investigation, many which affect the day-to-day prescribing practice of both GPs and hospital doctors. Although this was an extreme and distressing example, it highlights the importance of asking questions, and being prepared to be questioned, as a way that change may be made to medical practice (Smith, 2005).

Thinking and Discussion Point

You may be aware of 'incident forms' at your own hospital that are intended to flag up problems that can be addressed before they become more serious. How are such things done in general practice?

Practical Exercise

Think of a time when a decision you have made has been called into question by colleagues, friends, family or tutors. How did you feel? What was your initial response? Why was the question raised in the first place? Was there a protocol that you were unaware of? Think about positive outcomes that have arisen due to this questioning, medical or otherwise.

Tutor quote

Speak to the person directly and find out what went wrong; apologize and use the complaint to change your ways.

Good practice and the moral stranger

If we want to be good doctors and deliver the best practice, every single contact between one person and another has the potential for improving things, or the reverse, and so has a moral component. It is almost as if each consultation has its own little textbook of medical ethics waiting to be written about it.

Ethics means 'how people should live'. One of the earliest writers (outside religious books) was the Greek philosopher Aristotle. He often used the work of a ship's captain to illustrate his thinking. There is the tide, the wind, the condition of the boat: even with the latest computer, all who venture to sea have to use all their knowledge, skill, experience and intuition to get the best out of the voyage and return safely to land.

It is the same in the consultation. We may have the charts, but it is the rest that may drive us onto the rocks. What is uncharted may be very extensive, especially in general practice. Patients bring so many different things to their GPs. It is likely they will be wondering, too, what sort of person they are going to meet and what his or her approach will be. Even if patient and professional know each other well, the tide and weather of anxiety, exhaustion or excitement may overwhelm the usual responses on either side. One of the fascinations of medicine (and law) is that when private lives become more public, what actually happens in private is often very different from what the outside world might expect. The bouncer who listens to Mozart, the social work manager who goes on gambling holidays, the vicar who beats up her husband, the doctor who seems the model medic but is struggling to keep up: life is full of surprises. Pluralistic modern society raises further problems. It might be possible in very settled societies to be clear about what the 'rules' are, or how each family would 'play it', but in a modern urban society people have multiple identities, and signposts are few or may even point in the wrong direction at times of crisis. People of different generations and with different experiences may make choices for themselves outside their ethnic, religious or family tradition.

So each patient comes to us as what has been called a 'moral stranger'. We do not know how they will approach a particular problem. As doctors, we have to get to know not only our patients' medical problems, but also the choices they intend to make and why – their moral responses. We have to make a values diagnosis as well as a medical one; and we need to do it swiftly and surely and without compromising our own moral position.

🏴 Alarm symptom

'I know what to do, and just what this patient wants.'

Moral antennae: paying attention to the issues

Some moral issues we meet in a patient encounter might be absolutely obvious. However, it may not be quite so easy to see everything that could go wrong without paying particular attention. You may see when sitting in that the patient is looking uneasy or trying to talk about something that the doctor, because of the focus on the physical symptoms or on teaching, has not noticed. A question from the clinician may catch the patient off guard, and the patient may start to unburden him- or herself about something deeply personal; it may be clearly inappropriate for the student to be involved and the student may feel the need to withdraw.

All of these observations may be part of the skill that some have in abundance, but others may need to develop: of being sensitive to moral and psychological issues and responding appropriately. It may not always be easy to give a name precisely to all of these issues. We may just have a feeling. The importance of noting that something is going wrong or that there is a hidden problem needing to be addressed cannot be overstated. Our natural moral antennae link to our emotional awareness, and it is this as much as anything else which helps us to find our way on the moral chart. Unnoticed or unaddressed, the issue may act as a trap for all involved, and the emotional feeling, instead of being a signal for reflection or for going carefully, may burst out. Someone may become upset. Responses may be inappropriate; the treatment may be poorly directed or key issues may be held back and missed. A patient may complain or leave the list, a doctor may go home dispirited or go off to do some other type of work. So one of the important things to notice in medical work is a change in the emotional climate, within oneself, in the patient, or in the interaction. It signals, usually, a moral problem; one that is unidentified or unaddressed and desperately needs attention.

Roles, rules and duties

Case study 12.3

During a teaching session, an enthusiastic GP called the student away from her teacher's surgery to show her the physical signs of shingles in the patient he was seeing next door. The patient was a young man and clearly had no option but to raise his shirt to the student and show her the lesions. The GP then began to teach the student, and, without talking any more to the patient, bundled him out of the room, leaving a very embarrassed student with a self-satisfied GP.

One thing that commonly causes a consultation to stall is confusion about the task in hand. With the best will in the world, clinicians may find themselves changing what they are doing or being asked to do without realizing it.

We see above a role conflict for a doctor between duty to an individual patient and to teaching, but even within one consultation, roles may suddenly change. A patient may reveal something that may challenge the doctor as a fellow citizen, such as a crime. Either party may start a conversation that owes more to friendship or more intense feelings than to a professional relationship. Other conflicts of role may simply be built in and unrecognized. Country doctors may have to look after their staff's medical problems, or those of their own family. The counsel of perfection would be to avoid the situation, but if that is not possible we should at least be aware of these conflicts even if they are not made explicit.

One of the main reasons for keeping a close check on the task in hand is that each role may carry its own rules, formal or informal and separate from those of clinical practice: a teacher may be bound by one set of regulations, a researcher by another; a friend may feel bound to act, or a neighbour be inhibited from doing so. These rules may seem to get in the way, designed to trip us up, but in reality they are to protect us from making mistakes. They look ahead, as it were, to the job to be done and say: 'If you are to do this sort of job or to be in this sort of position, you must be prepared to be the kind of person who acts in this sort of way.'

For other people involved, as a doctor you make implied promises about what you are going to do and how you are going to do it, and these promises become part of broader duties that we undertake. Without them, others don't know what to expect, and how to trust us in difficult situations. Without them, we as professionals would not know how to resist other desires or outside forces that come to frustrate these promised actions. We are only human, and get tired, distracted; our concentration goes elsewhere. Our promise in practice keeps us at the task until we have completed it. Our duties define what else we could or could not do in the course of our work.

Duty

Case Study 12.4

A public problem

You are a GP registrar in an inner city practice. You often see young people who have been caught up in criminal activity – drug offences, petty theft and antisocial behaviour. You know that in the community your practice serves a large number of children under 16 who have been victims of knife crime. Your practice has contributed to an audit addressing long-term outcomes for those seen in the local trauma centre with stab wounds. It is a major public health concern. Several young lives, including practice patients, have been lost or spoilt due to knife crime.

It is something that you feel passionately about. Primary care can play a vital role in helping to reduce the numbers of lives destroyed by crime, and you are very active in your practice in helping to promote services like your teenager's drop-in clinic.

An individual's concern

One morning, a 13-year-old boy comes to see you. He hasn't been to the surgery for over 5 years, and never on his own before. He complains of acne over his upper back and face. It's getting him down. He's stopped swimming because of it. While you are writing a prescription towards the end of the consultation, you ask 'is anything stressing you out at the moment?'

The real reason?

After a long silence, fiddling, he mutters that it's his elder brother. 'He got arrested for carrying a knife … like all the kids on the estate.' His brother has finished his community service but can't find a job. He's always around, after food or cash. They get on alright, discussing games and girls. But he's never stopped carrying a knife, despite his conviction: he says 'You'd be stupid to walk round here without some form of protection.' He's going to get his little brother a knife too, to get him used to it.

Your patient says he'd seen his brother in a bad mood, and how angry he gets. The blade is serrated, 5 inches long. He can't stop thinking about his brother using it. He's afraid just walking around the estate, afraid his brother won't get off the next time he's caught carrying a blade, afraid of what his brother might do when he's angry at home.

The patient is suddenly aghast at what he's done. 'You're not going to tell my mum, are you? You're not going to tell the police?'

A duty to whom?

This case presents you with lots to think about:

- *Confidentiality*: The threat is not specific. If he had said his brother is going to kill this named girl and he told you so this morning that he will do it tonight, that would justify breaking confidentiality to the police, with or without consent. General threats and potential concerns are much harder to evaluate, and we must be able to clearly explain the gravity of our immediate concerns if we do break confidentiality.

- *Competence*: What about his parents? Doesn't his mum have the right to know one of her sons is coming into her home with illegal weapons? Would the patient discuss it with his mum himself? Perhaps she would rather know from her own family rather than waiting for a catastrophe, and her response may not be negative. What is his response to this suggestion? Does he understand the information you are giving him? Do you think the consequences are clear to him?

- *Age of responsibility*: Sometimes, is it necessary to decide whether a child under 16 can be given responsibility for decisions, with or without parental consent or even parental involvement. This is where we refer to 'Fraser Competence' (see Box 12.2).

- *Wider issues*: What are the possible consequences in this situation? Might you risk alienating your young patient, lose his precious trust? Might an offer of subtle intervention with the mum or the family from an impartial adult be a welcome relief from the burden of the stress he is under? But are you getting too involved? Is public safety more important than your relationship with your patient? You are not a law enforcement service: should the police simply be informed?

Box 12.2 Fraser Guidelines

'Fraser Guidelines' (or 'Gillick Competency') refer to situations where the competence of a child under 16 to make their own decisions about their healthcare without parental consent is being assessed. Mrs Gillick took her local health authority to court in 1982 to challenge the fact that children under 16 may receive treatment without parental consent. She lost her case. Appeal found in favour of the initial judgment:

'Whether or not a child is capable of giving the necessary consent will depend on the child's maturity and understanding and the nature of the consent required. The child must be capable of making a reasonable assessment of the advantages and disadvantages of the treatment proposed, so the consent, if given, can be properly and fairly described as true consent.'

Although the initial case was about contraception, the judgment has come to have a broader application. The Fraser Guidelines provide a framework for judging the competence of a young person.

A doctor in this situation should take the following questions into account:

- Can the young person understand the information given to him or her?
- Can they retain that information?
- Do they have an insight into the consequences of their decision? (i.e. Do they have capacity to make a decision?)
- Are they unlikely to be persuaded to inform their parents or guardian?
- Is the decision in their best interests?
- May withholding treatment cause them harm? (e.g. the young person will continue to have sexual intercourse whether they are prescribed a contraceptive or not).

An absolute duty?

Duty is a word with rather a heavy feel to it. It is something we owe because we said we would. People then have a claim on us to deliver. They have a right to expect something from us. But we must try to be consistent as well as reasonable. We cannot pick and choose. Because that consistency is so basic to professional lives, such duties (and, reciprocally, other people's rights) are often thought of as absolute. To go back to the issue of confidentiality, patients might not be as open as they would otherwise be to doctors when discussing some conditions if they did not know that what they describe or relate will be kept in confidence between them and the doctor.

Where there is some other reasonable but conflicting claim on us, however, the idea of an 'absolute' claim starts to lose its meaning. Confidentiality is not 'absolutely absolute', after all. It can, indeed it must, be broken in some situations. We have to negotiate these new and difficult waters and decide what to do.

Thinking and Discussion Point

By coming into a consultation as a student to learn, you have already broken into the confidential relationship between the doctor and the patient. How can we then view that confidentiality? How does your teacher view it? What do you think patients will think? How can you find out? Are there any rules you must make yourself?

Case Study 12.5

After conducting a family interview in depth at a patient's home, written up in long hand as it had to be, the medical student left his notes by mistake on the bus. He never found the notes again. His presentation was spoilt, but worse he worried that someone has found all the notes, with his name on them and the patients all identified and their address given, and that one day all this will burst into the open or the patients will come to harm. He still does.

This case raised an obvious issue before it all went wrong: the student was to share this information with a teaching group. Did the patient know this, and consent? What if a doctor needs to write a letter to a specialist and so has to put the letter on a tape to be typed by a secretary? What about a receptionist making a phone call about the patient, or the doctor consulting a colleague about the best form of referral? From inside the system, we can see that all of these situations may be necessary for effective care and proper teamwork,

so all these people – student, group teacher, secretary, receptionist, professional colleague – are still bound by the same duty of confidentiality, and that this formed a cordon around this group of people. Researchers have found that the general public does not understand confidentiality like this (Carmen and Britten, 1995), so there is probably a lot more work to be done.

The case of the young man and his brother raised another duty; in this case, to protect vulnerable people in danger. Society expects us to deal with medical harms, but we also have to deal with some harms unearthed in the consultation that go beyond the strictly medical.

Handling duties and consequences

When we make a promise to people we are close to, we may not have foreseen all the possible situations that may arise which may challenge that promise. But in medicine, we should know enough at least about the possibility of conflicting demands and so should think ahead. If we think there is even the outside chance that we might have to break confidentiality, we should not make a promise we know we cannot fulfil.

However, duties do not only face competition from other duties. Medicine judges itself in scientific terms or in terms of evidence assessed largely by outcomes. Is this treatment better than that? What should we do in order to improve lives or reduce suffering? In some situations, where one outcome would clearly be the best ('best' in the limited sense of best for the immediate people we are concerned with), duties prevent us from overstepping the mark. The daughter in Case study 12.2 could clearly see where things might lead. There might be many options – an old people's home, extensive daycare services or whatever would enable both mother and daughter to live reasonable lives in their different ways. But sometimes getting the balance right may seem difficult.

Case Study 12.6

Before the elderly mother in Case study 12.2 developed her dementia, a routine blood test demonstrated that she had some leukaemic cells in her white cell series. These were mildly aggressive, and certainly not likely to threaten her life more than other things: the specialist advice was to do nothing. She asked whether her blood test was all right. The doctor took a deep breath and told her it was fine.

Thinking and Discussion Point

Telling a patient that she 'had leukaemia but that I am going to do nothing about it' hardly sounds like the recommended communication. But it is the truth. What would you say? Does it matter that doctors don't tell lies? If the old lady, or her relatives, eventually find out, what would happen to their trust in you or their view of doctor's veracity? Does that matter?

There may be many ways round this problem by thinking about how we might express ourselves, but at this stage, this case pits a clear duty that the doctor has – to tell the truth to the patient about issues which concern her health – against a consequence – telling her about something that might cause major anxiety, and possibly blight the rest of her life.

Thus we find ourselves trying to balance things that not only are not similar, but are not even measured on the same scale. These are incommensurable, and we just have to accept that. We are left to make a moral balance. Outside groups are unlikely to have the answer. It is just that professionals tend to act in one way, while perhaps our intuitions or conscience may point in another, and so we may be left confused. The culture of our society may be in transition, or people may differ. We need a way of assessing the options and coming to a decision.

At least three different ways have been advanced to help us try to bring incommensurable things to a balance. In the first, we can analyse what principles underlie different arguments, and bring them together to create a way forward. As another way of thinking, we can focus not so much on what to do as on what sort of person we should be, and try to act in that way (looking at virtues and values). Finally, we could examine the different perspectives of the actors in each drama and combine them into a type of story, turning our responses into a narrative, and try to 'tell our way' through the problem.

In the paragraphs that follow, we look at each of these approaches. One may be more appealing than the others; one may fit the circumstances better than others. There may be yet other ways of looking at things that may be important for individuals, or may help particular branches of the healthcare professions. Probably, however, the best (or better) option requires us to use at least all three of these approaches as part of the 'ethical circuit' of thinking (Figure 12.2).

Four principles and scope

Benefit and harm

At work we are obviously trying to help or benefit people, and to reduce things that may be harmful to them. The principle of doing good for people – often called in medicine a 'duty of care' – is known as *beneficence*. There is a contrast with commerce; however 'ethical' a company, the bottom line in business is profit for shareholders, not benefit or care for customers. (However, even in business, a

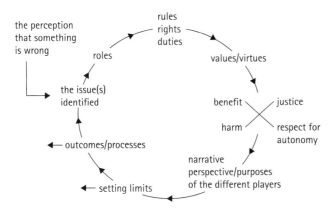

Figure 12.2 The 'ethical circuit' of thinking.

company might get into trouble if it caused harm to its customers.) In medicine the imperative to minimize or avoid harming people is very strong. This principle of reducing harm is called *non-maleficence*: it has defined our decision that we might break confidence if a consultation revealed abuse or danger to others. Sometimes even more important is the idea that in order to help people we actually have to do things that, outside medicine, would be considered as harms: the surgeon has to cut; the medicine has side effects. So doctors usually cannot avoid the possibility of harm, but must reduce it as much as possible and set it against the good to be achieved. Thus we have to balance benefits and harms, just as politicians or economists balance these ideas.

Thinking and Discussion Point

Take five patient situations you have been involved in. What did the patient want? What could be achieved? Was there a clear difference? If there were harms of various possible actions, where might the harms fall? How were these balanced? Was all this made explicit in the consultation? If not, why not?

Respecting autonomy

In Western societies recently another idea has become important. Even if the doctor can see what is best done to help a patient, what about that patient's own view of what should be done? Even if the doctor knows best in general, second guessing a patient's own personal choices or preferences is not the right way to work. People should be able to choose what happens to their own bodies and lives. Overriding their decisions, with the best of motives, is likely to lead to a poor outcome and may actually disable the individual into being a 'permanent patient'. It may simply be illegal. Helping people to achieve their own goals is a great benefit in itself. Doing something that seems like the best medicine at the time but which the patient does not want could be a major harm.

These sorts of ideas lie behind keeping medical secrets and getting people's permission before we do anything that affects them directly. This thinking about individual choice grew out of the political arena in Europe and America over the last 400 years (the earlier part of which is sometimes called 'the Enlightenment' because it opposed the traditional but unscientific approaches of mediaeval times). The words used were similar to those used in political discussion about countries wishing to rule themselves. Each individual was seen as his or her own sovereign in matters of personal choice. Each person should be treated as an autonomous individual. Autonomy means ruling oneself or oneself providing the laws for oneself. That could be interpreted as each person doing what he or she liked, but that freedom is, of course, constrained by other people's freedom, so some of the boundaries are clearly set. As one Enlightenment thinker, Jeremy Bentham, said, 'your freedom to swing your stick ends where my nose begins.'

Every person should acknowledge the importance of the choices individuals make about their own lives: we should respect their autonomy in being able to think, desire and actually do what they wish whenever we can if that is not in conflict with the autonomy of other people.

That freedom to make choices about things that concern our own personal lives has been translated from the grand political scene into that of personal politics in some sectors of modern life in the West. Between consenting adults in private, for instance, their sexual preferences are their business and theirs alone, much as choice of clothes, music or flowers to put in a windowbox are theirs (in our ideal world!) and no one else's. Where there are clashes, in home or at the workplace, we prefer shared or negotiated decisions to someone simply being told what to do. We believe that people should achieve their potential and should, wherever possible, as adults, be empowered to make their own decisions and choices.

Thinking and Discussion Point

In those five situations you thought about above, whose decision was it that was done? Was it the doctor's, the patient's, or someone outside the room? Was it a shared decision or one sided?

It has often been said that 'doctor knows best'. One of the reasons why individual choice is difficult to apply is that people often cannot easily make medical judgements about themselves. Patients cannot easily examine parts of their own bodies. If they can, they may not know what that examination means or what to do about it because they lack the medical knowledge. That drugs are dangerous poisons as well as potential cures means that most important ones are available only on a doctor's prescription. So, until the middle of the last century, most healthcare practice was paternalistic in style: the patient's duty was to obey orders.

Thinking and Discussion Point

Are there situations in medicine today where it is still vital that the doctor makes the decision for the patient? What justifies that?

Even with improving self-diagnostic aids, more access to medical knowledge for lay people and over-the-counter medicines, patients are still often not able to express their choices properly. They may be disabled by anxiety, too ill to think straight or actually unconscious. If the healthcare worker is to act properly, the autonomy of the patient has to be respected even if it cannot be expressed. This may be done by acting as the person would choose to act, or we know did choose to act before they became ill, by working to get patients into a situation in which they can really make their own choices again, or by avoiding going beyond certain sorts of boundaries in decision making – unless there are overwhelming reasons to do so, defined by obvious benefits or harms. This is important whether the concerns are major or the decisions are everyday ones.

Case Study 12.7

A retired sailor, Mr Mason had been treated successfully for renal and liver failure after a major road accident when he was 75, and now, coughing away on his own in the old people's home at 92, with all his close relatives and friends dead or distant, the doctor was faced with telling him that his tests showed he had lung cancer. Mr Mason almost looked relieved. 'Let me go doctor – I've had a good voyage, you know it. I'm tired out. Death holds no horrors for me like being stuck in four walls would. I want to see and smell the west wind. Just keep me out of pain as much as you can. You're the last friend I've got; I trust you.'

The same sort of thinking or reasoning should help doctors through difficult minor choices, like a patient refusing a 'flu jab or wanting to use complementary medicine, as it did with brave old Mr Mason. By all means doctors should explain, inform, try to persuade, to act as an advocate, as it were, of the choice that seems better to the medic but not to the lay person. But ultimately, by not listening to the patients' decisions or choices, healthcare workers can treat them like children. This is not only wrong in itself, but sometimes delays recovery.

Justice

Thus three important principles contribute to resolving a conflict – doing good, avoiding harm and respecting autonomy. However, our choices may be limited not only by what we know, but also by what can be afforded. A practitioner in Somalia may have a different range of options from one in Southwark or Saskatchewan. We may regret that, but it is reality. Equally, in different countries the healthcare system may have made different decisions about what type of care takes priority for funding, or how one chooses between two people with the same condition when only one can be treated. These are issues of justice.

We are all brought up in our families to have a view of what is fair, and how to address the situation when something is unfair. Many political movements are driven by similar thoughts writ large. These ideas of what is fair or just permeate healthcare too, whether it be to deal with a problem when someone has overstepped the mark and done something really wrong (retributive justice), or in circumstances in which there is not enough of something to go round (distributive justice).

Thinking and Discussion Point

Some people think that there is a natural ceiling for healthcare demand, when everyone has enough for their needs. Do you agree?

The National Health Service (NHS) in the UK was planned with that last idea in mind: it was assumed that as people got healthier, calls on the service would be reduced. For whatever reasons, however, most people now do not think it works that way. It seems as if, however much is put into any healthcare system, it will be inadequate for everyone's wants and for improvements in healthcare. Distributive justice in this view will always be with us. This approach not only sees a problem of how to distribute resources, such as curative drugs or doctors' time, but also (whether funding comes from the state or some commercial system) detects a general shortage of what is needed to satisfy the needs of the population overall. If the majority are right, or if the political will to correct an overall deficiency is not found, people working in healthcare will always have to make awkward decisions about how to allocate resources, not only on the expanding edge of bioscience but also in the centre of routine medical work. There will be conflict facing students and busy teaching GPs concerning how to make sure each patient's needs are properly addressed and the other calls on the student's and doctor's time are attended to. Good communication and time management skills will help, but something more is needed: choices have to be made.

Student quote

'When I was a kid I was often upset because things didn't seem to be fair, and my parents were good at trying to explain it or make it right. There seems a lot that's unfair in health and illness, though; and still in healthcare too. I hope I'll be able to see my way through this when I get to practise on my own.'

Scope

Some progress may be made to solve problems by looking at the scope or limits of the issue under discussion. A patient may present a concern, such as a dispute with a neighbour, which is quite properly not in the doctor's province. Someone else may want to talk so extensively about a psychological problem or has such a complex complaint that specialist help is needed. Perhaps the student should have prepared for his or her afternoon session the night before, or the doctor not allowed the management demands of the practice to impinge on his or her afternoon visits. Drawing lines in anticipation may be common sense but also may need clear thinking. Even the time given to thinking things through has limits!

Virtues and values

We all have casts of character that are quite obvious to our friends and family, if not to us. We may be good timekeepers or decision makers, excellent at listening to people, open and honest about our opinions, and so on. These we conventionally call *virtues*, and we prize them. They may make us effective in certain circumstances, and prone to make certain sorts of choices. Some of these will have led us into doing medicine: others may take us into particular branches of care. Neurosurgery and community psychiatry may share many things, but the virtues required of doctors and nurses in each area are likely to be very different. This in turn is in part because the outcomes expected and the processes used are different: but in these two areas of work, the balance is struck differently between tolerance and active inquisitiveness or intervention. (Perhaps this is in part due to the different dangers that each area of work poses for its patients.)

The moral challenge may thus be about what sort of person (or professional) we should be. To the degree that we change this – and we can probably all change our professional practice a lot more than we might think – we have to identify the important attributes to develop in a certain area of work or to display in a certain situation. Thus a particular approach may prevent problems arising (or the reverse!). The doctor facing the elderly patient with an incidental and probably irrelevant blood test abnormality may have less of a problem if he or she is always open and honest with patients. They have grown to trust her truthfulness and judgement.

Thinking and Discussion Point

What do you think are your particular strengths of character that may impinge on your work as a doctor? Do your friends agree?

What applies to individuals can, to a degree, apply to groups. In this context we usually talk about a deliberate choice of values. A particular service, say an oncology department or a group practice, may make a conscious decision to take a particular approach for the benefit of patients, or to reduce or stop their commitment elsewhere in order to give their work a particular focus. There may be local factors that are decisive. There are likely to be trade-offs. The same practice above involved in adolescent work might find it difficult when patients from a part of the locality that has gone 'upmarket' come in with internet printouts and complain about being kept waiting past appointment times. So both values and virtues are on a spectrum: the tolerance the above practice may have developed will be a menace for a busy executive superwoman who just wants her pills and to get home to take over from the au pair. Someone appearing to be brave in one situation may in another appear simply foolhardy. If we value choice, we also need to value choice of values, and each of us may have made particular choices of our values because of experiences we have had, or new goals we now need to achieve.

Perspective and narrative

We saw that each encounter with a new person could be a meeting between moral strangers. Understanding one person's relevant aims and goals may be quite a task, but understanding the experience or culture of a group or family, and how one individual blends with or differs from that group, gives a special extra dimension to family practice. It makes decision making, when there is dissonance, a real skill. Respecting the patient's choice may be supported by the law, regulating bodies and principles, and is unlikely to be far from the value set of most modern practitioners or service groups. However, within families these concepts may begin to unpeel like an onion, as illness or distress upsets a previously established and artificial harmony between different people's expectations, needs and experiences. Choice implies that there is also something that is not chosen; so the path not taken, the unvalued expectation, an unmet need or a negative experience may need to be addressed before progress is

made. Each person who has a stake in a difficult moral decision ideally should have the opportunity to offer his or her own perspective where it is appropriate to do so. This is (partly) the theory behind case conferences.

In practice, whereas professionals may be expected to present coherent options and the justifications for and against a particular approach, most people are more concrete thinkers, and express their preferences in other ways. Some of this is demonstrated in the desire to tell and hear stories. While most of us respond well to people telling interesting stories, the imperative in modern medicine to look for scientific evidence in treatment evaluation has led to some clinicians insisting that such things are 'mere anecdotes'. This seems not only to misrepresent what some patients are doing when they are telling stories, but also to underestimate the importance that such stories may hold at their heart. We are probably used to the idea that a religious leader may use a narrative to illustrate a moral point or clarify a particular belief, but modern novelists or soap opera directors are often doing the same. Though writers usually have several ideas they want to get across, the point is the same: telling about events is usually the vehicle for presenting the clash between ideas. When this happens in the consultation, there is usually a purpose to the story told; perhaps to help define what sort of person is consulting and why they are like that, and how the patient can help the doctor make sense of what has and is happening, separately or together.

Some may prefer to stick to the concept of perspectives. Understanding where each person in an interaction is 'coming from' is not the only aim of modern ethical practice – we still have to put each point of view together and reach a reasoned and reasonable conclusion – but it is certainly a good starting point.

Putting it all together

Much professional medical ethics derives from philosophical thinking down the ages, and law is made by judges and juries deliberating at length. No one would want to make a virtue out of work pressure, but the passage of time means something different in medicine. For the clinician, the patient is there in front of him or her and is likely to remain so unless some sort of decision is made. Other problems clamour for attention in the waiting room. Medical practice worldwide would grind to a halt if clinicians took time out to think deeply and extensively through each dilemma that came their way. Equally, even the most strident political advocate of patient choice would not expect clinicians to act like a dispensing machines, simply waiting for their buttons to be pressed. The practice of medicine is complex, but many of the difficult decisions have already been made. These decisions may be made by the people who set up the service, or by the GMC or the government. They may be based on the choices that patients or relatives have made before they arrive. They may be affected by the place in which the encounter occurs, or by the way two people interact.

Where difficulties remain, two things at least stand out. One is that patients spend quite a lot of time after consultations ruminating about what happened, and so doctors should too. For doctors, thinking through or discussing the ethics of an encounter afterwards is a professional imperative, so that in follow-up, or the next time something similar happens, our thinking may be clearer and our responses more coherent.

(Ancient Greek) tutor quote

If treatment is good, treatment after thought must be better.

The other marker we need to lay down is that we should try our best not to be pressed into doing something that we know, in our heart of hearts, is wrong. This is even more so if the pressure is simply of routine or workload. Medical ethics and law are often annoyingly short on prescriptions, and we may not find it easy to know what we should do, but it is extraordinarily obvious, in most cases, what we should not do.

Thinking in medical ethics and law can be exciting or challenging, and can take us to some unusual places. However, the 'bottom line' is that it helps us to practise well and stay out of trouble.

SUMMARY POINTS

To conclude, the most important messages of this chapter are as follows:

- You should be clear what laws and regulations govern your work before you start to practise medicine, especially in primary care, which can be either very supportive or isolating, depending on your approach to your work.
- You should keep alive your own sense of right and wrong in all aspects of your work, and particularly be alert to unusual or unexpected emotions that may arise, as these may indicate that there is a moral problem for you to think about.
- Emotional reactions are not enough, however, and your moral intuitions need to be subjected to scrutiny through some or all of the approaches suggested here to keep your healthcare in good shape.
- Doing that thinking or discussion and coming to conclusions that you feel are justified, respecting the wishes and needs of people you work with and protecting them from harm, will enable you to feel good about your work and sleep in peace at the end of the day.
- Having conversations with other colleagues within the cordon of professional confidentiality can be very helpful, so it is important to find careful and responsive colleagues who can help you to think through difficult issues that may arise wherever you work.

References

Carmen, D. and Britten, N. 1995: Confidentiality of medical records. *British Journal of General Practice* 45, 485–8.

Gillick v. West Norfolk and Wisbech Area Health Authority [1986] AC 112 1ALL ER.

Smith, Dame Janet 2005: *The Shipman Inquiry – The Sixth Report*. London: HMSO.

Further reading

The General Medical Council (www.gmc-uk.org) publishes on good medical practice, consent, confidentiality, doctors in management, and other issues of importance that arise. These are required reading for all doctors who intend to practise within UK or related jurisdictions.

The *Journal of Medical Ethics* (www.jmedethics.com) is the leading journal that discusses ethical issues, and this site provides a list of classified websites, articles from the journal and abstracts of many articles published in the last decade.

Her Majesty's Stationery Office (www.legislation.hmso.gov.uk) provides publications detailing UK statutes.

Boyd, K.M., Higgs, R. and Pinching, A.J. 1997: *The new dictionary of medical ethics*. London: BMJ Publishing Group.

Blackburn, S. 2001: *Ethics: a very short introduction*. Oxford: Oxford University Press.

As it says, very short, but extremely readable introduction to modern ethical thinking and writing.

Brazier, M. and Cave, E. 2003: *Medicine, patients and the law*. London: Penguin.

Campbell, A.V. and Higgs, R. 1982: *In that case: medical ethics in everyday practice*. London: Darton, Longman and Todd.

Dickenson, D., Huxtable, R. and Parker, M. 2010: *The Cambridge medical ethics workbook*. Cambridge: Cambridge University Press.

A very wide-ranging explanation of approaches to bioethics that is designed to be used in a similar way to this book.

Gillon, R. 1986: *Philosophical medical ethics*. Chichester: John Wiley and Sons.

Glover, J. 1990: *Causing death and saving lives*. London: Penguin.

This is the classical study of this area, which has never been surpassed.

Harris, J. 1985: *The value of life: an introduction to medical ethics*. London: Routledge.

This is an exciting and challenging book about many of the issues at the expanding frontiers of medical science.

Hope, T., Savulescu, J. and Hendrick, J. 2003: *Medical ethics and law: the core curriculum*. Edinburgh: Churchill Livingstone.

Kuhse, H. and Singer, P. 2009: *A companion to bioethics*. Oxford: Blackwell.

This and its companion volume, *A companion to ethics*, are very useful gateways to the range of modern writing.

SINGLE BEST ANSWER QUESTIONS

12.1 A man of 75 on a simple anti-hypertensive drug regime comes in to ask you, as a locum, if the drugs he is taking could cause impotence.

a) There are many possible side effects of most drugs and you should tell him to leave it to his normal doctors to sort out which are important

b) No one at 75 has decent sex anyway, and most men of that age would be impotent regardless

c) Everyone has an absolute right to know all about their treatment

d) You should inform him as much as you can in words he can understand about the possible side effects of his medication, help him make sense of that information to decide what to do, and ask him if he wants to discuss sex or any other personal problems while he is here

e) You should give him details of where to look it all up on the internet, as that would fully empower him to make his own decisions and save time for others in what might be an over-running consultation.

SINGLE BEST ANSWER QUESTIONS CONTINUED

12.2 A man of 75 who is on an expensive new anti-hypertensive regime is found to have widespread and treatment-resistant (and so terminal) cancer.

a) Don't tell him the diagnosis as it will upset him: he has enough to cope with in this shocking situation

b) All drug treatments should be reviewed in that situation: he may not need some, but he may now need specialist terminal care regimes

c) The expensive treatment should be stopped because it is now a waste of resources

d) His relatives should be reminded to persuade him to make a will

e) It is only fair to tell him exactly how long he has to live.

12.3 A man of 85 who is hypertensive, but with no other abnormal physical signs, begins to be vague and confused at the time it has been planned for him to move from home to sheltered accommodation.

a) He is likely to be dementing and an assessment of competence should be done to cover his last years of life

b) His drugs should all be stopped as it might be a side effect

c) His decision-making capacity is important at the time of a potential move, but is related to that decision and that time

d) If his confusion were caused by an infection, he would be pyrexial

e) Everything possible should be done to prolong his life, as if he were a younger man.

12.4 A shy young woman of 15 comes in to see you with her mother. The mother, who does all the talking, explains the daughter has a urinary tract infection.

a) When you get a urinary sample to test you should also quietly test for pregnancy

b) You should accept the situation with gratitude as at 15 she is too young to make her own decisions

c) You should tell the mother her daughter has the same right as anyone else to be seen on their own

d) When the daughter is on her own, she should be given what she wants without telling her mother, just like with anyone else

e) After talking with both, you should suggest that the daughter might like to talk to you a bit on her own or with a chaperone, and ask the daughter if she would like that.

12.5 The 'four principles and scope' approach to medical ethics may be best defined as follows:

a) Respect for autonomy means doing what the patient wants, whatever you think right as a doctor

b) Benevolence means doing the best for the patient, an alternative way of expressing 'the duty of care'

c) Non-maleficence means doing nothing whatsoever that might harm the patient

d) Justice is only about retribution, not about how to best distribute the 'goods' of healthcare

e) Scope covers the question of to whom or to what these principles apply.

CHAPTER

13

QUALITY ASSURANCE IN GENERAL PRACTICE

- There is plenty of scope for improvement
- Unexplained variation and value for money
- Rising expectations and patient choice
- What is quality in general practice?
- Practical approaches to quality assurance in general practice

- Clinical audit
- Summary points
- References
- Single best answer questions

Medical knowledge and technology change at an ever-increasing rate, making it very difficult for general practitioners (GPs) to keep up with the latest best practice and patient safety information. Economic constraints and the demands of patients make the cost efficient and clinically effective use of resources vital. Ensuring that the risks to patients in this rapidly changing environment are minimized, that new and effective treatments become available to patients quickly and that the experience of using services is improved requires good managerial strategies and clinical skills. This chapter will provide you with an understanding of three common and practical approaches to quality assurance to equip you for this.

LEARNING OBJECTIVES

By the end of this chapter you will be able to:
- understand that you and the healthcare systems you are a part of are fallible and sometimes something will go wrong;
- understand that there are quality assurance systems that help minimize the chances of things going wrong;
- understand the basics of three common and practical approaches to quality assurance used in general practice.

Thinking and Discussion Point

So you want to be a doctor. Brilliant! I hope that you make it. In this chapter you are set a challenge that hopefully will stay with you for the rest of your chosen career.

- How will you know if your practice is safe?
- How will you know that you are providing the most clinical and cost effective care to your patients?
- How will you know whether your patients value the healthcare that you provide?

The challenge for you is to be able to answer these three questions and back up your responses with clear evidence at any point in your future.

There is plenty of scope for improvement

Medical error

About 300 million patient consultations take place in general practice every year. This huge volume of workload is matched by the huge variation in patient presentations, which range from routine coughs and colds to the complex management of long-term conditions and the delivery of specialist procedures, including surgery. The National Patient Safety Agency (NPSA) reports that 'medical error occurs between five and 80 times per 100 000 consultations, mainly related to diagnosis and treatment' (NPSA, 2011). This is an intriguing statistic for two reasons. First, the range 'between five and 80 times per 100 000 consultations' shows that the data are not very precise and that reporting mechanisms are possibly not as accurate as they might be. Second, it shows that the vast majority of consultations pass without a hitch but the sheer number of consultations presents plenty of opportunity for error. At the higher end of the range the incidence of medical error in general practice is higher than the 2007 reported incidence of lung cancer in the English population, at 61.8 per 100 000 (Cancer Research UK, 2011).

Of course not all medical errors or 'untoward incidents' lead to or cause patient harm although these may be those most likely to be reported. The National Health Service Litigation Authority (NHSLA) the organization that manages clinical negligence claims against the UK National Health Service (NHS), reported that there were 6652 new claims made in 2009/10 and that they paid out £659 973 000 against claims in the same year (NHSLA, 2010). These sorts of statistics prompted Professor James Reason to declare that 'If Patient Safety was a disease it would be the top public health priority' (Reason, 2010).

Unexplained variation and value for money

The problems facing general practice are not just about safety issues, however. In the UK, and indeed the rest of the world, demand for healthcare, driven by advances in medical technologies, ageing populations and rising public expectations, has risen faster than the ability of governments and private insurance companies to provide sufficient funding. The Ford Motor Company in America once famously announced that it spent more on healthcare for its employees than it spent on sheet steel. The NHS website informs us that the NHS budget in 1948 was just £437 millions 'roughly £9bn at today's prices'. By 2008/09 the budget had increased to over £100 billion, 'a rise of more than 4% per year over and above inflation'. It is widely considered that this year-on-year growth is no longer affordable and the most recent two UK Governments have asked the

NHS to make efficiency savings of between £15 and £20 billion by 2014, equivalent to 5 per cent productivity gains year by year. This is a massive challenge for the NHS and can only be achieved by improving the clinical effectiveness and cost effectiveness of patient services.

Research has shown that there is wide variation in the delivery of effective care in general practice (see Case study 13.1 for an example from the King's Fund). Only part of this variation can be explained by differences in patient case mixes and by socio-economic factors. We know this to be the case in part because research has shown that the variation is not always just between general practices but within individual general practices too.

Reducing this variation to improve quality and productivity has become a central concern for general practice in the NHS and for healthcare systems around the world. As in all industries, quality assurance in healthcare is therefore also about improving productivity or cost and clinical effectiveness.

Case Study 13.1

In 2011 the King's Fund published a report into a major inquiry they had commissioned called *Improving the quality of care in general practice* (King's Fund, 2011). The key messages from this inquiry summarized the current state of quality in English general practice. The inquiry found that there was significant room for improvement and highlighted the need for more accurate data.

Diagnosis
'A variety of factors can lead to delays and errors in diagnosis, but there is not enough evidence to ascertain the scale of such problems in general practice.'

Referral
'There are wide variations in the rate of referrals between practices. The evidence suggests that a significant proportion of referrals made in general practice may not be clinically necessary. However, the appropriateness of a referral is specific to the context, and it may be difficult to decrease unnecessary referrals without also decreasing necessary referrals.'

Prescribing
'Variation in the level of prescribing between general practices is common and widely reported. Much of the practice-level variation in prescribing [but not

all] results from differences in the clinical case-mix of patients and socio-economic factors.'

Acute illness

'The evidence suggests that GPs are more likely to make a misdiagnosis of acute illness compared to non-acute illness.'

Long-term conditions

'[…] the evidence suggests that recommended care is not reliably delivered to all patients – especially to those with multiple long-term conditions.'

Health promotion

- *'There is a need to target childhood immunisations at those groups where uptake is low.*
- *Most general practices meet targets related to smoking cessation advice, but there is evidence that a more proactive approach to supporting patients may help people to quit smoking.*
- *Approaches to the management of people with obesity are inconsistent, and obesity is often seen as a lifestyle issue rather than as a priority for general practice.*
- *More evidence is needed for appropriate interventions in general practice.'*

Rising expectations and patient choice

It has become a truism in recent times that patients' expectations of the services that they receive from general practice and the NHS more widely have risen and continue to rise rapidly. It is thought that a number of factors coming together are driving these increased expectations. These include the wide availability of easily available information to patients, the introduction of patient choice, the ever increasing tax burden required to fund healthcare and a cultural change in attitudes.

In the past, GPs commonly told stories of 'heart sink' moments when patients arrived at the surgery with the latest copy of their daily newspaper, seeking explanations and changes to their treatment regime often as a result of poorly researched and sensationalist news stories. Today the internet provides patients with easy access to reliable sources of information which includes recognized treatment protocols, comparative outcomes data

and even patients' reviews of services and individual doctors. Patients and patient advocate groups have made great use of this information to demand better local services for themselves and their loved ones. Much of this information comes directly from the NHS itself as successive governments have tried to open up the NHS to market forces and use competition amongst service providers as a lever to drive up quality.

In recent years the Government have published details of a national GP patient survey in a form which allows patients to compare the results of their own practice with any other in the country (Department of Health, 2011). The survey asks questions about access, choice, continuity of care, the doctor–patient relationship and outcomes and has become a key performance indicator for English primary care trusts. Overall, the results suggest that patients are very happy with general practice services but again there is marked variation. This variation was highlighted by the King's Fund in 2011 (see Case study 13.2).

Case Study 13.2

In 2011 the King's Fund published a report into a major inquiry they had commissioned called *Improving the quality of care in general practice* (King's Fund, 2011). The key messages from this inquiry summarized the current state of quality in English general practice. The inquiry found that there was significant variation in the 'non-clinical aspects of general practice'.

Access

'Most people, most of the time, report good access to care. However, there are wide variations across all dimensions of access.'

Continuity of care

'Enabling patients to see the same doctor and other clinical staff with whom they build a relationship over time is regarded as a priority by GPs and patients alike. There is evidence to show that in recent years it has been more difficult for patients to see a preferred GP, raising concerns about continuity of care.

There is a need to improve co-ordination of care – particularly for those patients with complex and long-term care needs. Greater priority needs to be given to continuity of care and care co-ordination, and innovative ways need to be found to assess the quality of such care in practices, and between practices and others providing public services.'

Engagement and involvement of patients

'Patients report high levels of confidence and trust in general practice, but patients' experiences of involvement in decisions about their care and treatment vary. Overall, patients and carers remain poorly engaged in making decisions about their own health. More effort and attention in general practice needs to be placed on enabling patients to be engaged in decision making, and in supporting people to care for themselves.'

Thinking and Discussion Point

How does your practice compare with others locally and nationally? Log on to the GP Patient Survey website (www.gp-patient.co.uk/). Choose an indicator where your practice seems to be doing better than the average and ask yourself and colleagues why this might be the case. What could other practices do to improve? Now choose an indicator where your practice seems to be underperforming compared with the average and again ask yourself and colleagues why this might be the case. What could you do to improve your practice?

As patients and the public have become more aware of the range of treatments and services that are available and the costs to taxpayers of these services, they have become more demanding for better and fairer services. In tandem with this the generations that were born before the introduction of the NHS in 1948 are now in a minority. Few of us can remember what it was like before the introduction of universal healthcare and few of us are prepared to wait in long queues for second best healthcare services.

The movement to open up competition between service providers is particularly important for general practice providers who find themselves right at the heart of this emerging world. The vast majority of general practices are private, for profit, business partnerships working under contract to the NHS and now face very real competition from new and innovative service providers. GPs are therefore under increasing pressure not only to provide good clinical care but also a good patient experience.

What is quality in general practice?

Before we move on to discussing how to measure and assure the quality of the care that we provide, it is important to first have an understanding of what we mean by 'quality in general practice'. This has already been the subject of debate in a great many textbooks, lectures, research papers and, indeed and unfortunately, in the law courts. For the purpose of this chapter, however, there are two definitions that fit nicely together and although they do not tell us the whole story they give a satisfactory working definition for our purposes.

Thinking and Discussion Point

- How would you define 'quality' from the point of view of a GP?
- Discuss with your colleagues and peers. What does 'quality' mean to them when applied to healthcare?
- Discuss with your friends and family who are not doctors or training to be a doctor. What does 'quality' mean to them when applied to healthcare?
- How do the different views compare? Is there any agreement?
- Try to define what 'quality in general practice' means to you without using the word 'quality'.

In 2008 the NHS celebrated its 60th anniversary and the Government at the time published a series of reviews written by Lord Darzi to set out a vision and a plan for the development of the NHS over the next ten years (Department of Health, 2008). Central to this vision was to put quality at the heart and as the driving force of the NHS. For the first time the Boards of NHS organizations were asked to account for the quality of services that they provided or commissioned with the same rigour and accountability as they had previously for financial accounting and a duty to provide quality care was enshrined in law.

Darzi defined quality in three domains (see Case study 13.3):

- patient safety;
- clinical effectiveness; and
- the experience of patients.

Patient safety, according to Darzi, is about 'first causing no harm' and you will recognize this statement from the Hippocratic Oath. For Darzi, patient safety was to be measured in terms of medical errors, prescribing errors, infection rates and other avoidable harm. Clinical effectiveness was described by Darzi as the success rate of different treatments for defined clinical conditions and was to be measured by focusing on clinical outcomes such as mortality and morbidity rates, and by patients' own views of the success of their treatments – so-called patient-reported outcome measures (PROMS). For Darzi, the patient experience was all about the 'quality of caring' in terms of compassion, respect and dignity and was to be measured using patient satisfaction surveys of real patients' real experiences.

Case Study 13.3

In 2008 Lord Darzi in his next stage review, *High quality care for all* (Department of Health, 2008), defined quality from the perspective of patients and identified three key domains:

'If quality is to be at the heart of everything we do, it must be understood from the perspective of patients. Patients pay regard both to clinical outcomes and their experience of the service. They understand that not all treatments are perfect, but they do not accept that the organisation of their care should put them at risk. For these reasons, the Review has found that for the NHS, quality should include the following aspects:

- *Patient safety. The first dimension of quality must be that we do no harm to patients. This means ensuring the environment is safe and clean, reducing avoidable harm such as excessive drug errors or rates of healthcare associated infections.*

- *Patient experience. Quality of care includes quality of caring. This means how personal care is – the compassion, dignity and respect with which patients are treated. It can only be improved by analysing and understanding patient satisfaction with their own experiences.*

- *Effectiveness of care. This means understanding success rates from different treatments for different conditions. Assessing this will include clinical measures such as mortality or survival rates, complication rates and measures of clinical improvement. Just as important is the effectiveness of care from the patient's own perspective which will be measured through patient-reported outcomes measures (PROMs). Examples include improvement in pain-free movement after a joint replacement, or returning to work after treatment for depression. Clinical effectiveness may also extend to people's well-being and ability to live independent lives.'*

Some 20 years earlier Avedis Donabedian in a series of lectures and papers addressed the question 'The quality of care. How can it be assessed?' He wrote:

'There was a time, not too long ago, when this question could not have been asked. The quality of care was considered to be something of a mystery: real, capable of being perceived and appreciated, but not subject to measurement.

The very attempt to define and measure quality seemed, then, to denature and belittle it. Now, we have moved too far in the opposite direction. Those who have not experienced the intricacies of clinical practice demand measures that are easy, precise, and complete – as if a sack of potatoes was being weighed.' (Donabedian, 1988)

Donabedian died in 2000 but his words will ring as true today to doctors and healthcare managers swamped with targets and regulatory returns as they did in 1988. Of course, academic theory of quality in care and the science of measuring quality have developed a great deal since then and he left us with two foundation stones (amongst much else) that are vital to our understanding of quality in general practice today.

For Donabedian, there were two elements to the performance of practitioners: (1) technical performance and (2) interpersonal performance.

Technical performance is judged in terms of comparison with known best practice at the time: that is practice that is known to or believed to produce the greatest improvement in health. It is important to note that Donabedian was very clear that this element of performance was time-specific, and related to what was regarded as best practice at the time care was delivered. He said: 'Even if the actual consequences of care are disastrous, quality must be judged as good if care, at the time it was given, conformed to the practice that could have been expected to achieve the best results.'

Interpersonal performance was important for Donabedian because it 'is the vehicle by which technical care is implemented and on which its success depends.' He described the process of the interpersonal relationship as the patient provides information on which a diagnosis can be made and the physician provides information on the nature of the illness and its treatment and motivates the patient to collaborate. The success of an episode of healthcare is therefore dependent on both elements – technical and interpersonal – of practitioner performance. The continuity of thought revealed in Darzi's *safety*, *effectiveness* and *patient experience* domains of quality is clear to see.

Donabedian also guided us on approaches to measuring the quality of care that remain vital to our understanding today (see Case study 13.4). These approaches include:

■ structure,
■ process, and
■ outcome.

Structure refers to the settings in which care is provided. Are the facilities appropriate? Are healthcare teams properly qualified, reimbursed and resourced to provide care? Is there proper review of the services provided? *Process* refers to what is actually done in the provision and receipt of care by the practitioner and the patient. *Outcome* refers to the effects of care on patients and populations and includes improvements in the patient's knowledge and behaviours. This approach, Donabedian tells us, is possible because 'good structure increases the likelihood of good process, and good process increases the likelihood of a good outcome.'

Crucially, the links between structure, process and outcome in any given healthcare setting have to have been determined previously. Today there is a great emphasis on measuring outcomes as the key to defining and assessing the quality of care in general practice. We ignore structure and process, however, at our peril.

Case Study 13.4

In 1988 Donabedian wrote a series of seminal lectures and papers defining quality in care and approaches to assessment that underpin our thinking today (Donadebian, 1988).

'The information from which inferences can be drawn about the quality of care can be classified under three categories: "structure," "process," and "outcome."

■ *Structure* – Structure denotes the attributes of the settings in which care occurs. This includes the attributes of material resources (such as facilities, equipment, and money), of human resources (such as the number and qualifications of personnel), and of organisational structure (such as medical staff organisation, methods of peer review, and methods of reimbursement).
■ *Process* – Process denotes what is actually done in giving and receiving care. It includes the patient's activities in seeking care and carrying it out as well as the practitioner's activities in making a diagnosis and recommending or implementing treatment.
■ *Outcome* – Outcome denotes the effects of care on patients and populations. Improvements in the patient's knowledge and salutary changes in the patient's behaviour are included under a broad definition of health status, and so is the degree of the patient's satisfaction with care.'

Practical approaches to quality assurance in general practice

Quality assurance is a management process used in all industries to help organizations meet their strategic goals by ensuring that products and services are safe, meet customer needs and provide value for money. Good quality assurance programmes combine quality control, the need to meet minimum standards and continuous quality improvement, and the need to encourage development and innovation.

In this section we will look at some of the different ways that approaches to quality assurance have been applied in general practice. By adopting some or all of these quality assurance methods in your own practice, both personally and within your practice team, you will begin to be able to meet the challenge set at the beginning of this chapter.

The General Medical Services Contract Quality and Outcomes Framework

The Quality and Outcomes Framework (QOF) for general practice was introduced as part of the new 2004 General Medical Services (GMS) contract (see also Chapter 14 on management and Chapter 16 on being a GP). It is a voluntary quality assurance programme but is linked to strong financial incentives and has been described as the first attempt to introduce 'performance-related pay' for doctors working for the NHS. The Framework is based on a set of agreed standards that form four domains: clinical, organizational, patient experience and additional services (Table 13.1).

Table 13.1 The Quality and Outcomes Framework domains and indicators 2011/12

Domain	Indicator
Clinical domain	Secondary prevention of coronary heart disease
	Cardiovascular disease – primary prevention
	Heart failure
	Stroke and transient ischaemic attacks
	Hypertension
	Diabetes mellitus
	Chronic obstructive pulmonary disease
	Epilepsy
	Hypothyroidism
	Cancer
	Palliative care
	Asthma
	Dementia
	Depression
	Chronic kidney disease
	Atrial fibrillation
	Obesity
	Learning disability
	Smoking
Organization domain	Records and information
	Information for patients
	Education and training
	Practice management
	Medicines management
	Quality and productivity
Patient experience domain	Length of consultations
Additional services domain	Cervical screening
	Child health surveillance
	Maternity services
	Contraception

Payments are made to practices for meeting target thresholds and in some instances are calculated according to the number of patients treated, known as the 'practice prevalence'. There are 19 indicators in the clinical domain and each of these have a number of criteria. Most of the clinical indicators have a criterion that requires the practice to have a relevant disease register, an essential first step in delivering structured care to all appropriate patients. There are criteria within the domains that cover the 'structure', 'process', and the 'outcomes' of care, and incentive payments are made for many of the criteria at two levels, a lower threshold to set a minimum standard and a higher threshold to encourage continuous quality improvement.

There is general agreement amongst commentators that the Quality and Outcomes Framework has resulted in improvements to services provided in general practice. However there has been some criticism that improvement has only come in those areas covered by the various indicators and innovation elsewhere has been stifled. The Quality and Outcomes Framework has also been criticized for being too easy to achieve and has rewarded practices for implementing only the minimum standards that patients had a right to expect anyway. Partly as a response to this criticism, indicators have been regularly updated or replaced with new, more challenging criteria.

Royal College of General Practitioners Practice Accreditation

In 2008 the Royal College of General Practitioners (RCGP) launched a voluntary scheme of practice accreditation called the Primacy Medical Care Provider Accreditation (PMCPA), which aims to support general practices to provide patient-centred care and to improve the quality of their services (Table 13.2). The accreditation scheme has three key stages: a pre-entry stage that includes criteria that are legal requirements of all providers, a set of 30 core criteria and a set of 80 developmental criteria. To become accredited over a three-year period, practices must first qualify for the pre-entry stage and to receive accreditation the practice must meet all 30 of the core criteria and at least 40 of the development criteria. External assessment, by the RCGP, at entry to the scheme and annually thereafter will ensure that practices continue to develop and improve as in each year they must demonstrate that they have met more of the developmental criteria.

The accreditation scheme is divided into six domains and each domain has a number of core and developmental criteria that were developed by the RCGP and the National Primary Care Research and Development Centre at the University of Manchester:

- Health inequalities and health promotion
- Provider management
- Premises, records, equipment and medicines management
- Provider teams
- Learning organization
- Patient experience/involvement.

It is too early to know if the scheme will be a success but a pilot of 40 practices in 2008 showed promising results.

Thinking and Discussion Point

The Quality and Outcomes Framework and the RCGP Primacy Medical Care Provider Accreditation can be seen as examples of what is known as 'total quality management' approaches to quality assurance. That is, they attempt to define and measure quality across the whole organization and not just one part of its activities.

What do you think of them? Do they measure what you and your friends defined as quality in general practice in the thinking and discussion point above? What do they miss and what do you think might be added to improve them?

Ask your practice manager if your practice takes part in either scheme. If so, ask him or her to show you how the practice has implemented the quality assurance work into routine practice life. How does your practice fare? Where does the practice do well? What are the difficulties and what could be improved?

Table 13.2 RCGP Primacy Medical Care Provider Accreditation: domains and number of criteria per domain

Domain	Number of summative criteria	Formative dimensions	Number of formative criteria
Health inequalities and health promotion	2	Health needs assessment	11
		Children	
		Patient responsiveness	
		Supporting parents	
		Specific groups	
Provider management	6	Roles and responsibilities	13
		Team member records	
		Infection control	
		Managing performance	
		Policies and procedures	
Premises, records, equipment and medicines management	5	Medicines management	13
		Branch surgeries	
		Information for team members	
		Records	
Provider teams	7	Home care	15
		Patient responsiveness	
		Patient safety	
		Team values and team working	
Learning organization	6	Continuous quality Improvement and audit	17
		Training and professional development	
		Patient complaints	
		Relationships with other organizations	
Patient experience/ involvement	4	Patient responsiveness	13
		Specific groups	
		Interpersonal continuity	
		Information for patients	
		Patient and public Involvement	

From Lester and Campbell (2008).

Clinical audit

The term 'medical audit' was first described as being an expected part of the professional duties of all doctors in the Government White Paper *Working for patients* published in 1989 (Department of Health, 1989). Since that time, the term 'clinical audit' has taken its place and reflects the fact that audit is now a multiprofessional activity, involving many clinical profession-

als and managers within their respective teams. The White Paper contained two definitions of clinical audit:

'The systematic, critical analysis of the quality of medical care, including the procedures used for diagnosis and treatment, the use of resources, and the resulting outcome and quality of life for the patient.' (Department of Health, 1989)

'[Clinical audit involves] looking at what you do in a way that allows you to see how you might do things better, making appropriate changes and then looking again to assess improvements in clinical practice.'
(Department of Health, 1989)

In recent years, the basis of clinical audit has developed to be much more focused on the agreement and subsequent implementation of realistic plans to improve patient care. Such change plans, rather than being in the form of vague recommendations, can take on the rigour of plans familiar to the business community and be informed by a variety of professionals, managers and, increasingly, the patients themselves.

The basis of audit is that incorporated within the audit cycle, an example of which is shown in Figure 13.1. This shows a simple model for undertaking audit. Within it, however, lies a variety of complexities if professionals are to respond to an audit by being willing to make changes to their clinical practice.

An audit consists of a group of criteria – measurable statements about the clinical topic – together with an agreed standard for each aspect of care under review. Criteria are arrived at by discussions within the team and may be influenced by external information such as research evidence, local or national guidelines, and other audits performed or designed elsewhere. Each criterion is agreed by the practice team and represents an important measurable aspect of care that can be influenced within an appropriate time scale by the practice team. Criteria are constructed specifically to allow them to be judged as present or absent when data are collected.

In practice, criteria can be devised to look at clinical care from a range of perspectives. A frequent classification for criteria follows Donabedian and divides them into *structure*, *process* and *outcome*. Examples of criteria classified in this way, for an audit of patients with known ischaemic heart disease, are shown in Case study 13.5. Structural criteria concern the structures needed to be in place for care to occur effectively. Process criteria concern actual events in clinical practice that have or have not taken place. Outcome criteria concern whether those events have resulted in a positive effect on the health of the patient.

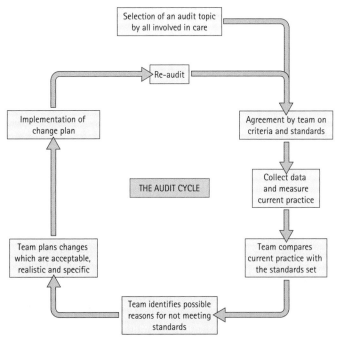

Figure 13.1 The audit cycle.

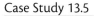

Case Study 13.5

Structure	A register of all patients with ischaemic heart disease exists/does not exist within the practice.
	A recall system is/is not in place to review all patients with known ischaemic heart disease at least annually.
	The practice has/does not have agreed guidelines for risk factor management in patients with ischaemic heart disease.
Process	The records show that patients eligible for aspirin therapy have/have not been prescribed aspirin.
	The records show that a serum lipid result is/is not present.
	The records show that for patients with abnormal serum lipids, dietary advice has/has not been given.
	The records show that a patient's blood pressure has/has not been measured in the last year.
Intermediate outcome	The records show that patients with abnormal lipids prior to one year ago now have/do not have a lipid measurement within the target range agreed.
	The records show that the last blood pressure reading for patients with hypertension diagnosed prior to one year ago was/was not below 90 mmHg diastolic.
Long-term outcome[a]	The mortality rate of patients with known ischaemic heart disease.
	The incidence of strokes in patients with known ischaemic heart disease.

[a]This is not usually appropriate within audit: see text.

The last 3–4 years have seen a greater emphasis on trying to define outcome criteria for our patients. However, within general practice any use of long-term outcome measures is severely hampered. Let us consider a major goal in clinical care: to reduce the mortality rate of certain groups of patients with ischaemic heart disease. The meaningful demonstration of this rate is impossible within a single practice due to the small numbers of patients concerned and the general turnover of patients who change practices. The same would be true for blindness or renal failure in diabetes.

However, intermediate outcome measures (or proxy outcome measures) can be used where research evidence has shown that a specific intervention can result in health gains for the individual patient. Research supports the assumption that our patients' health may well gain if we can show that patients with hypertension have their blood pressure controlled.

The setting of standards is an important step in audit as this defines, following agreement by the team, what is an appropriate level of performance in delivering clinical care. A standard is set specifically for each criterion in the audit. The actual level of standard set can be influenced by a number of factors. It is meant to be a realistic target of the level of care you feel is appropriate at a particular time, given the resources and systems you have in place. It follows that as a result of audit, these resources and systems may change, and so realistic standards may well increase in subsequent audits. Standards can also be informed by external factors such as research evidence, other audits and recommendations from organizations such as the British Diabetic Association or the British Hypertension Society. Examples of standards are shown below for an audit of patients with known ischaemic heart disease. (The particular percentages given here are arbitrary.)

Structure

- A register of all patients with ischaemic heart disease should exist within the practice.
- A recall system should be in place to review all patients with known ischaemic heart disease at least annually.
- The practice should have agreed guidelines for risk factor management in patients with ischaemic heart disease.

Process

- Eighty per cent of patients eligible for aspirin therapy should have been prescribed aspirin.
- A serum lipid investigation should have been carried out for 80 per cent of patients with ischaemic heart disease.
- Seventy per cent of patients with abnormal serum lipids should have been given dietary advice.

- Eighty per cent of patients should have had a blood pressure recording in the last year.

Intermediate outcome

- Sixty per cent of patients with abnormal lipids prior to one year ago should have a lipid measurement within the target range agreed.
- Eighty per cent of patients with hypertension diagnosed prior to one year ago should have a blood pressure reading below 90 mmHg diastolic.

Thinking and Discussion Point

Of necessity, clinical audit frequently involves making changes to our clinical behaviour. The factors involved in successfully changing our behaviour, or indeed the behaviour of others, are not straightforward. Think about the last time you changed some aspect of your social lifestyle (e.g. joined a club, started exercise):

- What motivated you to change?
- What did you need to enable you to make the change?
- In what way did you gain from the change?
- What were the costs for you or others?
- What did you need to maintain the change?

You may wish to discuss aspects of your thoughts with other students. Hopefully you will have been reminded of some of the important factors that influence changes in our behaviour.

Once clinical audit criteria and standards have been set and data have been collected, the results for each criterion are compared with its corresponding standard. Implicit in clinical audit is the assumption that where the criteria do not meet the standards a quality improvement plan is agreed and implemented and a re-audit is performed to check that the changes made have had the desired effect and that all criteria now do meet the standards.

Clinical audit has been and will continue to be a core component of quality assurance in general practice. There are two key benefits of the clinical audit cycle for use in primary care. First of these is its scalability: clinical audits can be of the whole practice or of an individual doctor's practice and can be of one or a great many criteria. The second key benefit of clinical audit is the built-in assumption that the cycle includes a process of improvement and re-evaluation.

SUMMARY POINTS

To conclude, the most important messages of this chapter are as follows:

- The huge volume and scope of general practice provides plenty of opportunities for things to go wrong.
- Overall the quality of general practice services is good but there remains unexplained and unacceptable variation.
- Quality in general practice can be defined in terms of patient safety, effectiveness and the patient experience and in terms of practitioner's technical and interpersonal performance.
- Quality in general practice should be assessed in three categories: structure, process and outcome.
- Good quality assurance programmes have two elements: quality control to ensure minimum standards are met and quality improvement to encourage development and innovation.
- There are three common and practical approaches to quality assurance in general practice.

References

Cancer Research UK 2011: Lung cancer – UK incidence statistics. http://info.cancerresearchuk.org/cancerstats/types/lung/incidence/ (accessed 21 April 2011).

Department of Health 1989: *Working for patients*. London: HMSO.

Department of Health 2008: *High quality care for all. NHS Next Stage Review final report*. London: The Stationery Office.

Department of Health 2011: GP patient surveys. www.dh.gov.uk/en/Publicationsandstatistics/PublishedSurvey/GPpatientsurvey2007/index.htm (accessed 21 April 2011).

Donabedian, A. 1988: The quality of care. How can it be assessed? *Journal of the American Medical Association* 12(260), 1743–8.

King's Fund 2011: *Improving the quality of care in general practice. Report of an independent inquiry commissioned by The King's Fund.* www.kingsfund.org.uk/publications/gp_inquiry_report.html (accessed 21 April 2011).

Lester, H. and Campbell, S. 2008: Accreditation of primary care providers. *RCGP News* June, 2.

NHSLA (National Health Service Litigation Authority) 2010: Report and accounts. www.nhsla.com/NR/rdonlyres/3F5DFA84-2463-468B-890C-42C0FC16D4D6/0/NHSLAAnnualReportandAccounts2010.pdf (accessed 21 April 2011).

NPSA (National Patient Safety Agency) 2011: General practice. www.nrls.npsa.nhs.uk/resources/health-care-setting/general-practice/ (accessed 21 April 2011).

Reason, J. 2010: *Patient safety in primary care* (DVD). TVC Films Ltd, London.

Acknowledgements

Thank you to Dr Steve Smith who was co-author in previous editions.

SINGLE BEST ANSWER QUESTIONS

13.1 What do we know of the current state of 'quality' in general practice?

a) There are insufficient reliable data to be able to say whether the current state of quality in general practice is good or poor
b) Overall the current state of quality in general practice is good but there is plenty of opportunity for error
c) The current state of quality in general practice is marked by widespread and unexplained variation within and between practices
d) In the main the current state of quality in general practice is good; however research has shown that there are widespread and unexplained variations
e) Research has shown that there are widespread variations in referral rates that put patients at unnecessary risk and do not provide taxpayers with value for money.

13.2 How did Lord Darzi define 'quality in healthcare'?

a) Lord Darzi in his 2008 review of the NHS defined quality in health as having three key dimensions; patient safety, the patient experience and clinical effectiveness
b) Darzi believed that quality in healthcare should be defined from the patient's perspective
c) Darzi defined quality in healthcare in terms of clinical and cost effectiveness
d) Darzi thought that patients should be treated with dignity and respect
e) For Darzi, quality in healthcare is all about ensuring that patients are not harmed by their healthcare.

13.3 How did Donabedian recommend that quality in healthcare be assessed?

a) Donabedian recommended that quality in healthcare be assessed in terms of technical performance and interpersonal performance
b) For Donabedian quality of care was something that could not be easily measured
c) Donabedian thought that healthcare should be assessed in terms of clinical outcomes for patients and populations
d) Donabedian recommended that healthcare should be assessed in terms of structure, process and outcomes
e) Donabedian recommended that quality in healthcare should be assessed by clinical audit.

SINGLE BEST ANSWER QUESTIONS CONTINUED

13.4 What is quality assurance in general practice?

a) Quality assurance is a management process used to ensure that general practice is safe, effective and improves the patient experience
b) Quality assurance is external, independent assessment of general practitioner's performance
c) Quality assurance was introduced in the 2004 General Medical Services contract as a way of rewarding doctors for good practice
d) Quality assurance is a form of clinical audit
e) Quality assurance in general practice is a framework of clinical and non-clinical indicators of good practice.

13.5 What is clinical audit?

a) Clinical audit is a process of measuring clinical performance against agreed standards
b) Clinical audit is a process that involves looking at what you do in critical way so that you can see how you might do things better, making appropriate changes to your practice and then looking again to see that you have made things better
c) Clinical audit is about setting standards of care against agreed criteria and measuring the difference
d) Clinical audit is a tool for improving patient care
e) Clinical audit is a process for measuring clinical performance in terms of structure, process and outcomes.

CHAPTER

14

THE MANAGEMENT OF GENERAL PRACTICE

- Organizational structure
- Contract with the NHS
- Practice income
- Strategic planning

- Summary points
- Reference
- Further reading
- Single best answer questions

The management of a general practice is complex. To all intents and purposes it is a business like any other which gets paid for the service it provides. However it has to balance the needs of patients, comply with numerous regulations and meet government targets all whilst remaining financially viable. It requires planning for the future as well as managing the present. The owners of the business have a responsibility to its customers/patients and also a duty to its employees. How well an organization performs is down to how well it is managed. The majority of general practitioners (GPs) employ a practice manager or business manager to help them to run their business.

LEARNING POINTS

By the end of this chapter you will be able to:
- outline the key responsibilities of the management team;
- discuss the different types of contract a general practice can have with the NHS;
- describe why strategic planning is important;
- identify the main functions of management within general practice;
- understand the different operational aspects of the practice manager's role;

Organizational structure

A general practice is 'owned' or contracted by self-employed practitioners. The 'owner' or 'contractor' could be an individual GP or a partnership where two or more individuals form a partnership, one of whom must be a medical practitioner. A third option could be a limited company whereby one of the shareholders is a medical practitioner.

A general practice is an organization and, dependent on size, will have a number of individuals working for that organization with varying skills and knowledge. Most partnerships will employ a practice manager or business manager to work with them on the strategic aspects of running their business, but also to manage all of the operational aspects. As most GPs have had very little training in business management skills, it is important to bring those skills into the business.

Management team

Typically the management team is made up of the partners and the practice/business manager. In larger practices the management team may also include an assistant practice manager and/or a finance manager and/or a patient services manager.

In the past, general practices have been run by partners who have shared all of the clinical work. The profits of the practice are split between the partners. Since the 2004 General Medical Services (GMS) contract was introduced there has been a move away from increasing the size of partnerships. One of the reasons for this has been that it has become more cost effective to employ salaried GPs as opposed to reducing the profit share between the remaining partners.

The management team will determine the strategic direction of the practice. In many practices each partner will take a lead role in a particular area. For example this could be a clinical area or a management area such as human resources (HR) or information technology (IT). As with any business, the owner has to take ultimate responsibility for the way that business performs. Having said that, the practice manager plays a key role in influencing and implementing the way the business is run. A practice manager will have the added knowledge and experience of managing a business which a GP may not.

Workforce

The size and structure of the workforce within a general practice is dependent upon a number of factors, including:

- the number of patients on its list;
- the availability of doctors and nurses in the local area;
- the skills and experience of the current workforce;
- the demographics of the local population;
- the staffing budget in relation to income and overall expenditure.

It will be up to the management team to determine how the skills within the practice are split. A typical general practice might employ the following categories of employee:

- salaried GP;
- practice nurse;
- healthcare assistant;
- receptionist;
- administrator/medical secretary.

Additional skills can be bought in by employing counsellors, therapists, bookkeepers, etc. Some of the workforce will not be directly employed by the practice but will work closely with the team. This group includes health visitors, midwives, dieticians and drug and alcohol counsellors. This list is not exhaustive. (See more about the roles of some of the team members in Chapter 2 on general practice and its place in primary care.)

Such a vast range of skills all housed under one roof makes the task of managing and utilization of all these skills a challenging one. It requires careful strategic planning, good communication and excellent organization. The design of such an organization is crucial to its success.

Most importantly, a general practice is in place to provide a service to its customers/patients. It has to be aware of its customers' needs and tailor its approach to meet those needs. Just like any other business, a general practice needs to fulfil its contractual responsibilities. A general practice is a private business that has its biggest contract with the NHS!

Practical Exercise

List the different categories of employee within your practice. Find out from the practice manager who is directly employed by the practice and who is not. How does the practice integrate those that are not directly employed?

Contract with the NHS

Each general practice has a contract with the NHS to provide medical services. Each GP contractor has a choice of whether to sign up to a nationally agreed standard contract, a General Medical Services (GMS) contract, or whether to agree to a locally negotiated Personal Medical Services (PMS) contract (see also Chapter 16 on being a general practitioner).

Primary care trusts (PCT)

The primary care trust is given authority by the National Health Service to commission services for its local patients within agreed budgets. It pays hospitals a national tariff based on the services they can provide to the local population. The tariff is agreed as part of an overall contract. The job of the

PCT is to ensure that care is provided to the whole community. The PCT may directly employ people to deliver that service, for example health visitors and district nurses. The PCT provides support and funding to general practices for service development and will performance manage practices that are not meeting the requirements of their contract. If a GP contractor has a GMS contract the role of the PCT is to ensure that the contract is implemented. If the GP contractor has a PMS contract the role of the PCT is to negotiate that contract but also ensure that it is implemented correctly.

At the time of writing, the coalition Government has outlined its proposals for the future within a White Paper, *Equity and excellence: liberating the NHS*, published on 12 July 2010 (Department of Health, 2010). Primary care trusts will cease to exist from 2013 and in their place will be small local health authorities and an NHS Commissioning Board. Most of the services commissioned will be commissioned by local GP consortia. This will change the mechanism for paying practices. A full review of the GP contract will also take place over the coming year/years.

General Medical Services contract

In 2004 the General Medical Services (GMS) contract was introduced. At the time of writing this contract is about to come under review.

A GMS contract is a standard national contract which general practices can choose to work under. The contract states that GP contractors must provide essential medical services. These services are to treat patients that are sick, terminally ill or who have a chronic disease. This is the basic service that all GP contractors must provide. Practices can offer additional services such as immunization of children, child health surveillance, maternity services, contraceptive services, cervical screening, vaccinations and immunizations, and minor surgery. Practices can opt in or out of these services on a temporary or permanent basis. They can also subcontract these services.

The GMS contract is nationally defined but locally implemented by primary care trusts.

Personal Medical Services contract

A Personal Medical Services contract is slightly different. Whereas a GMS contract is defined nationally, a PMS contract is defined locally. This gives primary care trusts the ability to tailor services to the needs of its local patient population. There are many similarities to the GMS contract. Both contracts must provide the basic services described above. A PMS contractor has a wider choice of additional services that it can offer which are agreed locally with the local PCT.

A PMS contract gives GP contractors more flexibility and its funding is distributed in a different way to allow more flexibility, in particular for employing salaried GPs and nurse practitioners.

Practical Exercise

Find out which type of contract the practice has. Discuss with a member of the management team their thoughts on the practice's current contract. How much flexibility does the contract offer?

Practice income

The main source of income that the practice receives is from the contract it has with the NHS. There are other ways in which a practice can generate income but there are restrictions on how much private income is generated.

NHS income

Global sum

Practices are paid money based on the number of patients that they have on their list. An amount per patient is given to the practice and a practice's list size is reviewed every quarter to take into consideration any variation. This is called the 'global sum'. The global sum can be adjusted up or down during the year accordingly. A practice can increase its income by increasing its list size. This sounds simple but an increased list size will also generate additional costs based on more demand from patients. The practice has to ensure it gets the balance right.

The global sum incorporates money for certain items of expenditure which in the past had been separated out. For example, the global sum will include monies to pay for out-of-hours services which the practice may or may not have deputized to an out-of-hours provider. It could also include money to fund protected learning time, which the practice can use to hold team learning events on a regular basis.

Enhanced services

In addition to the global sum, a practice can decide to provide additional or enhanced services. Some of these services are directed nationally and some locally. An enhanced service commands additional payment. Each enhanced service will have its own service level agreement which stipulates the criteria that have to be met before payment is made. It will also outline monitoring arrangements and reporting requirements to which the practice has to adhere. It is therefore important for the management team to read the small print before signing up to a new service. Practices can be caught out by the additional work involved in meeting all of the requirements of the service level agreement.

Directed enhanced service

The Department of Health determines areas for priority and gives national guidelines on how certain services should be carried out. Examples of these types of directed enhanced service are:

- flu immunization;
- minor surgery;
- childhood vaccines and immunizations;
- improved access (e.g. extended opening hours).

These services would be commissioned by primary care trusts following national guidelines.

National enhanced services

These services are additional services which any practice can sign up to. They are services which have been initiated nationally and sign-up is voluntary. Examples of this type of service would be:

- fitting of intrauterine devices;
- provision of drug and alcohol services.

Local enhanced services

These are services which the local primary care trust has determined would help to meet the needs of the local patient population. Practices can choose whether or not to provide these services. Examples could include:

- providing GP services to local nursing homes;
- sexual health clinics;
- chlamydia screening;
- talking therapies;
- governance;
- end of life gold standard care.

This list is not exhaustive.

Quality and Outcomes Framework

In addition to the global sum and enhanced service payments a practice can earn income by ensuring quality across clinical and organizational indicators. The Quality and Outcomes Framework (QOF) is a points-based system split into clinical and organizational domains. Each area has a list of indicators. The more a practice reaches a target within an indicator the more points they are awarded. The points are worth money. Primary care trusts pay practices an aspiration payment based on the expected achievement against the QOF. Seventy per cent of the expected achievement is paid up front, split into monthly payments. At the end of the financial year the practice and the primary care trust agree the total number of points actually achieved and the difference is paid or taken back from the practice.

As part of the July 2010 White Paper, a new outcomes framework is being introduced. At the time of writing, the National Institute for Health and Clinical Excellence (NICE) has been tasked with the development of the new Framework.

Practical Exercise

Find out what QOF points the practice achieved in the last financial year. How do you think a practice can improve upon its results? What do you think the impact would be if these points were not achieved?

Non-NHS income

In addition to the income generated by the GMS/PMS contract, practices can carry out private services which generate additional income. There are many different ways a practice can increase

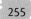

its level of income. The following list gives some examples of how this can be done:

- Medical examinations, for both registered and non-registered patients
- Medical/insurance reports, often requested by insurance companies and solicitors
- Provision of GP services to a local prison
- Provision of GP services to a nursing home
- Occupational health services provided to local businesses
- Data collection for research projects. In addition, practices can participate in research projects and earn additional income from this
- Acting as medical referees for the local crematorium
- Sports club GP
- GP with a specialist interest – GPs can provide specialist services to patients within the locality (see Chapter 16 on being a GP).

As you can see there are many different ways a general practice can earn extra money. There is a cap on how much private income a practice can earn. This is to ensure that the requirements of the PMS/GMS contract can be met. The management team need to ensure that any additional services do not put too much pressure on the practice's core service. This requires careful planning and regular reviews of the services that the practice provides.

Strategic planning

As part of the process of managing a general practice it is important to consider not just short-term plans for the practice but also long-term plans for the future. This will help the practice meet the needs of patients both now and in the years to come. This is called strategic planning. Strategic planning looks at where we are now and then where we want to be in the future. The gap is the journey or actions that will be required to get there.

Business plan/practice development plan

Many practices have business plans or practice development plans that analyse the present in terms of resources, skills and infrastructure, and forecast changes in these areas based on goals that have been set for the future. A plan is typically spread over a five-year period broken down into actions for the next 12 months. It is the responsibility of the management team to drive this plan and review it on a regular basis (e.g. every 6–12 months). Environmental factors will require that the plan adapts as and when needed. The plan is normally cascaded to the rest of the team; good practice would be to involve the practice team in the development of the plan. It is important for the team as a whole to have bought in to the plan and have individual performance objectives that are linked in to the plan.

Vision for the future

When determining the future direction of the practice a good starting point is to consider what the vision is for the future. The vision is about visualizing what you want the practice to look like in the years to come and is about determining the goals for the future. This should take into consideration the values of the partnership/management team. If a vision for the future is at odds with the personal values of one or more of the management team, this will mean the vision is distorted and will be difficult to achieve. This will need to be discussed and a way forward agreed.

The vision can then be broken down into achievable SMART goals: specific, measurable, agreed, realistic and time related.

Environmental factors

The management team will need to consider if there are factors that could prevent or change the goals that have been set. These could be a change in government or change in government policy. They could also be changes to services provided in the local area or the impact of staff leaving.

Strategic planning is about planning for the future based on what you know now. Good practice would be to hold a team event whereby the practice as a whole carries out a SWOT analysis, which looks at the practice's strengths, weaknesses, opportunities and threats that could affect the future direction of the practice. This process can help to determine how to overcome difficulties but also aids the practice's ability to be more alert to opportunities.

When planning for the future we have said that we need to consider where we are now and where we want to be. A good idea is to break this down into different management areas within the practice. Those areas could be patient services, human resources, finance, IT and marketing/communication. We explore these areas in more detail below.

Practical Exercise

Find out from the practice manager if your practice has a business plan or practice development plan. Ask to see this and then list what you perceive to be the key priorities for the next 12 months. Discuss with a member of the management team.

Patient services

What services do we currently provide?

A good starting point would be to review the services a practice currently provides. Are those services effective and do they make a difference to the patient? For example, a practice could offer a phlebotomy service to patients. Do many patients use the service? Are the clinics always full? A patient survey would give valuable insight into how well that service is delivered and received. Another important consideration is whether the service is cost effective (i.e. does the money received to run the service pay for all of the costs associated with that service?).

Once all of these factors have been taken into consideration, the management team can decide if it is justifiable to continue providing that service. Eventually the management team will have a clear list of the current services that it wishes to continue providing.

What services do we need for the future?

Is there a particular service that the practice is not currently providing but that would be of benefit to patients? A first point would be to consider whether the service is needed. That need could be provided by the closure of a local service or a new service that has been put out to tender by the local commissioners.

Currently the primary care trust commissions the majority of services that are provided by hospitals and community teams. As a result of the White Paper brought out by the coalition Government in July 2010 this responsibility will move from primary care trusts to local GP consortia. This will open up a wealth of opportunity to provide new services which have traditionally been provided by the hospitals. A GP practice could potentially provide a service for a local population which costs far less per patient than that of a local hospital. This then provides savings in order to provide more services in the locality. The additional benefit for patients is in that they could have more services provided to them on their doorstep, with a shorter waiting time to be seen. The management team would also need to identify who they have within the team to deliver that service. If they do not have the required knowledge or skills then this resource could be bought in and new skills employed to deliver that service. Of course the service has to be cost effective and a full financial review of the new service would need to take place.

Determining the need for new services requires analysis of data (e.g. a practice could look at the number of patients that require the service by reviewing and analysing referrals made to similar services). Data can be collected from the practice's clinical system but also from secondary care data held by local trusts. GP practices now have access to these data along with information about money spent on outpatient and accident and emergency care for their patients. Through careful analysis, a practice can see where savings can be made by providing services in the community.

Case Study 14.1

Town Road Practice carried out a financial review of its phlebotomy service. The money that the practice received to pay for the service was slightly less than the cost of employing a phlebotomist. The practice held a management team meeting and decided to close the service, giving patients one month's notice of the change. Notices were put up in the practice to inform patients. When the patients read the notices many were unhappy that they had not been consulted and would now have to travel a few miles away to the hospital to have their tests done. One month after the practice had closed its phlebotomy service the practice administrator noticed that the number of tests required to be carried out for the Quality and Outcomes Framework had fallen. The practice was not meeting its QOF targets as there were considerable delays at the hospital phlebotomy department. This led to delays in carrying out patients' chronic disease reviews.

What other factors should the practice have taken into consideration before deciding to close down a service? What was the impact of not taking these things into consideration?

Patient surveys also provide useful data on which to determine what and how a service is provided. For example where a practice wanted to set up an online booking service for patients the practice could identify how many people currently use their website by reviewing the number of clicks made to the site and also could place an online survey on to the website to determine how many people would want to use the service. Data analysis has become a key tool in supporting managers in their decision making.

Many practices now have patient groups which they can use to gain feedback and suggestions on how to improve patient care and pathways into certain services. Another useful tool is through patient complaints. Patient complaints can identify common problems and reinforce and influence the reasons behind changing a current service or introducing a new one.

Human resources

A business is as good as the people that it employs. None more so than the business of general practice. Careful planning of a practice's workforce will enable practices to succeed in delivery of those all-important goals.

Resource planning

Good practice would be to carry out a 'manpower analysis' based on the current workforce. This analysis looks at the skills and knowledge within the current team; it also looks at where there may be staff turnover in the future (i.e. forthcoming retirements and leavers) based on previous levels of staff turnover or known career aspira-

tions obtained from annual appraisals. 'What if' scenarios are also a good way of preparing contingencies and succession plans. For example, what if the nurse who sees all of our diabetic patients leaves? Who would take over that clinic? Would we still be able to provide that clinic? If the answer is 'no' then a contingency plan must be put in place which could mean training someone else to do that job even if it is just for an interim period while you recruit to replace. When someone leaves it should not be automatic that they are replaced by a new recruit. Proper consideration should be given to the team as a whole as this could be an opportunity to restructure the workforce or elements of it.

Once you have your current plan in place, the management team can then determine their ideal manpower plan. The difference between the two will be the steps you take to get there. Whenever an opportunity arises (i.e. someone leaves or is promoted), the management team should take action to move closer towards their ideal manpower plan. If it is thought that this will take too long then a restructuring exercise should take place. Restructuring can mean that the way in which people currently work will change and this requires careful consultation with individual employees. Legal advice should be taken prior to taking this option.

Training and development

One way in which to obtain new skills and knowledge within the practice is to train the current workforce. Individuals may have an interest in a particular area which also meets the needs and aims of the practice. The practice can then enable the individual(s) to be trained in a particular area, which will mean the goals of the business are met. A training needs analysis can clearly show where there are gaps in skills which can then be addressed. Training of all practice staff is vital to ensure that the practice's approach remains fresh and generates new ideas for improving current working practices and also introduces new ones. It also helps to motivate teams and individuals. Clinicians and managers have a professional responsibility to continuously develop. Practices therefore also have a responsibility to ensure that they continuously update their skills as a team which will help them meet the goals within their business plan.

Employee engagement

Most practices will have a meeting structure in place which allows them to make decisions. It is important to gather the views of the team. By taking on board everybody's ideas there is more chance of a good idea being suggested and improvements made. In addition, appraisal systems are a good method of gaining the views and aspirations of individuals. This can help with strategic planning by identifying manpower opportunities, training needs, ideas and suggestions for the future. If people feel that they are listened to they will engage more with what is going on in the practice. Employee engagement and involvement is motivational. Motivation means that people will care about what they do and how they do it.

Most practices will have a meeting structure in place whereby members of the team can discuss issues and share ideas and suggestions for improvements.

Financial planning

Many practices use the services of a bookkeeper to manage the financial transactions of the practice. It is also important that someone within the practice has a good understanding of the management of the finances and not simply the process within which they are collated. This will be about understanding where the practice stands financially at any given time. In some practices a partner will take the lead on this, in others the practice/business manager will.

To enable the management team to make accurate decisions, finance reports should be produced to show projected income and expenditure and how the practice is performing against set budgets. Budgets should be set for both income and expenditure. Past years' performances can be used to do this as well as having a good understanding of what could happen in the coming year. By having a clear picture of the practice's financial situation on a monthly/quarterly basis the management team can make adjustments during the year. This could be by reining in expenditure or by chasing new contracts. If there is a potential loss of funding on the cards, the management team may be able to plan ahead for this by finding alternative sources of income or by cutting costs to take into consideration the cut in income. Good financial information will enable the management team to see whether a new project is likely to be feasible. If the management team are unaware of the business's finances then they will be unable to make informed decisions.

The practice may wish to expand in the future: expansion will mean an increase in income but will also mean an increase in costs. If a practice already has a detailed picture of its finances it is able to produce feasibility reports for any changes to how the practice operates.

Information technology

Clinical system

Practices have a wealth of information technology at their fingertips to aid them in the work that they do. A practice typically has a clinical system which holds records for every patient that is registered or has been registered with the practice. Within these records treatments, tests and diagnoses can be 'Read coded' so that information can be retrieved and used to determine future treatment or the development of new services. Data management and analysis therefore becomes a key component to determining the direction of patient services. Local primary care trusts will have a data-sharing agreement in place with general practices.

Many clinical systems now have the ability to transfer patient data from one practice system to another. The NHS is currently developing a 'summary care record' which will mean that NHS organizations can share patients' information. Initially this will only include basic details about allergies, current prescriptions and any bad reactions to medicines. Gradually more information will be added and will include details of any health conditions, notes of any diagnoses, treatments or operations and plans for care in the future. Patients are able to opt out of the system if they wish.

Appointment system

A practice will also have an appointment system. The appointment system has the ability to produce reports and statistics based around how and when patients access practice services. This is another important management tool which can be used to make decisions around how a practice meets patient demand for its services.

Online services

Most practices will also have their own website which can inform patients about the services available and how they can access them. Online booking systems for appointments are becoming commonplace and the ability to order repeat prescriptions and register with a practice online provides a convenient way in which patients can access the practice without adding to the considerable pressure already placed on the receptionists and telephone system.

Operations management

The role of the practice manager

As well as being involved in the strategic direction of the practice, the practice manager is there to ensure that the day-to-day operation of the practice runs smoothly. The manager is responsible for ensuring that tasks are allocated effectively and that all processes and procedures are adhered to. The practice manager line manages the staff within the practice and has to ensure that the service provided by the practice is carried out in line with what has been agreed as part of the contract or service level agreement. Each manager will have his or her own management style. Management style describes the way in which managers set about achieving results through people. Some managers have an autocratic style, others a more democratic approach. Managers have their own style based on the value systems of the organization and their own natural inclinations and past experiences. All will have the responsibility to guide and support staff as required.

People management

The management of people involves encouraging, motivating and developing teams and individuals to carry out their individual job roles efficiently and effectively. The practice manager will manage all aspects of the employment relationship, which encompasses the following:

- recruitment;
- induction;
- training and development;
- communication;
- performance management;
- decision making;
- team building;
- discipline and grievance.

Each person will have a job description for their job role. The practice manager will manage the process of recruiting staff into the practice. This will involve advertising to attract people to the vacancy and putting a process in place to ensure all of the required checks are carried out and individuals communicated to at every stage. The practice manager will also be part of the interview panel and ensure that the correct process is adhered to. Once an offer has been made the practice manager has to ensure that contracts of employment are given to individuals. It is therefore important that the practice manager has continuous professional development to ensure his or her management skills, especially in the area of employment law, are kept up to date.

The practice manager is responsible for carrying out appraisals and assessing individual training needs. This will be carried out in conjunction with a GP partner when carrying out clinician appraisals.

The management of people also involves having difficult conversations from time to time. This could be around someone's performance if perceived to be below what is expected. It could also mean dealing with disciplinary situations and grievances. It is important that the management team have the right skills to be able to deal with these situations. Practices can make the mistake of focusing on administration skills in their practice manager over and above management skills. This is not advisable. Good managers can make the difference to how people feel about their working environment. A good manager will have the skills and experience to deal with some of the complexities of managing people.

The practice manager has to ensure that the practice is providing a good service and meets the targets that have been set. Some decisions will have to be made on the spot; others can be made in advance when planning ahead. Action planning is a useful tool when organizing specific events such as the annual flu campaign or implementing a new registrations process. In that respect the practice manager also becomes a project manager, managing projects in addition to the day-to-day routines. The practice manager works as part of a team and must take time to listen to staff views. Being a manager does not mean that you are the only person to ever come up with a good idea. A good meeting structure is a good way of doing this. Regular meetings held with the whole team or smaller teams and individuals encourage debate and discussion which then generates ideas. The practice manager plays a key role in facilitating this as they will normally be the person to chair practice meetings.

Core service

A practice's core service is the delivery of medical care and treatment to those that are ill. The appointment system within any practice is vital to the delivery of this service. Managing the appointment system means having adequate resource to meet patient demand. It will require careful planning of rotas and shift patterns for clinicians and support staff. Working patterns will be agreed when a person joins the practice; this will be based on the current need to meet demand at certain times.

Case Study 14.2

A practice decides to recruit a new salaried GP. The successful applicant makes a request to work on Mondays, Tuesdays and Wednesdays. The practice agrees to this. However after the GP joins, the practice manager realizes that there is a considerable shortage of appointments on a Friday. The practice manager asks the new GP to change to work on a Friday instead of a Wednesday. The new GP refuses as she does not have any child care on Fridays. What do you think the practice manager could have done to avoid this problem in the first place?

A practice will have to audit the demand for appointments on a regular basis and adapt to changes in that demand. An individual within the practice would typically manage/administer the appointment system and regularly review the numbers of appointments available on a daily/weekly/monthly basis. It is the role of the manager(s) within the practice to ensure that changes are planned for well in advance. The practice manager has to ensure that there are protocols in place which outline clearly the process in which people can book time off away from the practice.

Case Study 14.3

One of the GP partners decides to take annual leave in the first week of June. Two other GPs have already booked this time off and booked according to the practice protocol of six weeks in advance. The GP partner decided to take this holiday anyway as his wife had already booked this leave with her employer some weeks before. What do you think the impact will be to:

- the number of appointments offered to patients during that week;
- the morale of the other GPs left in the practice during the first week of June;
- the future enforcement of the annual leave protocol?

If a clear process is not in place and not enforced it will be impossible to meet the demand for appointments and can also prove very costly. If changes are not planned for, short-term fixes have to be used (i.e. locums employed at the last minute often with little or no knowledge of the practice). In some situations it may be impossible to get cover at short notice which will have the impact of not providing adequate appointment numbers to enable patients to access medical care when they require it. Patients would also much rather see a GP that they are familiar with rather than someone they have never met before.

Patient involvement and communication

Information is provided to patients on a number of things, posters and leaflets on a range of healthcare issues in addition to information about opening and closing times and services available. Different media are used to communicate to patients which can include utilizing the waiting room to sufficient effect, via a website, signage outside of the practice, and newsletters. The practice manager has to ensure that the information displayed is relevant and has the desired impact.

Many practices have patient groups which meet on a regular basis to discuss ways in which services can be improved. Focus groups are also a good way of gaining insight into how a particular group of people perceive the way certain services are run, or whether a new service would be of use; for example, a practice could decide to hold a focus group for diabetic patients to see if they would use the services of a dietician.

Patient complaints

The practice must have a complaints procedure in place which gives clear guidelines as to how complaints should be dealt with. All complaints have to be taken seriously, which requires investigation and changes implemented if appropriate. The practice team as a whole can learn from complaints made. It is good practice to hold an annual complaints review where complaints are discussed and learning points agreed.

Premises management

The premises may be owned by the partners or leased from the primary care trust. Either way the practice is responsible for reasonable upkeep. Maintenance costs have to be factored into budgets. Many practices have buildings which they have outgrown and this means thinking creatively about the space available and how it can be used. The premises have to be accessible, clean and welcoming and meet infection control standards. A practice manager will need to be clear with cleaning and maintenance contractors on the standards required. This will require regular monitoring.

Health and safety

All businesses are required to meet specific health and safety standards. All practices must have a health and safety policy: staff should be trained in the key areas of health and safety, for example, dealing with hazardous substances, manual handling, infection control, what to do in the event of a fire and how to report accidents and to whom. Regular risk assessments need to be carried out to identify potential hazards. The practice must also carry out training for staff with regular updates.

Financial control

The practice manager has to ensure that income due in comes in and that the bills are paid on time. The practice manager has to keep a keen eye on cash flow to ensure that there is enough money in the bank to cover expenditure. Planning ahead using budgets and income forecasts enables the practice manager to do this affectively. The practice manager also has to ensure that employees are paid accurately and on time.

It is vital that credit control is carried out on a regular basis and that the practice is aware of every item of expenditure. A protocol should be in place which details the flow of cash in and out of the business and the controls in place to account for every transaction. The protocol must also identify who the signatories are and authorization rights. An audit should be carried out periodically to check that everything is as it should be.

SUMMARY POINTS

To conclude, the most important messages of this chapter are as follows:
- The management of general practice is complex and requires a strong management team and organizational structure.
- Strategic planning is about determining key priorities and about planning for the future as well as the present. A business plan, or practice development plan, will aid this process.
- The management team has to monitor the demands of the business and put plans in place to meet those demands.
- Patient feedback is important and must be included when determining future direction.
- A practice manager has many different areas of responsibility: strategic planning, operational management including patient services, finance, human resources, and premises management and information technology.

Reference

Department of Health 2010: *Equity and excellence: liberating the NHS*. London: The Stationery Office.

Further reading

Armstrong, M. 2009: *Armstrong's handbook of human resource management practice*, 11th edn. London: Kogan Page.
Drury, M. and Hobden-Clarke, L. 1994: *The practice manager*, 3rd edn. Oxford: Radcliffe Publishing.
First Practice Management: www.firstpracticemanagement.co.uk.
  A comprehensive resource that provides guidance on all aspects of managing a general practice.
Gilbert, M. 2009: *Managing money for general practitioners*, 2nd edn. Oxford: Radcliffe Publishing.

Acknowledgements

Thank you to Sue Fish who authored this chapter in previous editions.

SINGLE BEST ANSWER QUESTIONS

14.1 What is the difference between a GMS and a PMS contract?

a) A General Medical Services contract is a nationally agreed contract which is predominantly given to GP practices with smaller patient populations. A Personal Medical Services contract is a locally agreed contract predominantly for practices with a larger patient population

b) A Personal Medical Services contract was awarded to practices if they achieved certain targets. If they did not achieve this they were awarded a General Medical Services contract which pays less per patient

c) A General Medical Services contract is a nationally agreed contract with standard terms and conditions. A Personal Medical Services contract includes much of the same standard terms but is negotiated locally so that it can tailor its services to the needs of the local population

d) A General Medical Services contract only provides essential medical services whereas a Personal Medical Services contract can provide additional services

e) A General Medical Services contract gives GP contractors more flexibility to offer different types of services. A Personal Medical Services contract has less flexibility and is limited with the types of services it can offer.

14.2 What is a practice's main source of income?

a) Income from QOF
b) Global sum
c) Directed enhanced service payments
d) Private income
e) Local enhanced service payments.

14.3 Why is it important for a practice to plan strategically?

a) To ensure that a practice can raise enough funds to pay staff wages in the future
b) To plan for a major policy change within the NHS
c) Strategic planning helps a practice to meet the needs of patients both now and in the future. The plan is the actions to be taken in order to achieve that aim. It is about planning in both the short and long term
d) Strategic planning helps a practice to look at the year ahead and plan for known changes
e) A practice would do this when deciding whether to set up a new service

14.4 What should be included in a practice development plan?

a) Vision and goals for the future including plans for services, staffing, technology and finances. It would also look at where environmental factors could impact on these plans

SINGLE BEST ANSWER QUESTIONS CONTINUED

b) An income forecast for the future

c) Learning and development plan for the practice

d) Planned changes to patient services in the future

e) Manpower succession plan.

14.5 Why is it important to gain patient views?

a) It enables a practice to determine whether there is a need for a new service

b) So that you can see whether you are providing a good service and plan improvements based on feedback from patients

c) It enables the practice to tailor its existing services to include unmet patient need

d) In order to furnish you with information about how to rebut patient complaints

e) It provides patients with broader insight into why services are provided in the way they are.

CHAPTER

15

PREPARING TO PRACTISE

- Introduction
- Adopt consultation and reasoning modalities appropriate to the clinical situation and the patient
- Demonstrate good written communications skills
- Demonstrate good working relationships with members of a primary healthcare team and other agencies
- Show evidence of good time keeping and organizational skills
- Implement strategies for managing uncertainty

- Demonstrate an awareness of your own limitations and an understanding of when and where to seek help
- Accept and utilize constructive criticism, be willing to reflect on your own strengths and weaknesses, and act upon them
- Maintain sound professional conduct
- Adopt strategies for lifelong learning
- Summary points
- References
- Further reading
- Single best answer questions

A placement in general practice offers opportunities for learning that are relevant to your development as a practising clinician whatever your final career choice. The variety inherent in the cases you will deal with should encourage you to look beyond the immediate case to the common elements; the thinking and learning processes you employ will be generally applicable to all types of medical practice. This chapter considers some of the practical ways in which you can use these opportunities.

LEARNING OBJECTIVES

This chapter is based around nine selected learning objectives, and springs from experience gained designing and running a course for senior undergraduates called 'Eight Weeks in General Practice and Primary Care', at King's College London School of Medicine.

By the end of this chapter you will be able to:

- adopt consultation and reasoning modalities appropriate to the clinical situation and the case;
- have good written communication skills;
- maintain good working relationships with members of a primary healthcare team and other agencies;
- show evidence of good timekeeping and organizational skills;
- implement strategies for managing uncertainty;
- operate within your own limitations and seek help when appropriate;
- accept and utilize constructive criticism, be willing to reflect on your own strengths and weaknesses, and act upon them;
- maintain sound professional conduct;
- adopt strategies for lifelong learning.

Introduction

'I was able to work independently and had real responsibility for the first time in medical school. The GP had an excellent balance of allowing me to work independently and still being on hand if I needed assistance. This improved my confidence and made me more aware of the limitations of my knowledge.'

(A final year medical student)

The nine learning objectives consider aspects of your learning that are all achievable in the general practice setting, and are designed to be as relevant to those who will not eventually specialize in general practice as to those who will. The sections can be considered separately, but they do interrelate, and there are cross-references. Much of the activity leading to the achievement of these learning objectives is based in clinical practice (i.e. seeing and consulting with patients yourself, ideally in a separate room from your tutor but in close proximity, and with supervision and sanctioning of your decisions by your tutor). Reflection on your performance in those consultations will yield interesting and useful information, so we encourage you to keep a log diary of your clinical sessions. Reading the chapter, especially the thinking and discussion points and practical exercises, will indicate the sort of information you could record in your diary.

Log diaries can be updated between consultations with patients or by reviewing the notes at the end of a clinical session. Sometimes it is useful to use different techniques, recording immediately after a consultation is more influenced by the emotional impact of the individual consultation (an important factor that has to be considered in its own right), whereas recording at the end may illuminate how one consultation affected others in the same session.

Take opportunities to discuss more than individual patients with your tutor; consider how your performance is changing, evolving or getting stuck. Ensure you consider the big picture as well as individual scenarios; take opportunities to see common ground, similarities between patient scenarios or between management strategies, as well as the differences – this will enable you to generate ideas within a consultation even when the case itself is not one you have encountered before,

Don't worry, no one knows all the answers to everything, you are here to learn, and your supervisor will check your consultations. Try to use a problem-solving approach, to be prepared to justify your thought processes, and to safety-net and follow-up your patients.

You will already have developed or be developing your own personal style. An aspect of this individuality is that we do not respond in the same way to patients, and some consideration of the impact different patients have on us as individuals is necessary so we understand how this can influence our decision making. These are good areas for discussion in one-to-one tutorials, or group sessions with your peers.

In group sessions, everyone is a source of information, expertise and views, and all contribute; you are all responsible jointly for each other's learning. Functions of group sessions may include:

- sharing individual experiences, learning vicariously about unusual presentations,
- sharing ideas of expected levels of competence,
- providing support for each other,
- debating difficult or sensitive issues in a protected environment,
- practising peer review and receiving constructive criticism,
- working collaboratively on a particular topic,
- practising skills through role plays and group discussion,
- recruiting expert support in certain shared areas of learning need.

Thinking and Discussion Point

The general practitioner (GP) may know his or her patients well and over a long period. The apparent informality of this relationship might appear unusual to a learner; you might like to consider what the pros and cons of this might be. Where would be the best place to discuss this: with your GP tutor or with your group?

Adopt consultation and reasoning modalities appropriate to the clinical situation and the patient

About clinical reasoning

Many learners coming into general practice from a hospital environment notice the apparently very different consultation technique, and the speed at which consultations occur. First, it is important to put aside speed as an independent goal – it is easier to learn to do the job well and then speed up than to learn to do it quickly and then get better. Second, is this technique really as different as it seems?

Some words about clinical reasoning may shed light on this. Undergraduate medical students are taught to take a history, perform a physical examination and write up case notes with the differential diagnosis at the end, as though it could only 'appear' at that point. This linear model of thinking is known as inductive reasoning, which can be described as the completion of a comprehensive information-gathering programme before thinking begins (Figure 15.1).

Most experienced clinicians actually use a different model, hypothetico-deductive reasoning, which involves the postulation of an hypothesis during the consultation and the gathering of supporting or refuting evidence – sometimes known as 'guess and test' (Figure 15.2).

A necessary part of this thinking is 'pattern recognition', which depends on experience and which, at one extreme, may occasionally telescope the whole reasoning process (Figure 15.3).

Clinicians are able to use these models interchangeably, shifting emphasis according to the situation (Figure 15.4).

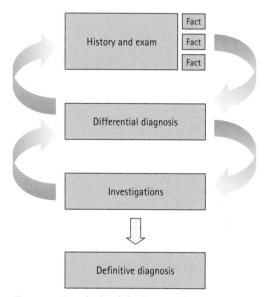

Figure 15.2 Hypothetico-deductive reasoning.

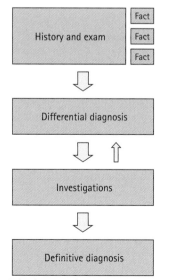

Figure 15.1 Inductive reasoning.

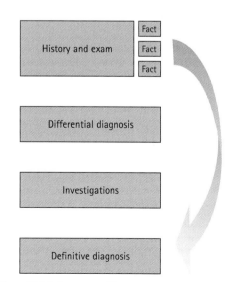

Figure 15.3 Pattern recognition.

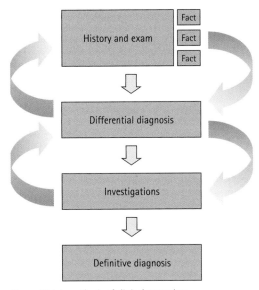

Figure 15.4 A synthesis of clinical reasoning.

Most trainee doctors use the inductive method, as it is thorough and tends to avoid error; experience makes it easier to use hypothetico-deductive reasoning. Different tasks can influence the reasoning approach used: the specialist must explore possibility, reduce uncertainty and marginalize error, so may make more use of inductive reasoning than the generalist, who explores possibility, accepts uncertainty and marginalizes danger. When diagnostic uncertainty is the reason for referral to secondary care, an inductive model is likely to be used, even by an experienced doctor, but many consultations in secondary and tertiary care, particularly in outpatients, are problem orientated and use a hypothetico-deductive base, just like the consultations in primary care.

The terms 'alarm symptom' or 'red flag' are often used to identify clinical features which need investigating (e.g. a cough with haemoptysis or abdominal pain with rectal bleeding). Whether or not a symptom gets 'red flag status' will depend on the patient's age, sex, lifestyle, etc. The recognition and response to red flag symptoms necessarily changes our consultation and reasoning processes.

The influence of the clinician's personality

Dangers lurk: there is an ever-present danger of fitting the evidence to the hypothesis, rather than the other way around – remember Procrustes and his comfortable bed.

Procrustes lived alone on a busy route between two towns, and there were no hotels nearby. He would invite tired travellers to stay, but he was most particular that they fitted the spare bed exactly. If they were too tall, he cut off their feet, and if too short, he stretched them on a rack.

We are not machines; we have individual personalities and our own foibles, all of which we incorporate into our thinking. It may be useful to consider how we rank the list of our differential diagnoses. Several factors influence how we order the diagnoses we have considered.

- *Incidence* – age, sex, race, job, lifestyle, etc. This is hard information, not dependent on individual personalities.
- *Expertise* – have you heard of it? You cannot diagnose something you have never learned about.
- *Seriousness* – how threatening is it? We tend to give higher priority to those diseases that cause major harm, e.g. is it carcinoma of the rectum or piles causing this person's rectal bleeding?
- *Treatability* – do we have any treatment? Conversely, we are sometimes slow to confirm the diagnosis if it is one for which we have no treatment, for instance dementia or one of the degenerative neuromuscular diseases. This is an inevitable corollary of doctors' need to be seen to have a remedy.
- *Novelty* – 'I read a paper in the BMJ last week.' Things stick in our minds – recent articles, striking cases, or sometimes something we missed once and are determined never to miss again.
- *Bias* – 'I don't believe that chronic fatigue syndrome exists.' If so, you cannot diagnose it.

So how should all this influence how you conduct consultations as a learner in primary care? If a possible diagnosis occurs to you during the consultation, follow it up, look for supportive or refuting evidence, do the relevant physical examination. If not, follow the inductive model until an idea emerges. You should not expect to perform as fast as your tutor, and you will almost certainly not have as many well-known 'patterns' in your head as he or she does. Remember, your own personality colours your choices, so you may have to 'correct' for that, and, above all, remember that when you hear hooves, think of horses, not zebras – common things occur commonly.

Practical Exercise

❏ Look at a list of patients you have seen in a morning surgery lately, and consider the diagnoses that you were concerned with. In how many cases did you order investigations in relation to diagnoses that were not actually the most likely but that you felt obliged to consider for other reasons. What were those reasons?

❏ How often were you able to shorten your consultation because the diagnosis became clear? How often did you perform a classical 'clerking' before you were clear what happening?

❏ Repeat this exercise after a few weeks – reflect on any changes and the reasons for them.

❏ Compare your pattern with that of the partners in your practice, or with a fellow learner.

Demonstrate good written communications skills

In writing notes, a report or referral letter, it is important to consider the purpose, the reader and what they need to know. What should be included, and what left out? Do any ethical or legal issues need addressing? (See also Chapter 12 on ethics and law.)

The purpose

This may be to provide information to optimize future decision making: withholding sensitive information may impair the patient's future care if another doctor is unaware or does not think to ask for it, but including it relies on clinicians behaving non-judgementally. Another purpose may be to record decisions made and actions taken, including postulation of strategies and future care plans,

with 'if, then' statements, especially if these have been negotiated with the patient. A further purpose is to enable self-audit and governance.

The reader

The reader may be another doctor or healthcare worker. General assumptions about confidentiality and professionalism are beginning to be questioned here, and even now some confidentiality walls occur between, say, psychological/counselling services and doctors, or between the genitourinary services and the rest of the National Health Service (NHS). Tension occurs between disclosure of unnecessary personal details and wish of some doctors to personalize the patient.

Some written documentation is for patients or their non-medical advocates, for instance applications for housing or other social support, or for employment, insurance or other purposes. Assume this information will be dealt with by a non-clinician unless otherwise stated.

Recorded information may be for use by one of the governance agencies in audit and resource planning. Therefore, likely but unconfirmed diagnoses are better recorded as symptoms, for instance wheezing (instead of asthma) or chest pain (instead of angina), until the diagnosis is confirmed objectively; likewise, once the diagnosis is confirmed, you should code it correctly (see more about coding below).

Inclusion/exclusion

The question of relevance is all-important. A useful guide is the need-to-know maxim; that is, to do the job requested, what does the reader need to know? The problem is that you may not be able to answer that, but there are some safety nets. First, if the letter/report is accompanying a clinical situation, the patient can be asked to supplement the information, but you should ensure that information that the patient may not be clear about is in your communication (e.g. medication history). Second, you can indicate how the reader should contact you for supplementary information.

Ethical/legal issues

A few comments may help to identify the commonest issues, but this list is not comprehensive.

Remember always, patients can have access to notes written about them.

- *Non-judgementalism.* Your language must be non-judgemental. We all depend on our colleagues being non-judgemental as well; if we are not confident about this, we will be unable to write what is needed. It is allowable to make 'I statements' if materially relevant. For example: 'I find it hard to understand what this patient says', rather than 'This patient doesn't speak clearly'.
- *Consent to disclose.* This is particularly important if you are writing to a non-clinician. Alternatively, you can give the letter or report to the patient, allowing them to decide whether or not to pass it on.
- *Third-party interest.* In whose interest is the information to be used? It may not be your patient's. The best example is writing to insurance companies. The patient should have consented, but may not be aware of what he or she has consented to. Remember, insurance companies are not altruistic; they exist to make money for their shareholders.
- *Honesty and truthfulness.* There is an important but often misunderstood difference between these. You can be honest and untruthful ('I saw you at the park yesterday' – believing this to be the case, mistakenly) or dishonestly truthful ('I go running regularly' – not mentioning that it is only once a month; that is to say, hiding behind words). You should aim to be both honest and truthful.
- *Governance issues.* Some patients become anxious about information in their clinical notes being used for governance. Issues about agglomerated and anonymized information are still debated; society's unresolved dilemma about individual autonomy claiming superiority over the common good (e.g. 'not in my backyard') is a problem here.

Issues about format

With clinical record keeping now computerized, issues about format are more charged. For some time there has been wide variation in how notes have been kept 'traditional'/problem orientated (e.g. using 'SOAP' – subjective data, objective data, assessment, plan – headings for your notes; Weed, 1969), the use of personalized shorthand or cues etc. There is the additional problem of free-text computer records being more problematic to search/analyse/audit than formatted or field-based records.

What to include

Notes need to be brief, giving a summary of the history and examination, any important positive or negative findings, a record of any 'red flags' that are present or absent, your impression or working diagnosis, management plan, and an idea of your follow-up plan with safety netting. Safety netting is:

- What you expect to happen if you are right
- What you expect to happen if you are wrong
- What you would do in both these cases.

Many note-recording systems use 'Read coding'. In the 1980s a GP, Dr James Read, developed a medical diagnosis coding system for use in general practice. It allows for audit trails and searches, and is almost universally used now when recording consultations electronically.

Some referral systems now use pro-forma letters. These inevitably constrain the referring clinician, particularly around personalization, but they do prompt for relevant information that might be forgotten.

Thinking and Discussion Point

How do you respond to the question 'Can I tell you something, but I don't want you to write it down in my notes?' What are the advantages/disadvantages to the patient/doctor of agreeing to this request?

Compare your notes with those of your tutor, and consider the advantages and disadvantages of both.

Does the content (thoroughness, competence, etc.) of the referral affect the timing and confidence of discharge back? Does the referral affect the nature, tone, interest of the consultation itself?

Practical Exercise

With a fellow learner, each write a referral letter about a recent patient, then swap letters and read the other letter as though you were the specialist receiving the letter. Ask yourself, 'What am I being asked to do? Can I do this? What information is missing? Will the patient be able to supply it?'

Practical Exercise

Interview members of your primary healthcare team to understand their roles and responsibilities. Find out which patients they feel should be referred to them and which not. Ask for examples of good and poor team working, and consider whether you agree.

Practical Exercise

After you refer someone to another primary healthcare team member, discuss with them the referral from their perspectives.

Demonstrate good working relationships with members of a primary healthcare team and other agencies

You will also find material relevant in the chapters on general practice and its place in primary care and chronic illness. In most disciplines/specialties, doctors work within teams providing a mix of knowledge, skills and experience, personalities and approaches to care. Teams share caseloads, decision making and the uncertainty of working with patients, therefore providing a professional safety net.

Teamwork can be challenging; in particular, communication and mutual respect are key elements in a team's success. As with hospital multidisciplinary team meetings, primary care teams often meet frequently to discuss patients and plan their care. You should know about each member's role and responsibilities and how best to liaise with them. Sitting in and observing them at work is a valuable way of beginning to understand their work, but you should aim after a short time to take an active role.

When working on the wards, planning a patient's successful discharge, you will find it very useful to have a practical knowledge of primary healthcare team members and community professionals – for instance, knowing that a speech therapist can be a vital help for someone with swallowing difficulties after a stroke. Understanding what services are really likely to happen in the community will help you avoid revolving-door readmissions, which are distressing for patients and relatives, and expensive and wasteful for the NHS.

Show evidence of good time keeping and organizational skills

Clinical work requires using time and resources efficiently. Importantly, before the placement begins, think about what you want to achieve by the end. Arrive punctually from day one, make a good impression and maintain that throughout the placement. These things form the evidence.

Setting priorities

First consider how you set priorities. One way is to use a system such as shown in Figure 15.5. You may need to set priorities within a consultation (e.g. the patient who presents a number of issues simultaneously) or within a session's work.

	Important	Unimportant
Urgent	(Red)	(Amber)
Not urgent	(Purple)	(Blue)

Figure 15.5 An example of a system for setting priorities.

At the end of a morning surgery, you may have several activities to juggle – letters or emails, phone calls, discussing patients with colleagues, house calls, writing repeat prescriptions, having lunch or going to the loo. (Remember that the last two are important, as you may not function effectively if you are physically uncomfortable or hungry/thirsty.) Thinking about which tasks to perform, when and how long they will take, will help you plan the next few hours.

Allowing time

Time expectations should not necessarily be the same for juniors as for seniors – you should expect to take longer over most consultations, letter writing, etc. If you get into difficulty, it is best to find a colleague to discuss it with or to ask help from. If you run constantly over time, it may be more appropriate to negotiate a different consultation period or insert frequent short breaks than merely to endure (and impose on others) the stress of running late.

Multi-tasking

Some people find multi-tasking easier than others. If you find it difficult, first acknowledge this to yourself and your supervisor, and adapt or find strategies to cope, such as taking more care with setting priorities and making sure others are aware of your working style.

Coping with distractions

Telephone calls and other interruptions occur continually. You need different criteria for allowing these, depending on whether or not you are the doctor on call. It is useful to have strategies for answering or deflecting requests for attention that do not offend or alienate the requester.

The opposite is important, too: how do you get and hold someone's attention without annoying them? It is useful to set ground rules with your tutor/supervisor about how you get their attention when you need it.

The way this learning objective is measured is primarily through in-course assessment, but don't forget that clinical examinations contain elements like coping with noise, time constraints, multi-tasking, prioritizing, etc.

Thinking and Discussion Point

With your tutor/supervisor, discuss their criteria for managing interruptions and try to develop your own sets of criteria for different situations.

Practical Exercise

Write a list at the end of morning surgery of tasks you have generated, and other tasks ahead in the day. Consider how you give them priority and whether that priority then remains fixed or continues to change as the tasks unfold.

Practical Exercise

With fellow learners, set up role plays of consultations interrupted by telephone calls or visitors. Practise the communications skills needed to deal with these both during 'ordinary' morning surgery and during a 'duty doctor' session. Get feedback from the people playing the interrupter and the patient.

Implement strategies for managing uncertainty

What is 'managing uncertainty'?

Our response to uncertainty has to include both our thinking (the 'decisions') and our behaviour.

Although one might divide uncertainty in the clinical situation into diagnostic and therapeutic uncertainty, the former is commoner. When a doctor is uncertain what to do, it is usually because he or she does not know precisely what the problem is; management dilemmas occur less frequently.

Differentiation between uncertainty and ignorance/incompetence

Because of the high premium put on knowledge both by society and by traditional medical education (and thus doctors), not knowing is easily equated with incompetence; this is much more in the doctor's mind than in the patient's. However, clinical problems present in a multitude of ways (as each patient is unique) and at a multitude of points in the natural history of the problem, so it may not be crystal clear to every doctor at every consultation what exactly the problem is. Consequently, handling uncertainty is the stuff of medicine, and general practice is where you can learn about it.

Being a junior

Although we are all learning all the time, you are in the lucky position of being junior, so expectations should be lower, and asking for help should be easier. Also, you may have come to expect that most clinical situations can be resolved within the time frame of a hospital admission. Problems in general practice often continue to evolve over many consultations; even such things as childhood minor illness will evolve over time as the parents gain experience and confidence. The ability to decide what needs to be dealt with now, and what can be left, is often a major challenge to a young doctor, and depends on the ability to 'manage uncertainty'.

Use of time – as diagnostic aid or as therapy

Time is one of the major tools in managing uncertainty. Time enables the problem to evolve, such that either new features appear, making a diagnosis easier or the problem resolves itself. Time may also show the effect of other factors on the problem – self-help, over-the-counter (OTC) remedies or symptomatic treatment – which may illuminate the diagnosis.

Here is an example of how time can be used to manage uncertainty. A youngster with colicky central abdominal pain, and some nausea, without very marked abdominal tenderness, may be seen by the GP, who advises symptomatic relief with fluids and paracetamol, suggesting 'a virus' or 'an upset stomach' as the cause. Indeed, many times this will be the case and the patient will recover; but the GP will know that, once in a while, one such patient will go on to develop the classic history and signs of appendicitis. Does the GP alert the patient and family to this possibility, or does he or she think this is harmful alarmism?

The patient may turn up in the accident and emergency department later saying, 'My GP told me it was an upset stomach', as the casualty officer looks incredulously at a 'barn-door' diagnosis of appendicitis! Alerting the family involves 'admitting' uncertainty, but is more honest, more likely to enable the family to seek further advice if needed, and more likely to nurture the GP's reputation.

Practical Exercise

In June you see a 15-year-old with a febrile illness and headache without meningism. What would you advise the patient and family? What difference does the time of year make?

Other helping hands

This is all about safety netting.

- *Open door.* The security that the patient can consult again at short notice is a feature of general practice. This allows a sharing of responsibility between doctor and patient, relieving some pressure to sort everything out at one go. It places more of the locus of control with the patient, thus easing the doctor's responsibility.
- *Use of negotiation.* Discussing with patients the various options available not only shares some responsibility with them, but it may also articulate the choices for the patient and make the right decision more obvious. Patients may have views about how acceptable some options would be – our advocacy of an option unacceptable to the patient (i.e. lack of concordance between doctor and patient) often leads to a poorer outcome.
- *Appropriate goal setting.* We cannot assume that the endpoint of treatment we have in mind is the one that the patient shares. Some patients accept levels of risk that we might not; others might be looking for a goal beyond that which we can achieve with current medicine. Being honest and explicit about these things may help in setting shared, achievable treatment goals; this is another aspect of concordance.
- *Being explicit about expectations.* Distressed or needy people want answers; it is easy to fall into the trap of finding a superficially credible expla-

nation or treatment simply to assuage the distress. It might be better to deal with the distress, acknowledge the need for answers, but honestly admit to the uncertainty. Disappointment and disillusionment may occur, but in smaller doses than if an expectation is created and subsequently not met.

- *Referral*. This could be from the GP to the specialist, but the same process occurs (and might be equally useful) in the case of the learner asking his or her tutor, the registrar asking his or her trainer, the assistant asking a partner, or one partner asking another. It might also be appropriate to ask a specialist from another discipline – nursing or therapy colleagues, for example. Saying you need another opinion is not necessarily a sign of intellectual bankruptcy, but more a sign of recognition of your own limits (see below).

Demonstrate an awareness of your own limitations and an understanding of when and where to seek help

Central to the correct response to the awareness of one's own limitations is an honest view of what might reasonably be expected of you, and being open to feedback (see the section 'Accept and utilize constructive criticism', below). If you are not yet at the expected level of competence, some more learning is required (see the section 'Adopt strategies for lifelong learning', below).

Alternatively, you might be at the level of expected competence but be facing a problem that is outside it; this is normal for any clinician, whether generalist or specialist. Learning to respond properly is covered in the section 'Implement strategies for managing uncertainty' (above), but you do need to be able to seek help.

What kinds of help are there?

- Written information, e.g. in a book or on the internet.
- Information or a second opinion from a peer/colleague on site. This happens informally in hospital, on ward rounds, when discussions

take place without anyone 'asking for help' explicitly. In primary care, discussions at the time, with a partner (or with the learner in the room!), at coffee time, or days after the event, when someone else has seen the patient for a further consultation, are all ways of getting help.

- Advice from a specialist source on or off site. Seeking advice either instantly or by appointment (a 'referral') is easily sanctioned. However, when making the referral you might consider not only the patient's needs, but also your own (can you learn something from this referral?).

Checking information should be acceptable, but some students or juniors (and some seniors) find it embarrassing to open the *British National Formulary* in front of a patient. Consider which is more embarrassing – looking in the *Formulary*, or discovering afterwards that you made an error in prescribing. The manner in which it is done is important: if you feel uncomfortable or embarrassed (arising from a misplaced internal expectation of 'knowing' lots) it will show, and the patient will naturally assume that you are justifiably embarrassed, and his or her expectations of you and your colleagues will simply increase. You are at a stage where it should not be embarrassing to check information, so you have the chance to set healthy behaviours for the future!

Telephoning a specialist registrar may be helpful; they may be flattered that their advice is being sought, particularly if you are seeking advice about how you might handle the problem, and not just handing over the patient to their care, without trying. Not infrequently, an offer of an outpatient appointment may then come easily.

Unless one is in single-handed practice, there are almost always fellow clinicians around. As a learner in a practice, you may only rarely witness your tutor ask a colleague, although you may see him or her being asked. The reason is that while you are there, your tutor already has a colleague on hand – you! Otherwise, it is not that unusual for one clinician to ask another, informally, for a second opinion, either at the time or later. Doing it afterwards provides a sounding board, checking out what one has decided, and also helps the next consultation.

As you are a learner, your tutor will almost invariably check the outcome of every consultation, but you may be uncertain about the physical examination or about what a certain part of the history signifies, and so the enquiry ('referral') would be about these things. You should not be reluctant to ask for this help, as without it you may make an avoidable clinical error (for which the tutor would be responsible), and you would not benefit from the learning that might accrue. It is really important to learn healthy ways of asking for help before you get to your early years as a junior doctor.

Doctors help themselves learn by reviewing their own performance, in audits, SEAs (significant event analyses), practice meetings, grand rounds, etc.

Problem areas

For some people, asking for help with their skills can be easier than asking about knowledge; the techniques are the same, so whichever you find easier, apply the same technique to the other. It is often harder to ask for help if one's attitudes are causing problems, not least because these may be more difficult to see in the first place, and more difficult to admit. Sometimes people think that their attitudes are private, part of 'them', and therefore not on the agenda for change. However, our attitudes can affect our behaviour, and if this causes a problem, we must change it, even if we continue to hold our private underlying beliefs.

Asking for help when one is ill can be harder, particularly if help-seeking behaviour is not securely established. Doctors not infrequently fail to take time off when they are ill, and sometimes treat themselves (though this is unprofessional). Guilt about increasing our colleagues' workloads, and deeper seated beliefs about showing vulnerability, deny us the time and space we need, and that we would advise for our patients. This can lead to clinical mistakes, and can contribute to burnout.

One area where doctors are out of step with other professions is supervision. Nurses belong to supervision groups, and practitioners of almost any kind of talk therapy have a supervisor; but most GPs do not. Some GPs join peer-support groups as an informal form of supervision.

Practical Exercise

During or at the end of one morning session, look back and ask yourself what, if anything, caused most difficulty in the consultation. Was it something you didn't know? Something you couldn't do? Or something about yourself that 'got in the way' (i.e. your knowledge, skills or attitudes)? Make a note and discuss with your tutor how to deal with these learning needs. Reflect on how you would do this if there were no 'protected' time for supervision in your timetable, and/or how you might set this time up.

Accept and utilize constructive criticism, be willing to reflect on your own strengths and weaknesses, and act upon them

Contextualizing your own performance

As doctors in training, we need to identify whether our performance is above or below expectations, and to consider whose expectations those are and how realistic they are. You may appear to be asked to perform the same task as in previous firms or attachments, and not consider that a higher standard of performance or a greater assumption of responsibility is expected of you. Conversely, a tutor may sometimes overlook the fact that you are not yet a registrar. Try to discover the standards expected of you at your summative assessment.

Using methods of self-assessment may also be helpful, and the RIME model (Pangaro, 1999) provides a helpful framework for the senior undergraduate years, and beyond.

- *Reporter* – acting as the patient's mouthpiece
- *Investigator* – thinking about tests, referrals, etc.
- *Manager* – thinking about treatments
- *Educator* – thinking about explaining to patient/ peers.

Use this model to think about how, for a series of patients, you may take on several different roles, and how the prevailing role changes with time.

Another method of self-assessment is to notate your learning objectives with confidence ratings, comparing week-on-week or month-on-month improvements in confidence.

Obtaining and listening to feedback

Direct feedback on your performance can be incredibly helpful when it is expressed in a constructive way that you can hear, accept and use to change what you have been doing. It might sometimes contain direct suggestions about what you might do instead, although ideally without any element of obligation. It is entirely appropriate for you to ask for this kind of feedback.

One thing that many doctors in the UK find hard to accept is praise – often it is met with embarrassment and internal disbelief; as such it is not 'useful', though what needs to change here is the attitude of the recipient. It seems to be part of the medical mind-set that praise is base currency; perhaps, if punitive criticism were less the norm, praise could be rehabilitated.

It is important to accept criticism in a constructive manner. By unlinking criticism from judgementalism, one can 'hear' it, consider its truthfulness, accept it and act on it.

Use of recording

This can be a powerful adjunct to another's critique: you yourself are the observer and can see your own performance. It can be challenging, sometimes disturbing, even embarrassing, but it can also be powerfully affirming. Video is ideal, but audio is useful and may be technically easier to achieve; patient consent is essential. Suitable guidance and a downloadable consent form are available from the General Medical Council (GMC, 2011a).

Personal reflection

The biggest obstacle to personal reflection is the allocation of protected time. Since it appears to be entirely selfish, it is often demoted in importance, but it is vital to the preservation of quality.

Some learners are uncertain how to reflect. The process is quite simple and unthreatening.

Practical Exercise

Think about something you have experienced.
- ❏ Start by writing down what actually happened; consider what you felt confident about and what you felt uncertain about.
- ❏ How did it make you feel?
- ❏ What do you think other people felt?
- ❏ What did you learn?
- ❏ What might you have done differently?
- ❏ Draw up some action points to work on so you can feel more prepared for the next time.

Aids to reflection may help: using open question sheets, generating lists or writing full significant event analyses. The process should embrace honesty, both in the narrative and, ideally, also in the emotional underlay (the reflector's emotions).

There is an important link here with the use of a portfolio (see below), which aids reflection as well as forming a record of evidence.

Johari Window

Feedback, self-assessment and reflection on our work can illuminate issues that we wish to develop or change. However, problems can arise if we are unaware of or wish to hide some of our weaknesses, deficiencies or 'black holes'.

The Johari Window, named after its developers, Joseph Luft and Harry Ingham (Luft, 1969), shows clearly the various states of self-knowledge (Figure 15.6). The idea of self-assessment, feedback and reflection is to expand the 'open' box and minimize the other boxes. If you and your tutors become more aware of your problem areas, you are in a better position to change them. The relationship between learner and tutor can play a central role in expanding the open box. A trusting and supportive relationship can provide a safe environment in which to discuss sensitive issues.

Need for change

There is an active process that precedes change happening: first an acknowledgement that things are not right, and second an acceptance that

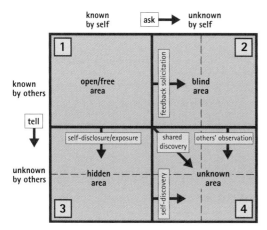

Figure 15.6 The Johari Window. This version Alan Chapman 2003 www.businessballs.com.

change is necessary; this is akin to the shift from pre-conceptual to conceptual thinking with which you may be familiar in the context of behaviour modification.

Grounding

Key to knowing how much change is necessary is having an understanding of expectations (see the section 'Demonstrate an awareness of your own limitations', above). Being grounded with your peers is of inestimable value; in this context it means having an understanding of what your peers are able to do in similar situations, and having similar expectations of yourself. The best way of being grounded with peers involves, either formally or informally, some kind of small group activity, such as:

- undergraduate seminars,
- journal club,
- significant event analysis discussion,
- half-day release groups,
- young (or mature) general practice princi-pals groups.

In discussions, you will gain an idea of where the common standard of competence is, and be able to establish whether that standard is sufficient for the expectations of your course/job.

Practical Exercise

At the end of the week/course, think back over what you have seen, experienced and learned. Use one of the suggested Thinking and Discussion Points, or generate your own.

Practical Exercise

Evaluate your RIME score for the last ten patients, and consider how you would have improved your score in each case. Re-evaluate your score a week later.

Thinking and Discussion Point

Reflect on the consultations you have under-taken on your own.
- Which one has affected your own personal thoughts and feelings most?
- Why did it affect you?
- What did you learn about yourself from this experience?

Thinking and Discussion Point

Reflect on your learning experience in gen-eral practice.
- What would be the one most important point of feedback you'd like to give to your tutor/supervisor?
- What have you learned in this course that has changed or consolidated your approach to medicine?
- What do you perceive are areas of weakness that you have not addressed on this course and would like to build on in the future?

Maintain sound professional conduct

It is recommended that you read the guidance on good medical practice on the GMC's website (General Medical Council, 2011b). In particular, you must know the duties of the doctor that the GMC has defined:

'Patients must be able to trust doctors with their lives and health. To justify that trust you must show respect for human life and you must:

- Make the care of your patient your first concern
- Protect and promote the health of patients and the public
- Provide a good standard of practice and care
  - Keep your professional knowledge and skills up to date
  - Recognise and work within the limits of your competence
  - Work with colleagues in the ways that best serve patients' interests
- Treat patients as individuals and respect their dignity
  - Treat patients politely and considerately
  - Respect patients' right to confidentiality
- Work in partnership with patients
  - Listen to patients and respond to their concerns and preferences
  - Give patients the information they want or need in a way they can understand
  - Respect patients' right to reach decisions with you about their treatment and care
  - Support patients in caring for themselves to improve and maintain their health
- Be honest and open and act with integrity
  - Act without delay if you have good reason to believe that you or a colleague may be putting patients at risk
  - Never discriminate unfairly against patients or colleagues
  - Never abuse your patients' trust in you or the public's trust in the profession.

You are personally accountable for your professional practice and must always be prepared to justify your decisions and actions.' (General Medical Council, 2011b)

You will already notice how many of these resonate through the subjects of this chapter. Getting feedback is essential for monitoring your behaviour, informally, or formalized in ways like a 360 degree appraisal. Keeping a reflective diary is a way of self-monitoring. At all times, remember attendance is a proxy for commitment, and punctuality for reliability.

Adopt strategies for lifelong learning

Purpose

Why is lifelong learning important? Medicine is changing and developing rapidly; you cannot expect your present knowledge to be up to date for long. As professionals, we have a responsibility to keep up to date to ensure we provide good care to our patients (see also the previous section on the GMC's guidance on good medical practice). We need to be safe practitioners and analyse and learn from our mistakes; to enjoy our work, we need to remain enthusiastic by stimulating our own interest. The public, through our governing body the GMC, needs to be assured that we are maintaining high standards of care: annual appraisals with revalidation every 5 years in the UK is now the norm. Doctors need to meet an established minimum competence level to be relicensed to work in the NHS in the UK.

As learners and doctors, we must ensure we continue to learn and to develop strategies on how best we learn so that this learning is sustainable throughout our careers.

What is it?

Incorporating adult learning principles is important for lifelong learning and continuing medical education.

Adult learning is deciding what we want to learn and using our past experiences. What we learn needs to be relevant to what we do in everyday practice, so that we improve patient care. It involves:

- Identifying strengths and weaknesses: being able to say, 'I don't know about this'.
- Reflection (Kolb's cycle): putting learning into

action is very powerful, confirming the value of what you have learned and stimulating ideas on what else you would like to learn (see Figure 15.7; Kolb, 1984). There is more on reflection in the section 'Accept and utilize constructive criticism', above.

■ Setting realistic objectives and goals for yourself.

Lifelong learning is key to our professionalism, and a crucial part of this is the ability to reflect on practice and learning.

How to do it

There are many different ways that we can keep up to date. Some activities will suit you, others will not:

■ Update sessions/courses can be useful, but may not always meet your needs.
■ Journals and journal clubs: sharing information with peers includes grounding yourself and setting realistic standards of care in your practice or department. This can be a useful way of providing consistency of care within a team.
■ Electronic information is available while you consult, and can be shared with the patient; many websites are available.
■ Patients are an invaluable resource, particularly since the advent of the internet. Some doctors feel challenged by well-informed patients (does this threaten the role as keeper of 'secret professional knowledge'?) but actually we have the very important role of helping the patient understand how relevant/complete/accurate the information is.
■ Developing a special interest or responsibility within a team will necessitate you keeping up to date and being a resource to others.

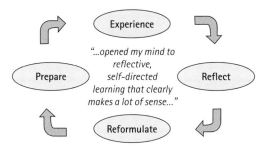

Figure 15.7 Kolb's cycle.

■ Keeping a log: we often come across areas of medicine that we are unsure of. By keeping a log of things to look up when seeing patients and following up what we are unsure of, we learn 'on the job'. Try not to be intimidated doing this in front of patients – it is much better to feel sure you are doing the right thing.
■ Peer groups offer support and an opportunity to reflect on your own practice, and set this in the context of the practice of others at your level (see also the section 'Accept and utilize constructive criticism', above).
■ Correspondence from colleagues can be a useful way of learning up-to-date management approaches.
■ Asking for advice and help from a colleague is a common method used when there is uncertainty in clinical decisions.
■ Television/media: hearing something on the news or even in a television soap can often be a learning point for us or to help us to understand patients' thought processes.
■ Developing a portfolio (see below).

Portfolios

These are increasingly prevalent in medicine but are common in other professions. Nurses have been using them for a number of years for continuing professional development and accreditation. They originate in graphic arts and consist of a collection of evidence that shows learning has taken place.

The learner decides what goes into the portfolio. Seeing a patient with a particular illness may spark your interest in finding out more about that illness; when faced with a clinical problem that you are unsure about, you can use the opportunity to include what you learn in your portfolio. The portfolio uses your clinical experiences as the starting point for your learning, so that when you next see a patient with a similar problem you are more confident managing them. It is relevant and usable for future clinical practice.

The portfolio's success depends on how much effort and time goes into it. Be careful not to embark on huge projects that become unmanageable. Try to be specific (e.g. instead of writing about 'ischaemic heart disease', consider focusing on, 'the pharmacological treatment of angina').

Reflecting on experiences is central to developing a portfolio. When thinking about clinical encounters, identify strengths and weaknesses – areas where you feel confident or unsure. Think of strategies you can use to learn about the areas you do not feel confident in (e.g. read a review article, go to an outpatient clinic, speak to a specialist, read a book). Then write about your learning and how it may affect your clinical practice in the future. For example, studying the management of urinary tract infections in general practice may increase or decrease your requesting of midstream urines, or your referral rate, etc. Thinking about your learning can spark ideas of other areas you would like to learn more about, which you can include in your portfolio.

It can also be useful to think about *how* you learnt: did you learn more by reading an article, going to a presentation, or discussion group? This helps you identify how best you learn, which should make it easier the next time.

Sharing your portfolio with a tutor or peer may be useful, particularly when discussing what and how you have learnt.

Portfolios can replace formal examinations as a form of assessment. Some medical schools have replaced the traditional final examinations with a portfolio that students develop in their final year. The advantages of a portfolio as a form of assessment include the following:

■ A portfolio can assess areas not easily assessed by other methods, particularly professionalism, because the ability to reflect is a key component of professionalism. This is useful, given the push from the public and the GMC to ensure professional standards are met at graduation and postgraduate levels.

■ Portfolios are authentic; they can chart what the learner actually does over a period of time. Multiple choice questions (MCQs) are useful for assessing knowledge, and objective structured clinical examinations (OSCEs) assess 'shows how', but this may not be what the learner actually does daily in practice when seeing patients.

Making a habit of it

It is our professional responsibility to remain up to date and skilled in our area of medicine. To learn effectively, we need to use strategies that suit us so that we can sustain our learning throughout our career.

Practical Exercise

Set your own learning objectives and start your portfolio; complete a self-assessment exercise or a reflective journal.

Practical Exercise

Write down how you found out about something you were not sure about – books/colleagues/internet.

SUMMARY POINTS

Things you learn while you are in general practice are useful whatever you do in medicine. To conclude, the most important messages of this chapter are as follows:

■ Being aware of how you think and make decisions helps improve how you consult with patients.
■ Reflective learning is easy and helpful.
■ Fostering and maintaining relationships with colleagues is crucial to clinical team working.
■ Organizing your time and resources helps in your working day.
■ Being honestly self-aware is healthy and productive.
■ Feedback from peers, colleagues and patients is a valuable resource.
■ There are a multitude of ways to keep learning.
■ Productive learning is satisfying and fun (Figure 15.8).

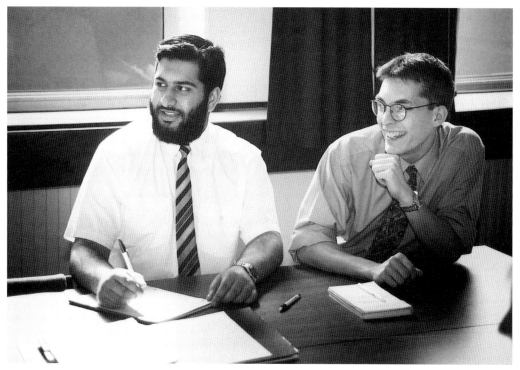

Figure 15.8 Learning can be fun.

References

General Medical Council 2011a: Making and using visual and audio recordings of patients. www.gmc-uk.org/guidance/ethical_guidance/making_audiovisual.asp (accessed May 2011).

General Medical Council 2011b: Good medical practice: duties of a doctor. www.gmc-uk.org/guidance/good_medical_practice/duties_of_a_doctor.asp (accessed May 2011).

Kolb, D. 1984: *Experiential learning: experience as the source of learning and development.* Englewood Cliffs, NJ: Prentice Hall.

Luft, J. 1969: *Of human interaction.* Palo Alto, CA: National Press.

Pangaro, L.N. 1999: A new vocabulary and other innovations for improving descriptive in-training evaluations. *Academic Medicine* 74, 1203–7.

Weed, L.L. 1969: *Medical records, medical education, and patient care. The problem-oriented record as a basic tool.* Cleveland, OH: Case Western Reserve University.

Further reading

Dowie, J. and Elstein, A. 1988: *Professional judgement. A reader in clinical decision making.* Cambridge: Cambridge University Press.

Royal College of General Practitioners 1993: *Portfolio-based learning in general practice*: Occasional Paper 63. London: Royal College of General Practitioners.

www.gmc-uk.org

www.nosa.org.uk

www.londondeanery.ac.uk

Acknowledgements

Thank you to Dr Cath Miskin who was co-author in the second edition.

SINGLE BEST ANSWER QUESTIONS

15.1 A patient whom you know very well tells you that they don't want what they have told you recorded in the notes. They only want you as their doctor to know about it. You feel that the information is relevant to the patient's care.

a) You agree to their request
b) You make a record using oblique or obscured language that only you will understand, in order to 'hide' the information from others
c) You explain the purpose of the notes is to record what the patient tells you and that you have an obligation to record everything they say, honestly and truthfully
d) You explain the purpose of the notes is to ensure the patient's care is optimized and that, if information is withheld from the notes, future care may be compromised so you cannot agree to their request
e) You explain, as in C above, and allow the patient to decide whether they want to take the risk of future suboptimal care.

15.2 At the end of a morning surgery, hungry and fretful, you still have some tasks to do. There is an urgent visit to do in the nursing home round the corner, a form for an MSU needs to be done before the pathology collection goes, and you promised a letter for a patient you saw yesterday morning but didn't have time for then. Then a junior student arrives wanting you to teach them something. You prioritise:

a) Eat, form, visit, letter, student
b) Form, eat, visit, student, letter
c) Visit, form, eat, student, letter
d) Eat, visit, form, letter, student
e) Letter, student, visit, eat, form

15.3 A patient, Mr Smith, challenges you in the consultation, saying, you gave me the wrong treatment two days ago for my... I looked it up on the internet, and there is some new treatment which you should have given me, called ...

a) You say "OK I will prescribe you the new treatment"
b) You apologise for making a mistake, and prescribe the treatment the patient has mentioned
c) You say that you don't know anything about the new treatment, so cannot prescribe it for them
d) You ask them to finish the current course of treatment to see if it will work and, if the problem is no better, to come back. You make a mental note to look up the new treatment in case they come back.
e) You say you don't know about the new treatment, and you can look it up, and check if it's suitable and available, and if so, it may be possible to prescribe it; when you know the answers to those questions you will contact the patient.

15.4 Later the same morning, you realise that the consultation with Mr Smith had irritated you more than you realised, you were grumpy and short with the remaining patients and made more referrals than usual.

a) You decide that you need to go on a refresher course to update your knowledge
b) You decide you are working too hard and that you should have a holiday
c) You speak to some other GPs the same as you, and ask them whether they would have done the same or different
d) You ask the receptionists what Mr Smith is like, and they say he is always rude and difficult with them. You ask them not to make Mr Smith any more appointments with you
e) You talk to the senior partner in the practice, who says he always refers problems like that, to keep his working life manageable.

SINGLE BEST ANSWER QUESTIONS CONTINUED

15.5 Your tutor has decided to offer you a tutorial on dermatology. This is your favourite topic about which you know quite a lot, as you have done a very good hospital attachment in this subject

a) You welcome the opportunity to show what you know
b) You are glad not to be challenged on an area of relative ignorance
c) You acknowledge the offer, and ask the tutor to concentrate on common dermatology issues in GP
d) You ask if your tutor can change the topic, as you don't need to learn any more dermatology
e) You phone in sick on the morning of the tutorial.

CHAPTER

16   BEING A GENERAL PRACTITIONER

- Introduction
- What is a general practitioner?
- Training for general practice
- The work of the GP
- A week in general practice
- The GP Surgery

- The changing face of illness in general practice
- Patient and public expectations of a GP
- Summary points
- References
- Single best answer questions

The work of a general practitioner (GP) necessarily reflects the health needs of the population, and the many changes in these needs, together with changing economics and social profiles in communities, means that in most parts of the world, general practice is a dynamic place to be in. No more so that in the United Kingdom, where radical changes to the National Health Service (NHS) are occurring in order to accommodate an ageing population, increasing prevalence of long-term conditions, and an urgent need to address prevention of illness – all in an increasingly constrained financial framework. In this chapter we explore the emerging new roles for GPs, and how they can be incorporated into traditional concepts, in order to preserve what is best in terms of patient choice and personal care, while moving forward into a sustainable high-quality health service for the future.

LEARNING OBJECTIVES

By the end of this chapter you will be able to:
- define what a GP is, and where general practice fits into the NHS;
- understand the training and career opportunities for GPs in the UK;
- describe the main aspects of work of a GP;
- know the structure and the team, and importance of teamwork, in general practice;
- understand the changing nature of general practice in the UK;
- identify key skills and attributes of GPs.

Introduction

General practice is the first place of contact for most patients with concerns about their health in the UK, and has been the backbone and one of the main strengths of the NHS since its inception in 1948 (Parliament of Great Britain, 1947). About a third of all doctors who qualify in the UK become GPs, dealing with more than one million consultations per day, and managing over 90 per cent of illness within primary care.

The role of GPs has expanded over the years and although traditional consultations in the surgery or patient's home remain at the core of the profession, new roles have emerged in response to increased demands and needs within the NHS as medicine and technology advance, and in recognition of the need to establish balance between costs and benefits. Thus public health responsibilities, leadership skills within an expanding primary care workforce, financial acumen to manage devolved budgets, and specialist skills as services move from secondary to primary care are just some of the new roles for GPs to embrace.

Significant work some years ago by the World Organisation of Family Doctors (WONCA) defined the key functions of general practice (WONCA Europe, 2002). Since then GPs have had to embrace, and respond to, change demanded by social and medical progress, while preserving the confidential and valued doctor–patient relationship which is central to the NHS's effectiveness in both clinical and economic respects.

What is a general practitioner?

When the NHS was established in 1948, GPs chose to retain their independence as there was scepticism about its likely success. This meant that, unlike hospital doctors, who became employees of the NHS, each GP entered into a contract with the Government which entitled them to claim fees for services provided under 'general medical services'. General medical services included what we today recognize as the core roles of consultation: diagnosis and management of patients. To these, over years and through contract revision, other specific services such as maternity services, contraception and minor surgery (to name but a few) were added. GPs were paid according to how many patients registered for their care (their list size) with additional payments for other specified services they contracted to provide. The importance of this is that we still have the legacy of this structure which impacts on current work.

GPs originally were responsible for their patients 24 hours a day, 365 days a year. Time off was a rare occurrence and relied on GPs, who normally worked alone and from home, finding someone to cover (a locum), or linking with a nearby colleague to provide mutual cover for patient care. As medicine advanced and workload increased it became increasingly difficult for GPs to sustain these long working hours. A crisis in the 1960s led to the first of many significant changes to working patterns of GPs, with the GP Charter of 1966 (British Medical Association, 1965) leading the way to the establishment of GP partnerships and improved premises. This enabled the concept of the general practice team to grow and flourish into

the multiprofessional environment that we see in general practice today.

Once GPs started to work collaboratively, they could not only introduce flexibility into their own working lives, but also look at employing others, including other GPs, nurses and administrative staff to help in the running of their practices. Most practices that you visit today will have a range of employed staff, including practice manager, receptionist, practice nurse and employed doctors. You can still find single-handed GPs, but this is increasingly uncommon, and even here the GP is likely to have a small team of employees around them.

Practical Exercise

When you are next in general practice, identify different professionals and personnel who work at, or visit, the surgery. How do they complement the role of the GP?

The description above provides the background to different types of GP you will find in general practice in the UK. Those who contract directly with the NHS will still be self-employed and will be GP principals, responsible for the overall performance of the practice against budgets and clinical standards in their contracts. Their income will depend upon profits after expenses (including paying their employees). They will often own their premises, but you may encounter some who rent or lease space from other agencies. They have seen a number of changes to their contracts over the years.

The central contract with Government for General Medical Services (GMS) was supplemented in 1998 by an option for an alternative contract, negotiated more locally with the primary care trusts to reflect local health needs – Personal Medical Services (PMS) (NHS Executive, 1997). The latter was easier to manage by practices as numerous claim forms for services were replaced by unified budgets to cover all costs, including staff salaries. However, discrepancies arose between remuneration for GMS and PMS practices, and in its drive for cost effectiveness, the Government is now seeking a new national contract that will be equitable and make all practices accountable for the resources they use for NHS services. Thus GP principals will increasingly need excellent negotiation and management skills and ability to work closely with neighbouring practices in order to secure the best care for patients.

With the development of larger practices, it has become possible for GPs to work in a variety of ways. As a GP principal it is now possible to work part-time, although overall responsibility for the practice remains, and a partner could reasonably be called to step in in any crisis. Those who want less responsibility for managing the 'business' of general practice can opt for salaried work. A salaried GP is employed by the practice for specified hours and duties, and has the protection in law of an employee. They may, however, have less flexibility if they wish to change aspects of their contract, and they will not necessarily have as much say in how the practice is run. Some GPs who take time out of practice for maternity leave or other activities may work in very limited capacity within the practice in order to retain their skills (the Retainer Scheme), or to regain lost skills (retraining after a period of absence), or to combine GP work with education and research. Many of these posts are part-funded by the GP deaneries which oversee the clinical education needs of the workforce and work closely with the Royal College of General Practitioners (RCGP) and General Medical Council (GMC) to maintain clinical standards and fitness to practise.

The other group of qualified GPs that you will encounter are sessional GPs. These include GPs who work in a locum capacity, responding to needs of practices to provide medical cover when regular GPs are away and internal cover is not feasible. They are trained in the same way as principal and salaried GPs but are self-employed, controlling their own working time by accepting work in different practices. The advantages in this type of work are flexibility and variety, but downsides include lack of continuity of care with patients and relative isolation without a regular team of support. To balance this many locums form local networks, as do salaried doctors, through 'non-principal' support groups.

The complexity of medical care and increasing patient demand has made it important that GPs work together to provide care for their patients. From the 1960s, many GPs have worked in groups to share responsibility for out-of-hours care (traditionally between 6:30 p.m. and 8:00 a.m., and at weekends and Bank Holidays), and in the 1990s formed larger groups of GP cooperatives. Primary care trusts took over this role employing sessional and salaried GPs to provide out-of-hours services, after GPs were given the opportunity to opt out of this in their contracts in 2004. However, as GPs take on greater responsibility for organisation and funding of services in the community, including extending their own availability within general practice, this area is likely to be revisited.

This brief overview of the evolving GP role through the lifetime of the NHS will hopefully give you some insight into the variety of general practice that exists within the UK. General practice or family medicine exists in some form within most healthcare systems, and although details may vary, they will be dealing with similar issues to those discussed in this chapter.

Practical Exercise

Explore the structure of another healthcare system and consider why differences are appropriate to different circumstances.

Training for general practice

Specific training for general practice was made compulsory in 1981, but had been optional since 1975. All medical graduates in the UK complete a Foundation Training Programme, currently over 2 years, during which time they gain full registration with the GMC and experience different specialities in primary and secondary care services, including general practice. Those intending a career in general practice then apply for Speciality Training Programmes of 3 years' duration. This includes 18 months in general practice and 18 months in approved hospital posts relevant to the needs of general practice. Throughout the training they have an educational and clinical supervisor who monitors their training and progress. When in general practice their supervisor is their GP trainer who has specialized in education and training for general practice. It is the trainer's responsibility to ensure that the trainee (often called GP registrar) has sufficient and broad experience to gain necessary skills for independent practice. The RCGP has developed a curriculum for training for general practice, which explores each clinical area and is a helpful aid to learning (Riley *et al.*, 2007).

The trainee is responsible for their own learning and is required to keep records in an e-portfolio of their learning, with internal assessments and reflection. This contributes to their six-monthly assessments with their educational supervisor, which are submitted to the RCGP as part of the accreditation process. In addition, the trainee has to pass examinations in knowledge (Applied Knowledge Test – AKT) and consultation skills (Consultation Skills Assessment – CSA). At the end of training the trainee applies for a Completion of Certified Training Certificate (CCT) from the GMC which then enables then to work independently as a GP.

The work of the GP

The core role of all GPs is to provide personal medical care to patients and families. Within this role they have to work closely with others in the practice team and collaborate with community and hospital colleagues, to ensure best care for their patients. In addition to their role in helping patients understand health issues and sharing options and decisions with them, GPs need to be aware of local and national health needs which influence how resources are used, and have to balance the needs of the individual with the needs of the wider community. These influences impact on the consultation and can cause a dilemma for the GP. In this respect, being part of a team and being able to discuss concerns and share decision making is increasingly important. Very few GPs now work without the support of a practice team, or a network of colleagues to share dilemmas with, in order to avoid isolation in decision making and risk management, and the stress that this can otherwise cause.

The consultation

The consultation forms the basis of the doctor–patient relationship and is the heart of general practice (see Chapter 3). It focuses on the personal interaction between GP and patient, where the patient is able to share concerns and problems, sometimes when they have not shared them with anyone else. This requires trust and confidence, not only in the GP's clinical skills but also belief in their integrity, honesty and desire to do good – beneficence (see Chapter 12). With this trust, GPs integrate past knowledge about the patient and family, medical knowledge and understanding of the context in which the symptoms are presented, and formulate possible diagnoses and management plans. By sharing these with the patient, GPs are able to involve the patient in the diagnostic and management process, gaining their ownership and commitment to the plan that is finally agreed.

Thus, the consultation model has moved from doctor-centred to patient-centred. Gaining the commitment of patients, their understanding of the problem and their involvement in treatment enables GPs to share responsibility and management with patients, who are the only people able to make sustainable changes in their lifestyle to affect outcome – whether by taking regular medication, regular exercise or other action.

Consultations have traditionally taken place in GP surgeries or in patients' homes, but as society's needs have changed and demands on GP time have increased, several things have happened to add variety to the types of consultation that occur:

- The length of average consultations has increased over time, currently to 10 minutes, and may increase further. This allows GPs to explore more problems and in greater depth, and also give health advice and gain information which forms the basis of decisions about public health issues in the community.
- GPs may engage services of other professionals to help in the consultation process, such as practice nurses to see patients with chronic diseases like asthma, diabetes and hypertension. Nurses manage illness within agreed frameworks and refer back to GPs only if management is not going well. In this way GPs

can use their skills for the more seriously ill patients, confident that others are being well cared for by others. For the consultation this means that patients learn to trust more than one professional in the practice, with transfer of trust from the individual GP to the practice team.

- Consultations can now occur by telephone and electronic means. The GP must still protect confidentiality and trust, and practices have developed ways of ensuring these issues are addressed, to protect patients and doctors, for example by recording telephone calls, which verify what was said in cases where there is any confusion.

- Home visiting is now less common, given the mobility generally in the population. Home visits are, however, retained for the housebound and terminally ill, and add an additional dimension for GPs to appreciate how patients cope with illness in their own homes. Although less popular, the availability of home visits is an important way for GPs to reduce unnecessary hospital admissions. By understanding a patient's home environment, GPs can mobilize community services, enabling patients with serious disease, including terminal illness, to choose to stay at home (see Chapter 10).

Case Study 16.1

Mrs Y is a 78-year-old woman with diabetes whose condition has been poorly controlled on oral medication. Her GP has persuaded her to start insulin, but she is anxious. She sees the practice nurse who spends time showing her how to give injections and test her blood sugar. The nurse calls her every day over the next week to see how she is doing. After a week she comes back to the nurse, happy with her progress and the support she has received. Insulin doses are adjusted and she begins to learn how to manage insulin independently. By the time she sees the GP in a month's time she is feeling confident and her diabetic control is improving.

Here the GP shares clinical responsibility with the nurse and also the patient. What are the advantages and risks in this management?

Decision making and risk taking

How do GPs decide what symptoms are serious, and what will resolve without intervention? One of the most difficult jobs for new junior doctors in accident and emergency departments is to decide which people to send home. The same is true of GPs in general practice. It is easier to investigate and refer to specialists as this avoids potential risk. However, this does not always lead to best care and means that when a patient really needs urgent help it may not be available if the system is overwhelmed by demand rather than need. So GPs have evolved as 'gatekeepers' to secondary care services, and are expected to manage risk and demand, to create a sustainable NHS.

GPs manage risk and uncertainty by several means. They use active listening skills in the consultation to explore symptoms and understand the meaning behind what patients describe. They use medical knowledge to develop differential diagnoses, weighing up the probability of serious illness versus self-limiting problems. They discuss the patient's underlying concerns and the reasons for these, and they use clinical examination skills to support or refute possible diagnoses. By these means GPs can share options with patients to plan a route of management which may or may not involve investigation or referral. Often GPs are able to explain why investigation or referral is not required and give advice which will help patients manage their own health. This may sound similar to activities of all doctors but GPs have an additional opportunity to test theories by reviewing patients. Provided the situation is not urgent, the GP can review the patient another time, for example later the same day for a vague abdominal pain which might be early appendicitis, or in a week to monitor treatment for a non-specific skin rash. In each case the GP demonstrates commitment to the patient through on-going care and also learns by directly seeing the progress of illness.

Case Study 16.2

Miss G attends surgery with a mole on her shoulder. She does not like its appearance and requests referral for its removal. There are no suspicious features and the GP knows the NHS will not remove lesions for cosmetic reasons. He also knows that removing moles at this site can leave significant scarring. He explains both issues to Miss G who is initially upset but then decides she would not want an ugly scar. The GP emphasizes the importance of taking care in the sun and Miss G leaves, satisfied without a referral.

GPs often have to negotiate with patients. Why do you think the outcome was satisfactory here?

Despite the above there can still be times when GPs feel anxious about particular decisions they have to make. In these cases being able to discuss them with colleagues, revising decisions where necessary, not only helps GPs manage the stress of uncertainly, but also improves care for patients.

Working in a team

We have already referred to the importance of the practice team in delivering comprehensive care for patients. When you visit general practice it will be hard for you to imagine that GPs originally worked alone from their homes with only their wives as support and general administrator. You are now likely to see a team of receptionists who can arrange appointments, organize recalls and carry out a range of customer services, including coordinating satisfaction surveys; a practice manager who will manage the day-to-day running of the practice, and manage staff, finance and rotas (see Chapter 14); administrative staff who will deal with correspondence and communicate with other professional groups to coordinate care on behalf of the GP; nurses who will manage chronic disease clinics as well as health promotion, immunization and general nursing (dressings etc.); healthcare workers who may be responsible for phlebotomy services and specific services like ECGs, spirometry and well person checks; and other GPs all working for the benefit of patients. Together they can deliver a range of services that a single GP would be unable to do.

When GPs appoint new members to their teams they will be acutely aware of the skills they need to recruit to enable the practice to enhance its services to patients – they may specifically look for a nurse who can manage diabetic patients, or a GP with information technology (IT) skills. In this way the practice competences are increased by the sharing of acknowledged resource and skills and

teamwork becomes vital for the patient to receive a smooth 'seamless' service.

Case Study 16.3

Mr F has lung cancer. His wife calls the surgery at 08:00 hours on Monday morning as he has become more breathless. The receptionist recognizes her and knows that breathlessness can mean an emergency. She immediately puts the call through to the GP who knows the patient. The GP agrees to visit at the end of surgery but gives advice on medication in the meanwhile. She also contacts the local hospice team whose nurse visits at 10:00 hours. The nurse and GP discuss the patient before the GP visit at 13:00 hours.

When patient and carers are worried, effective teamwork is vital. What do you think enabled this patient to receive effective care?

Teamwork has taken on new concepts, particularly in using IT to increase efficiency. Communication between professionals, as with patients, used to be limited to direct contact or telephone but can now be electronic. This is particularly effective in speeding the process of investigation and referral and enables clinicians, including GPs, to access information and advice easily. Patients can also access information about their health on-line and this allows them to be more involved in their own care and decisions, and effectively become members of the team when addressing their own health needs.

Working with patients

In addition to working individually with patients with their personal health, GPs and their practices now engage directly with patients through newsletters and patient groups, which are ways of seeking a wider view from the practice population about where the practice should be focusing to meet local needs. Satisfaction surveys have been used in recent years to give GPs and practices feedback about how services are perceived, and have enabled practices to become more receptive to patient suggestions, particularly in areas of access and opening hours.

Working collaboratively with patients also allows GPs to share dilemmas in balancing individual and population needs. Patients are now engaged in helping the decision process for where resources and NHS services should be focused. As GPs become responsible for managing NHS budgets and commissioning services from the rest of primary care and secondary care, this dialogue with patients will become even more important, and the GP's role in these discussions is likely to be a crucial factor in balancing wants and needs in a financially constrained system.

Working within the NHS

The working options for GPs and potential for diversity through variable personal interests in specialities that encompass all realms of medicine are both assets and risks in the NHS. As assets they allow patients choice in registration with a GP or practice which delivers care in the style they prefer, and choice of practice where services they most value are delivered. As risks, however, they enable variability in standards which might compromise patient care in a worst case scenario. This diversity is one reason why individual GPs and practices have different thresholds for referring to secondary care or other agencies. Regulatory bodies, including the GMC and the Department of Health, have sought various ways to retain the diversity that patients want, but to reduce variability in standards of care.

GPs were initially rewarded for attending a set number of postgraduate education hours (PGEA) per year, with the aim of helping GPs protect time for continuing medical education. This was beneficial but one of the most useful outcomes was that GPs met together to discuss their clinical concerns. You can imagine, if you were working as a single-handed GP or in a sessional (locum) capacity, you might be isolated from clinical dialogue with colleagues. This not only added to risks of clinical error (and failure to recognize this), but also to stress for GPs who might be managing levels of uncertainty and emotional burden that was detrimental to their own health.

Using guidance for best practice established through the National Institute for Health and Clinical Excellence (NICE), incentive schemes have been established to financially reward GPs for delivering care to specified standards. These have included specific incentives set nationally – Department of Health Enhanced Schemes (DES),

or locally – Local Enhanced Schemes (LES), to deliver specific services, for example sexually transmitted disease services in general practice. These initiatives tend to address areas where there is transfer of activity from another source to general practice, making them more easily accessible for patients. The second initiative has been the Quality and Outcomes Framework (QOF), which was a government initiative to improve standards of care across a range of clinical areas (Department of Health, 2000). By rewarding GPs for performance in managing specific diseases, and publishing results, the government was able to target areas of greatest need (ischaemic heart disease and smoking, as examples) and allow patients to see which practices were performing best. This had a dramatic effect on activity in general practice, with increased focus on prevention of illness and active management of chronic disease.

The QOF allowed the Government to increase the public health role of general practice, as some targets were related to collection of information about patients (e.g. height, weight, smoking, alcohol intake and exercise levels). GPs now need to incorporate collecting this information into consultations as well as dealing with the patient's agenda. This can cause conflict of interest in consultations, particularly where income of the practice is dependent on achieving targets, and is a new area of dilemma for the GP to address.

GPs will have a significant role in the future NHS in the use of limited resource to achieve the best clinical and cost-effective outcomes for patients. Traditionally, services have been purchased (commissioned) by local health authorities (primary care trusts in recent years) using public health data and historic patterns of referral from primary to secondary care as a base. Relatively little clinical engagement has contributed to this process and, with medicine advancing at an increased pace, using historic information is not encouraging new ways of working. Given the close relationships between GPs and patients, the Government intends to increase GP input into the commissioning process. GPs will be allocated budgets for their practices and will be expected to work through commissioning consortia with other GPs to purchase services for their patients.

In 1991, the Conservative Government of the time introduced a scheme called 'Fundholding' as part of their NHS reforms whereby individual practices could purchase services for their own patients (Rivett, 1997). GPs who took part in this voluntary scheme developed considerable commissioning skills and were able to retain savings they made from budgets. The scheme closed in 1998, with a change of government and on recognition of the imbalance of care emerging between fundholding and non-fundholding practices (Petchey, 1995). However, benefits in involving GPs in commissioning care were recognized in terms of innovation and efficiencies in care developed and the new scheme of GP commissioning, which will commit all GPs to be involved, will require GPs to work in groups (consortia) with savings from budgets being fed back into patient services. GPs will take a collaborative role in the development of the NHS and will need to agree where to prioritize services and how to work together to stay within budget (Department of Health, 2010). This will be one of the greatest challenges to face general practice since the beginning of the NHS. The concept of individual autonomy is likely to change to one of corporate autonomy within the profession, and represents an enormous opportunity for those GPs interested in taking a leadership role in the evolving NHS.

Running the practice

Most GP principals now employ practice managers to manage day-to-day activities of the practice, and accountants to deal with taxation liabilities, and advise on financial issues and practice investment (see Chapter 14). The GP principal's role in management is now in strategic direction. This role includes prediction of developmental needs within the practice and preparation for changes the practice might face. For example, if a practice is to deliver full diabetic care, it will need to ensure that team members are appropriately skilled by training of existing staff or recruitment of people with existing skills. The GP will need to budget for training and recruitment needs. Similarly, if the NHS undergoes substantial change, GP partners will need to identify who will take an active role in understanding how the practice might be affected,

and to ensure the practice is not caught unprepared for change.

Practical Exercise

Make a list of all the activities a GP principal might be involved in when running the practice in addition to consulting with patients. Go through these with the GP.

Despite delegating some management tasks, the GP principals continue to retain overall responsibility for activities of the practice, as would owners of any business. GP principals will normally have regular meetings within the practice to remain up to date with clinical, premises, staffing and financial issues. GPs working together will be advised to have a practice agreement as a legal framework to ensure that any disputes between partners are resolved in a satisfactory way. Regular meetings in the practice enable the practice to remain focused on identified goals in healthcare and share developments within the whole team. These meetings may involve any combination of practice manager, clinical team members, the whole practice team, and the extended practice team including attached staff such as health visitors and community nurses. In this way salaried and trainee GPs can learn about management and can engage in some decisions taken in the practice. These activities require GPs to have management and leadership skills which become more important the larger the practice becomes.

Although other clinically qualified staff will have membership of a defence organization for any clinical negligence issue, GPs need to retain an overview of the practice performance and will likely to be involved with dealing with, and resolving, any complaints.

Maintaining standards

The importance of keeping up to date in a changing world cannot be overstated. In general practice, as in other disciplines, the profession is facing the need for revalidation which is already in place in a variety of forms in many other countries. In the UK, the GMC is working with the RCGP to develop a process that is relevant but not unduly onerous. Since 2004 all GPs have had to undertake an annual appraisal with a primary care trust approved appraiser. This process requires GPs to record their activities in continuing professional development (CPD) with analysis of significant events and to reflect on their learning. The outcome includes production of a personal development plan (PDP), which forms the basis for future learning. The use of on-line facilities to record information, such as the NHS Appraisal Toolkit, RCGP portfolio, and the GP trainee's e-learning portfolios, has considerably helped this process and the annual appraisal is likely to be incorporated into revalidation.

Case Study 16.4

Dr S sees a 23-year-old female patient with a vaginal discharge. He realizes that he has not reviewed management of sexually transmitted diseases for some time. He speaks to a colleague in the next room for advice on managing the patient and records his own learning need. He subsequently attends an update course. With this knowledge, he reports back to the practice team, writes a practice guideline identifying the roles of nurses and GPs and when to refer, and records his learning in his appraisal file.

One way of keeping up to date is recognizing when we cannot help a patient. What was the significance of the action taken here in addressing a learning need?

The appraisal process recognizes that not all GPs learn best through traditional educational meetings and lectures and now GPs can accredit learning through reading, e-learning and meetings in a variety of situations. The important outcome is the learning achieved and how this is used to improve clinical practice.

Other activities

So far we have focused on the GP in clinical practice largely dealing with patients, and negotiations with others which directly support patient care. We have referred to the GP's role in teaching and also in work to support change in the NHS as in clinical commissioning. Here we consider these further, together with other options that GPs can undertake to extend their portfolio of skills and activities.

Teaching

Many GPs are involved in teaching in a variety of ways. Indirectly, GPs engage in teaching their patients when they give advice in management or avoidance of illness. In a more formal role some GPs become GP tutors and seminar leaders and have medical students attached to their practices for specific activities – to learn clinical skills, to learn about the consultation process or to explore the impact of illness in communities. With so much chronic disease now being managed in the community it is difficult for students to gain clinical experience for these illnesses in hospitals. Extending this role, GPs can be directly linked to universities and medical schools as lecturers linked with departments of general practice and primary care.

At postgraduate level, GPs can become GP trainers linked with GP deaneries to train future GPs through the GP Speciality Training Programme, take newly qualified doctors for training during their Foundation training, or supervise retraining of GPs returning to general practice.

In all cases GPs need teaching skills and are encouraged or compelled to undertake formal training. Many undertake Postgraduate Certificates in Education (PGCE) or equivalent, and some take this training further to Master's level. Universities and deaneries are responsible for ensuring their GP teachers are delivering postgraduate teaching to required levels, and use a variety of measures to ensure this, from structured curricula with student feedback, to three-yearly reselection interviews and practice visits for GP speciality and Foundation trainers. One advantage of this work is that it is largely practice-based. This means that GP teachers are still in the practice for day-to-day work, and that practices are also involved in the process, enabling the practice team to benefit from the enthusiasm and variety that trainees and students bring.

Research

Some GPs develop an academic career in general practice research, linking with their clinical work. While some do this formally through working with departments of general practice and primary care or deaneries, some carry out research projects independently in their practices. GPs have great opportunity to monitor patterns of disease and effects of intervention with largely stable populations they can follow over many years.

Working with local health organizations

There are many ways for a GP to engage with the political side of the NHS in primary care. GPs are represented by local medical committees (LMCs), and membership of this committee will give GPs good insight into developments that affect their working lives in the NHS. This committee feeds local views to the British Medical Association (BMA) which negotiates with government through the Department of Health. The LMC gives advice to local health organizations, currently the primary care trusts (PCT), as does the Professional Executive Committee, which is recruited by the PCT with GP members to offer strategic clinical input into local service developments. With the advent of clinical commissioning consortia, the PCTs may disappear, but clinical engagement will significantly increase, with GPs in the front line to help commission and redesign services within the NHS.

Developing clinical interest areas

GPs need sound knowledge in all clinical areas but many have areas they particularly enjoy and in which they gain advanced skills. They can pursue interest areas through study for higher qualifications, academic work in deaneries or universities, or sessional work as clinical assistants in hospitals working alongside consultants to gain practical experience. They may have expertise from prior work in other disciplines before entering general practice. With appropriate skills and experience, GPs can take the role of GP with a Special Interest (GPwSI) and you may recognize this term when you hear about services being moved from secondary to primary care, using GPwSIs and GPs with appropriate skills with consultant support. Other areas for developing clinical interest activities include working as a police surgeon or in occupational health for large firms. Some GPs also develop writing and journalistic skills, not only to publish research, but also to contribute in public debates in the media. All these, and other, activities provide interests which add to the variety and diversity of life as a GP, as well as providing additional sources of income.

A week in general practice

You might appreciate, from the range of career options within general practice, that it is difficult to describe a typical GP. I have worked as a GP principal for 25 years and have seen my role change many times. I now work as a teacher, at both undergraduate and postgraduate level, and as a clinical commissioning lead within the PCT. Before this I have spent time as an LMC and professional executive committee (PEC) member and have studied initially to be a GP trainer; then to gain a PGCE and finally Master's degree. During this time I have juggled family life, raised children and worked within the practice as a GP principal. Such experience and evolution of roles and responsibilities is common to many GPs, and is one aspect that makes general practice an exciting and excellent career choice for doctors with a variety of skills and interests.

Table 16.1 shows a week's activities for you to see how different activities can be incorporated into the week. The first thing I hope you will recognize is how important it is for GPs to work in effective teams. I could not spend time away from the practice if I did not have cover and support in the practice from colleagues. I am away from the practice for commissioning activities and I do most of my teaching in the practice. The whole practice is involved in training and teaching, particularly with GP trainees, and this is very enjoyable and rewarding for all – patients included.

Making time to debrief with the trainees and practice team is very important, in order to keep up with what is happening in the practice. For example I need to know if staff members are sick or having difficulties personally inside or outside the practice in order to coordinate support they might need and ensure the practice continues to run smoothly. I choose to do this through direct conversations and time with the practice manager, which works well in a relatively small practice. In larger practices you may find an administrative member delegated to take on these issues who then relates back to the partners.

My practice has weekly clinical meetings to review clinical concerns, discuss referrals and prescribing issues, and to learn about new NHS developments that will affect the practice. Here we share clinical uncertainty and the emotional burden that caring for the chronic sick and dying can generate. The more junior the clinician the more vulnerable to these stresses they tend to be, and I debrief at least daily with my GP trainee. However I admit I am also grateful to be able to share my concerns and sadness when a patient I have known for many years is taken ill or dies – we are all human and have natural feelings of loss, sadness and joy, which is one reason why patients value us so highly.

Practice meetings occur at six-weekly intervals and include attached staff such as community nurses, health visitors and counsellors. We also have six-weekly partnership meetings which are additional to daily meetings with the practice manager and allow for strategic decisions that have to be made and documented. Furthermore we meet six-weekly with our palliative community care team to review patients we care for who have chosen to die at home. This is a particular interest area for us, and we benefit from sharing information and knowledge. It may seem from this list of meetings that there can be no time to see patients – certainly meetings take more of our time than in past years, but benefits of close working relationships and consistency in care make this investment invaluable.

The GP Surgery

Table 16.2 illustrates a typical surgery on a Friday morning. The scheduled time is from 8 a.m. to 11 a.m., but I expect to finish by 12 noon. We run a 10-minute appointment system for attendances, but allow for 5-minute telephone calls which can be booked like consultations. Patients are given a time range for the call rather than a specific time. This allows for flexibility when surgeries are busy, so that those in the waiting room are not delayed if consultations overrun. You will notice that there is a 2 : 1 ratio of attendance : telephone call consultations. This is fairly normal, as telephone consultations are becoming more common, as are

communications by e-mail. Receptionists have guidelines for interrupting doctors for emergency calls but apart from this it is the doctor's decision as to how to balance telephone calls and surgery consultation time. I like to deal with calls as I go along but one of my colleagues prefers to take all his calls at the end of surgery.

I take time to review patients with my GP registrar as needed. If additional emergencies arise they are added to the end of the list – hence the usual finish at 12 noon. Patients are advised by receptionists if there is likely to be a delay of more than 20 minutes to give them the option of rebooking or seeing another doctor.

Notes from the surgery

- 08:00 Review of thyroxine dose post-thyroidectomy. Discussed obesity. Agrees to see nurse. I have my doubts about success here but offer encouragement.
- 08:15 Patient with osteoporosis, aggravated by steroids she takes for bullous pemphigoid. She fell as a result of osteoarthritis of her knees and clinically has fractured her coccyx. More important than pain were the psychological effects of immobility and loss of independence. We agreed she should see a counsellor. I refer to occupational therapist for practical help at home.
- 08:24 This lady had multiple problems associated with ageing. She had developed gout as a result of treatment of her heart failure with diuretic. She also had a painful shoulder from arthritis. The only relief she had from this was with an anti-inflammatory drug which aggravated her heart failure. I have to compromise between clinical best practice from guidelines and quality of life – the latter won, but the discussion with the patient meant she knew risks as well as benefits of using anti-inflammatory drugs.
- 08:40 Straightforward consultation with boy with ear infection who I gave a prescription for antibiotic. Grandmother tried to do all the talking – I had to interrupt to ask the boy what he thought.
- 08:52 Patient has a swollen leg following DVT. She had refused anticoagulation and presented

Table 16.1 A week in general practice

Monday	Tuesday	Wednesday	Thursday	Friday	Saturday	Sunday
07:50 Arrive at surgery	07:40 Arrive at surgery. Deal with messages; e-mails	07:45 Arrive at surgery	07:45 Travel to commissioning office	07:45 Arrive at surgery	Not my turn for Saturday morning surgery this week, chance for lie-in!	Afternoon spent reading preparing for meetings in coming week; prepared workshop I will run on facilitating group meetings for GPs; planned student teaching session on communication skills
08:00–11:30 Surgery – 15 patients; 11 telephone calls	08:15 Travel to commissioning office	08:00–09:00 Messages; letters; prescriptions; four telephone calls to patients	08:30–11:30 Meeting with other clinical commissioning leads re commissioning strategy	08:00–12:00 Surgery – 16 patients; 9 telephone calls		
11:30–12:00 Meet practice manager	08:45–11:30 Meet PBC manager to review clinical guidelines and arrange educational events.	09:15–11:00 Four visits to housebound patients. Follow-up telephone calls to hospice nurse and local pharmacist regarding medication and support		12:00–12:30 Meet practice manager		
12:00–12:40 Debrief with GP trainee	12:00–13:00 Practice visit – meet GPs and practice manager to review referral patterns. Established objectives for audit and review	11:00–12:00 Partners' meeting – agreed refurbishments and rewiring in surgery. Discussed receptionist training and new telephone system		12:30–13:00 Lunch		
12:40–13:00 Lunch	13:00–13:30 Travel back to practice – sandwich in car	12:00–13:00 Clinical meeting – referrals review and significant event – missed case of DVT in postnatal patient. New guidelines for headache management discussed				
		13:00–13:30 Lunch				

13:00–14:15 Two home visits – COPD and dementia reviews

14:15–16:00 Paperwork – prescriptions; letters; results; talk to colleagues

16:00–16:30 Six telephone calls

16:15–18:45 Surgery – 12 patients

18:45–19:30 Paperwork – letters, e-mails

19:30 Lock surgery. Home

13:30–14:15 Debrief with GP trainee

14:15–15:00 Joint visit with GP trainee to terminally ill patient

15:00–15:20 Meet practice manager

15:30–16:15 Paperwork and e-mails

16:15–18:40 Surgery – 12 patients and 4 telephone calls

18:45 Home

13:30–16:30 Reading – *BMJ* and new developments in PBC. On-line learning in child protection completed

16:30–18:00 Deal with results; letters and messages

19:00–20:00 Talk to community group on living wills

12:30–14:30 Meeting with PCT directors re service redesign

14:30–15:00 Travel back to practice

15:00–15:30 Debrief with GP trainee

15: 30–16:00 Paperwork and messages

16:00–18:40 Surgery – 12 patients and 6 telephone calls

18:40–19:30 Results; letters; e-mails

19:30 Lock surgery

Home

13: 00–14:00 Palliative care meeting – reviewed 7 terminally ill patients with hospice nurse, community nurses and practice clinical team

14:00–16:00 Tutorial with GP trainee – case-based discussion; discussed breaking bad news

16:00–16:30 One visit – elderly lady with chest infection

16:30–17:30 Results and e-mails

17:30 Home via supermarket for week's shopping

Table 16.2 A Friday morning GP surgery

Patients seen in surgery		Other activities during the surgery	
Time	Consultation	Time	Activity
08:00	55-year-old woman, post thyroidectomy	08:12	Reception query re prescription
08:15	71-year-old woman, fall 2 weeks ago	08:36	Home visit request – agreed
08:24	94-year-old woman, heart failure improving		
08:40	13-year-old boy – high fever; earache	08:48	Tel. call from 61-year-old patient with diabetes – insulin dose query
08:52	85-year-old woman – follow-up after DVT. Bereaved	09:04	Tel. call from 74-year-old with back pain
09:15	66-year-old woman with rheumatoid arthritis	09:10	Tel. call from 74-year-old with breathlessness. Known heart failure – arranged to see
09:28	77-year-old woman for dementia review		
09:42	42-year-old woman with menopause	10:15	Review patient with rash with GP registrar
09:52	75-year-old man with lung cancer	10:28	Assist nurse with difficult cervical smear
10:05	76-year-old woman with arthritis and obesity	11:00	Review patient with anxiety with GP registrar
10:20	88-year-old woman with temporal arteritis	11:05	Visit request – patient agrees to come to surgery this afternoon
10:35	5-year-old boy with attention deficit and hyperactivity disorder	11:07	Tel. call from community nurse – request for prescription
10:50	23-year-old woman 1st pregnancy	11:10	Tel. call – results of tests discussed
11:15	58-year-old woman – depressed – came as emergency	11:45	Supervise GP registrar with shoulder injection
11:30	64-year-old woman – lump in breast – came as emergency	11:58	Tel. call to patient with sore throat – advice given

late. She was grieving for her husband who had died a month earlier. We discussed how she was coping and she agreed to see the bereavement counsellor. It would have been easy to offer her antidepressants but grief and depression can appear very similar and she really needed to talk rather than take medication.

■ Emergency call at 09:10. 88-year-old man with gradually worsening breathlessness over last week. I checked that breathlessness was not severe, no chest pain, and was comfortable – arranged to see after surgery but advised that if worse to contact me again.

■ 09:15 Rheumatoid arthritis under good control but patient had had an episode of rectal bleeding. She is taking a non-steroidal anti-inflammatory drug as well as steroids and methotrexate. Her blood results were normal, as was examination. I could not exclude a more serious problem in the bowel and had to persuade her to consider referral for colonoscopy. We discussed the possibility of bleeding having been caused by medication, but that we should not always attribute everything to her arthritis. She wants time to think about referral and we agree to talk again on Monday. Being able to give patients time to consider what they want to do is a great advantage for the GP. [This patient was subsequently found to have a sigmoid carcinoma.]

■ 09:28 Reviewing a patient with dementia involves not only assessing their level of functioning (I use the Mini-Mental State Examination), but also general physical examination and assessment of social needs and how their carer(s) is coping. Many patients with mild or moderate impairment can still live in the community but need support. We have a carers' group in our practice to help support carers, which this patient's husband finds very helpful. This patient is having problems taking medication in the evening when she is tired and irritable. I went through medication with her husband and we changed all medication to be given in the morning.

■ 09:42 This patient has reached the menopause at an early age. She does not want hormone replacement as her mother had breast cancer. We discussed the value of exercise and calcium intake in the diet, and also the emotional impact of facing the ageing process – she was quite upset and I listened.

■ 09:52 This patient was recently diagnosed with lung cancer and is deteriorating rapidly. He is anxious, not only for his future, but also that of his wife, who suffers from dementia. He has become very breathless. We talk about managing his symptoms and I gently broach the subject of managing symptoms rather than cure. I talk to him about what might happen and what we can do to help and support him. We arrange to meet again on Monday to continue our discussions when he will bring his son. He leaves and I feel quite sad – I have known him for 20 years.

■ 10:05 This obese lady recognized her need to lose weight to help her joint pains. She agreed to see the nurse and join our weight reduction programme.

■ 10:15 My GP registrar sees a patient with pityriasis rosea. This is a common rash in general practice but not seen often in hospital, so was unfamiliar to him. I make a note to review common skin problems in our next tutorial.

■ 10:20 This patient with temporal arteritis unfortunately lost sight in one eye before diagnosis. She is coping well with her disability and has come for medication review.

■ 10:28 My nurse has a problem taking a cervical smear. Finding an anterior cervix is not always easy and I show her how to take a smear with the patient on their side.

■ 10:35 Mother and child came together to talk about the child's newly diagnosed attention deficit and hyperactivity disorder (ADHD). This was a difficult consultation as Mum had lots of concerns and questions while I tried to prevent the child from wrecking the surgery and from harming himself – not an easy task! I felt exhausted by the end of the consultation and I appreciated the stress that his parents were going through on a daily basis.

■ 10:50 I enjoy seeing patients with new pregnancies who are excited about the prospect of a baby. It is a good opportunity to talk about healthy living as well as explain the process of maternity care and who will be involved. She goes away with lots of literature to read and I make a note to make the appropriate referrals at the end of surgery.

■ 11:00 My GP registrar calls me, having reached an impasse with a patient with chronic anxiety. The patient has overwhelmed him with her list of complaints. Fortunately, I have known this woman for many years and am aware of her underlying cancer phobia which emerges when she becomes depressed. I ask some direct questions and we are able to avoid repeating investigations. She agrees to restart her antidepressants, and my registrar and I agree to discuss somatization, using this consultation as a base in tutorial.

■ 11:15 This patient came as an emergency, feeling life was no longer worth living. She was having relationship difficulties at home. I used a depression questionnaire with her, and as we explored her symptoms it emerged that underlying depression was contributing to arguments at home, together with financial worries since her husband's redundancy. She had no active suicidal thoughts (something that is not as difficult to ask about as you might think) and agreed to see the counsellor as well as visit the Benefits Office to review the family entitlements to state support. We arranged to meet again in two weeks.

■ 11:30 It is uncanny how the last emergency is often the most serious. This woman had noticed a breast lump several weeks ago but had only just decided to come. She knew that the diagnosis would be cancer and I was not going to deceive her. However, I was able to explain possible options for treatment and how the outlook for breast cancer had improved so much in recent years. She went away relieved – I think as much because she had shared her burden, as for what I had been able to explain about the next step. I sent an immediate fax for an urgent appointment to the local breast cancer clinic.

■ 11:45 This was a planned shoulder injection for me to supervise my registrar learning the procedure. Doing joint injections is a useful skill in general practice, saving many referrals to secondary care and very satisfying for the GP when the patient improves!

The changing face of illness in general practice

There is no doubt that the problems we manage in general practice are changing. At its inception, the NHS developed with the premise that as infection was treated so illness would disappear. This may seem naive in retrospect as there was no anticipation of the extended life that healthier and wealthier living environments would bring.

Living longer is a great achievement but we now see more age-related illness, such as cancers and arthritis, and also consequences of excess, namely obesity and alcohol- and smoking-related problems. Progress of medicine and the increasing range of medications available bring risks of illness through drug interactions and adverse effects of treatments (iatrogenic illness). These factors mean that GPs are often dealing with multiple health problems involving complex decision-making processes.

In addition, society is changing, with cultural and religious diversity influencing patients' health beliefs, patterns of behaviour and illness. GPs need to be sensitive and aware of their own behaviour to avoid causing unwitting offence and to obtain the best outcome for all patients. Increased travel means GPs can have to deal with tropical illness (e.g. malaria) and variable working patterns in society require GPs to offer services that are appropriate in time and place to meet needs. These factors make it more likely that GPs will choose to work in groups to share their skills,

resources and clinical concerns, to achieve the best care for their patients, and to enable their role to expand within the new NHS.

Patient and public expectations of a GP

When there was little on offer for treating illness, the main role of the GP was as the family friend and advisor. Although these traditional roles have remained, and are still valued through the concept of continuity of care, patients are generally well aware of advances in medicine, and expect their GP to be able to offer an educated opinion in almost all areas. However, no one can be expert in all areas, and perhaps more important than knowledge alone is the ability to be honest and admit to a patient when one does not know the answer. Honesty and integrity are vital attributes for GPs – many national scandals that have faced medicine in recent years have been where one or both of these attributes have been breached and trust has broken down. Government and the GMC have stepped in to increase regulations for the profession, but patients will judge their GP as an individual and will respect the doctor who can acknowledge their limitations as well as their strengths.

Seeking help when needed is not a weakness, and one of the challenges GPs face, as their role in the NHS increases, is to recognize the best and safest route of care for the patient – a traditional role modernized through the need to take on board issues of cost effectiveness as well as clinical effectiveness.

The GP needs to stay up to date with current best practice, as this knowledge has to be balanced against individual need. The final decisions and options should now be a shared process with patients but patients will expect that the GP's advice will be sound and based on medical evidence. This will become even more important as services move from secondary to primary care and GPs take more responsibility for management of illness traditionally managed in hospitals. At the same time GPs need to understand the facilities available in their locality. Many therapeutic options will involve a number of different

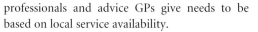
professionals and advice GPs give needs to be based on local service availability.

The GP's role continues to change in parallel with society's needs and demands. As public servants it is a huge privilege to share in the intimacy of patients' lives and be able to influence the future course of the NHS. I, for one, do not regret my career choice.

SUMMARY POINTS

To conclude, the most important messages of this chapter are as follows:

- General practice offers a wide range of career opportunities for doctors with different interests and skills.
- GPs are responding to changes in society and the NHS which are going to place them in the forefront of developing new services.
- GPs work within primary healthcare teams and collaborate with colleagues to deliver an increasing range of services for patients.
- The doctor–patient relationship and continuity of care remain fundamental to general practice, with focus on patient involvement in the decision-making process.
- A career in general practice is not static. Development is encouraged through continuing professional development and response to public need.

References

British Medical Association 1965: New contract for general practitioners; a charter for the family doctor services. *British Medical Journal* (Suppl. 1), 89–91

Department of Health 2000: *Quality and performance in the NHS. NHS performance indicators.* London: The Stationery Office.

Department of Health 2010: *Equity and excellence: liberating the NHS.* London: The Stationery Office.

NHS Executive 1997: *Personal Medical Services under the NHS (Primary Care) Act 1997. The contractual framework for PMS provider pilots.* Leeds: NHS Executive.

Parliament of Great Britain 1947: *National Health Service Act of 1946.* London: HMSO.

Petchey, R. 1995: General practitioner fundholding: weighing the evidence. *Lancet* 346(8983), 1139–42.

Riley, B., Haynes, J. and Field, S. 2007: *The condensed curriculum guide for GP training and the new MRCGP.* London: RCGP.

Rivett G. 1997: *From cradle to grave. Fifty years of the NHS.* London: Kings Fund, 424–7.

WONCA Europe (World Organisation of Family Doctors) 2002: The European definition of general practice/family medicine. www.woncaeurope.org/Web%20documents/European%20Definition%20 of%20family%20medicine/Definition%20EURACTshort%20version.pdf (accessed 10 June 2011).

Acknowledgements

Thank you to Dr Brian Fine who wrote this chapter in previous editions. Some of his ideas were retained in this edition.

SINGLE BEST ANSWER QUESTIONS

16.1 The best way to approach continuing professional development and new medical developments is:

a) To go on annual update courses for GPs, covering a range of recent medical developments

SINGLE BEST ANSWER QUESTIONS CONTINUED

b) To read reputable journals regularly and thoroughly

c) To identify learning needs through reflection on significant events; patient unmet needs (PUNS) and doctor educational needs (DENS), and practice development needs, and plan learning according to preferred learning style

d) To ask the GP appraiser to say where to focus learning for the future

e) To attend all education sessions arranged locally by the GP tutor.

16.2 Mrs Smith has been a patient of Dr Red's for 17 years. A blood result now suggests that Mrs Smith has developed type 2 diabetes mellitus. How should Dr Red approach the concept of continuity of care for Mrs Smith?

a) Dr Red should ask his nurse to call Mrs Smith and ask her to book into the diabetic clinic

b) The receptionist should call Mrs Smith and tell her to come and collect some literature before making an appointment to see the nurse

c) Dr Red should call Mrs Smith and tell her she has diabetes but that as it is not his area of expertise he is asking the nurse to see her

d) Dr Red should arrange to see Mrs Smith to give her the diagnosis and the opportunity to ask questions before exploring options for treatment and on-going management

e) Dr Red should refer her to the hospital.

16.3 Mr Brown attends his GP for review of his asthma. He has been more breathless and has put on weight since being made redundant. Peak flow has not changed and examination is normal. What should his GP do?

a) Tell the patient to go to the gym and lose weight and that this will sort out the problem

b) Explore the reasons for weight gain and discuss how Mr Brown might address this, offer-

ing support from the practice nurse and counsellor, and regular review of progress

c) Refer to the British Thoracic Society guidelines and increase medication

d) Explain it is normal to be more breathless if weight goes up and that he should focus on getting a new job

e) Pass Mr Brown on to the practice nurse who runs the asthma clinic to deal with.

16.4 The community nurse calls requesting a home visit for a patient with swollen ankles. How should the GP respond?

a) Speak to the community nurse directly to explore the problem, likely cause and agree a plan of action, including joint visit

b) Ask the receptionist to tell the nurse you will visit later today

c) Add the patient's name to the routine visit list for any doctor to do

d) Call the patient and say you can't visit today, but will call later in the week

e) Call the patient's relative and ask if they can bring the patient to the surgery.

16.5 The practice has a practice nurse vacancy. How should it approach filling this?

a) The practice manager should ask around local practices to see if a nurse is looking for a new job

b) The practice should identify skills it already has and those it needs to recruit, and develop a person specification to go with an advertisement, with subsequent interview and references

c) The practice should ask its remaining nurses to take on extra hours to cover the vacancy

d) The practice should streamline its services to get more out of the remaining nurses

e) The practice should advertise in a national forum and decide who to appoint when the applications come in.

APPENDIX

ANSWERS TO SINGLE BEST ANSWER QUESTIONS

2.1 The best answer is D. Primary healthcare provides over 90 per cent of healthcare in the UK. It provides healthcare in the first instance from a variety of community-based services and includes acute care, chronic care, rehabilitation and health promotion.

2.2 The best answer is E. Primary healthcare is aiming to achieve a service that is accessible to all, acceptable to the population, able to identify the health needs of a population, based on need rather than demand and able to make the most cost-effective use of its limited resources.

2.3 The best answer is C. The core activity of the majority of GPs is consulting with patients. All the other answers are flawed. Outpatient activities are part of secondary care. Practice nurses are registered general nurses with relevant nursing experience who can, if opportunities are available, take part in practice nurse training. District nurses manage care within the community outside of the general practice setting.

2.4 The best answer is C. The British Medical Association is the doctors' union and accountability of the practice is to the Secretary of State for Health for General Medical Services (GMS) practices and locally to the Primary Healthcare Trusts for Personal Medical Services (PMS) practices. In the UK patient participation can be through the practice, self-help and community groups, and Government-funded Local Involvement Networks. GPs are mainly accountable to their patients and their peers.

2.5 The best answer is B. Abuse of NHS staff is not acceptable and must be addressed in a way that supports practice staff and makes it clear to the patient that this is so. It is also important to talk through what led to the incident with practice staff and the patient in order to consider what might be done in future to make it less likely that this type of behaviour will happen again.

3.1 The best answer is C. This tells of behaviours within the consultation rather than the tasks that are achieved during the consultation (the content).

3.2 The best answer is A. For some patients and in some contexts (e.g. in an emergency) the patient prefers that the doctor takes control of the consultation. However many patients wish to take an active role in the consultation. Being patient-centred means that the doctor ascertains and acts on how active the patient wishes to be in the interaction.

3.3 The best answer is E. A good relationship is not possible with all patients although one must do one's best to foster this – it might take time and many consultations to build such a relationship. The reasons for a patient's attendance may not become clear until part way through or at the end of a consultation, later or never. Not every consultation requires a physical examination, for example where one is counselling a patient. Safety netting is making sure that no serious possibilities regarding the patient's health have been missed. Strong emotional responses are always important to reflect on as they affect the doctor–patient relationship and may lead you to better understand what is going on for you and the patient; they may affect the outcome of the consultation, and only you can accommodate or alter them.

3.4 The best answer is D. In such situations it is important to check out with the patient how they are in general. Patients often come with a physical symptom as a 'ticket of entry' when they

ANSWERS TO SINGLE BEST ANSWER QUESTIONS CONTINUED

wish to talk about something else that is happening in their life that they feel uncertain about divulging. Sadness and anxiety may make minor illnesses more worrying to the patient and recent research has shown that they may also have an effect on immune responses.

3.5 The best answer is C. All these options are helpful but you will meet patients from so many cultures and sub-cultures that the best way to learn is from the patients themselves. The trend these days is away from learning about groups of patients to learning about patients as individuals each with their own perspectives. Assumptions can often get in the way of communication and understanding.

5.1 The best answer is arguably A. The short history in a young woman is very unlikely to represent sinister pathology. Treating with a PPI is likely to be diagnostic as well as therapeutic (and so may obviate the need for investigations such as D and E). Stopping smoking and losing weight are both important but neither will relieve symptoms in the short term (though are of unquestionable importance in the longer term).

5.2 The best answer is D. The similarity to the previous question is deliberate. However a new symptom with weight loss in a patient of 63 makes sinister pathology far more likely. The best answer is D as excluding such a cause is vital. Advising on weight loss and smoking cessation are of course important and there is no reason to withhold treatment (such as PPIs) whilst other investigations proceed. Helicobacter testing would reasonably be deferred until there is evidence that this is a chronic problem.

5.3 The best answer is B. The brief story does not suggest organic pathology, and irritable bowel syndrome is high on the list of possible causes. What we don't know is why he should be getting psychosomatic symptoms at this point. Exploring the patient's beliefs (B) will reveal that his mother was recently diagnosed with stomach cancer at which point reassuring, as in D, becomes relevant and useful. General reassur-

ance (as in C) is not likely to be helpful (would it reassure you if you were in his situation?).

5.4 The best answer is B. Patients frequently request advice about alternative therapies. The time and attention (and sometimes elaborate investigations) lavished on patients will unquestionably have strong placebo effects, but by their nature these will be short lived. The GP has an important role in advising and educating patients about the claims of therapies and to do so may need to research them (so B is correct). Often alternative therapies have no research base, which does not necessarily mean they are ineffective. Some alternative therapies (of which celebrity nutritionists are a good example) make elaborate scientific sounding claims and couch their writing to look like academic papers which (deliberately) conceal an absence of any real scientific underpinning.

5.5 The best answer is E. Either A or B would represent current best practice as a choice of antibiotics for community acquired pneumonia. The simpler regime in B would certainly help the patient comply. Stressing the importance of taking the antibiotics properly (D) is important, but the interaction is all one way. On the other hand fluffy ideas of patient centredness (C) where you pass all responsibility over to the patient deny the patient your expertise. Taking A, B, C and D together, where you discuss the effective treatments, explore the patient's concerns and come to an understanding, as in E, offers the best approach.

6.1 The best answer is B. This is an example of an idiosyncratic reaction (B), which is quite uncommon but with potentially dangerous consequences so it is important to warn patients about taking prompt action when it arises.

6.2 The best answer is C. All these will help patients take their medication (although B can be a very patronizing way to achieve this). Keeping dosing regimes simple (D) is important, although a three times daily regime hardly meets this need. The doctor should always show empathy (E) and always stress the importance of

ANSWERS TO SINGLE BEST ANSWER QUESTIONS CONTINUED

the therapy (A), but to be effective these need to be combined into a shared understanding and agreement (concordance) (C).

6.3 The best answer is D. The elderly are relatively sensitive to drugs so reduced doses should normally be used initially (A). More than four drugs constitutes polypharmacy (B): many elderly patients are on more than this which should be a warning to prescribers. Fixed combinations of drugs may be inflexible, but the benefits of simple dosing regimes generally outweigh the disadvantages (C). Community pharmacists (D) have many roles and are an underused resource but to ensure compliance needs someone on the spot which is why relatives or professional carers are best placed to ensure the patient receives the support they need.

6.4 The best answer is E. You must state the age of children, but this is not required for adults (A). Milligrams (the commonest unit) may be abbreviated to mg, but avoid abbreviating micrograms, where it could potentially produce confusion. Latin dosage abbreviations are permitted, but discouraged (D). Patients frequently remember little of what has happened in a consultation, including, critically, instructions on taking drugs. Writing them onto the prescription (E) ensures they will appear on the bottle and is an aid to compliance.

6.5 The best answer is E. Arguably this is the most important message in the book: as a foundation doctor you can have a profound effect on your patients' outcomes by writing clear discharge notes. Write immediately (don't wait as in A). Give detailed information about each drug, so the GP understands the hospital's intentions and give clear guidance as to how long to continue each medication (B and C). Most hospital prescriptions last two weeks (hospital drug budgets are cash limited, so they try to transfer prescribing to general practice as soon as possible – foolish given it all comes from the same budget in the end) so a month (D) is too long. Giving your consultant's name and contact details legibly means the GP can contact the

right hospital team quickly if there is a problem. So the best answer is E.

7.1 The best answer is C. The concept of common symptoms refers to those symptoms which, in population surveys, are reported most frequently. Unfortunately, just because a symptom is commonly reported, it does not mean that it is always harmless and it does not mean that a doctor has no role to play in interpreting its meaning. Many common symptoms provide clues to the possibility of underlying disease.

7.2 The best answer is D. At 66, this man is quite likely to be newly retired and adapting to a new lifestyle. Headache is a common presenting symptom of depression. Brain tumours only rarely present with headaches even though this is often the first thing a doctor thinks of when seeing a patient with a headache. The other conditions are all possible, but less likely to be causes of headache in a man of this age, in routine general practice.

7.3 Probably the best answer is C, although these days, E is a close contender. It surprises most medically trained professionals that under half of all cases of new onset rectal bleeding ever get to present to the GP. The larger proportion of cases is just ignored, probably in the hope that they will simply go away (which most do, of course). However, the possibility of underlying cancer of the colon means that new onset rectal bleeding should always be taken seriously when seen by a doctor.

7.4 The best answer is D. Of course, the textbook answer is probably C but in the reality of day-to-day general practice, it is not feasible to offer a full medical clerking of all patients. A question such as 'why now' can often get to the bottom of whether a common symptom has more serious significance. In this case, it might be because the indigestion was no longer responding to simple antacids (suggesting the need for stronger treatments such a proton pump inhibitors), or he may have started to get dysphagia (a red flag symptom suggesting a possible carcinoma of the oesophagus) or the pain might be occur-

ANSWERS TO SINGLE BEST ANSWER QUESTIONS CONTINUED

ring on the slightest exertion (suggesting that the patient had interpreted their cardiac pain as 'merely' indigestion).

7.5 The best answer is A. Common symptoms are often medically unexplained. Perhaps surprisingly, there may be a few cases in which the patient would be helped by further investigation or even a laparotomy. However, longstanding, persistent and even quite disabling symptoms are not uncommon. Often there is no clear diagnosis although it is important to rule out serious underlying pathology. Perhaps the single greatest skill a doctor can offer is the skill of active listening. The patient who feels that they have not been listened to is likely to either become a frequent attender or to become disillusioned with their doctor and the primary care team. Whereas if the doctor is able to listen to the patient and explore their concerns, they may be able to address underlying concerns such as a fear of cancer, or a story about a family member who had a similar pain and then suffered a dreadful complication. For common medically unexplained symptoms, reassurance is usually of little help, whereas exploring the patient's concerns is more likely to lead to resolution.

8.1 The best answer is D. As a single person with no partner he is more vulnerable to suicidal acts anyway, but as a person with an alcohol problem studies show his risk multiplying hugely, well over ten times in some. A doctor may be a person those contemplating suicide do consult, and of course if he is frankly suicidal hospital admission may well be important, but he seems still far from understanding why he is so unwell. Seeing him every day may substitute one dependency (alcohol) for another, but there is no doubt that persuading him to stop drinking is a first and vital step, and local alcohol services and agencies such as Alcoholics Anonymous may be very helpful. A counsellor's help and insight will be helpful, but few would see him while he is still drinking. If you answered B, are you sure you are in the right career?

8.2 The best answer is E. Picking on a recurrence of the problem she had when she was 5 now she is over twice that age without eliminating or at least seriously considering the other possibilities would be very risky medicine indeed. A and D are easily tested for, but C may require specialist help: if rape is an issue, obviously from specialized police. The school health service (approached confidentially) may sometimes have access to exactly what is needed without stigmatizing Joanne or risking confrontation with her Dad (who remains a possible suspect as a perpetrator, horrible as we might think that idea to be). B needs exploration with someone who can develop rapport with Joanne, and this might be a school counsellor, a local teenage project or (we hope) it might be you.

8.3 The best answer is D. This is probably the main approach that unites professionals in the 'talking therapies', who work in differing frameworks. It is not a bad watchword for a general practitioner either, though more may be required on rare occasions, as when the health of someone else or the general public is at risk. Most counsellors work with practices on the understanding that what passes between them is confidential and is only shared with another person with the client's consent or in exceptional circumstance (like a real suicidal risk). Only rather domineering restrictive NHS management has placed the limit of six visits on counsellors, though it is often quoted. Few counsellors will see someone who is currently drinking (see Q8.1 – if you got that wrong, take a break and start again with a bit more concentration). B is a mistake that students often seem to make: the spelling is different.

8.4 The best answer is E. Don't conclude your first consultation without making another time to meet. A is not usually a helpful strategy in the circumstances, unless you sincerely want this patient to make sure she never sees you again. She may merit antidepressant treatment, but initiating that needs much more assessment and should be the other side of understanding

ANSWERS TO SINGLE BEST ANSWER QUESTIONS CONTINUED

together what has got under her skin. She may be unsafe with children, but D is a last resort if she insists on returning to work when she is still seriously ill. C would be considered by most people as just a stupid waste of resources.

8.5 The best answer is B. In all these examples the distress may be real. The symptom may be caused by loneliness, which is a common condition in some areas: so far no one to the writers' satisfaction has come up with a good strategy for loneliness in general practices, except the prudent thought that while rejection is cruel it simply may not be possible to become every patient's best friend, and we should beware appearing to promise that. The symptom should always be taken seriously but severe or psychotic mental illness should be considered if the patient reports that two people are discussing him or her in derogatory tones in his or her head. Anxiety may cause E: bereavement C and serious depression D (though it may be for some a common and annoying experience when their mood is normal – an 'earworm'), but none of these links are diagnostic or consistent except B.

9.1 The best answer is C. The GP's clinical responsibility begins when the patient registers. Any communication received thereafter, whether a test result, a letter, or face-to-face consultation, becomes the responsibility of the GP.

9.2 The best answer is D. Clear, truthful, and accurate information is always important. However information should always be given in a way that enables the patient to make best use of it, to incorporate it into their belief system, and to develop their understanding with time. Information and interpretations that directly oppose the patient's understanding and beliefs are likely to be rejected.

9.3 The best answer is C. Hypothyroidism is a relatively common condition which can occur spontaneously or which follows chemical suppression or surgical removal of the thyroid gland. Treatment is essential and lifelong and usually relatively uncomplicated. Thyroid replacement dosage often requires adjustment

in the early years especially after radio-iodine treatment. The best test to assess the appropriateness of levothyroxine replacement is thyroid stimulating hormone (TSH) which should be done annually in the absence of symptoms. The timing of testing is not critical and patients should not be put at risk of running out of their medication if they have not had the test done.

9.4 The best answer is C. Seventy-five per cent of the population in the UK attends their GP in any year. Raised blood pressure becomes more common in patients over 35 years. This is a good threshold at which to begin seeking raised blood pressure. Raised blood pressure is an important risk factor in cardiovascular disease but most people with raised blood pressure have no other comorbidities. Inviting by letter otherwise healthy patients to attend for blood pressure checks does not lead to better rates of blood pressure surveillance than taking the blood pressure of those who attend their GP for other reasons.

9.5 The best answer is D. The best person to assess the blood pressure in this patient and to make a strategy for its management is the GP. It is appropriate to assess the patient at home, if he is indeed housebound, because the strategy the GP develops should include an assessment of his ability to undertake appropriate investigations and where they should be done. After initial assessment involvement of healthcare professionals from other disciplines could be considered where appropriate.

10.1 The best answer is E. This patient is having chest pain that could represent a heart attack by virtue of its position and character. The main risk to the patient is the possibility of a fatal arrhythmia such as ventricular fibrillation or asystole. He should be taken to hospital by ambulance by a paramedic crew. The paramedics could intervene if he had a cardiac arrest. He should be assessed by the emergency medical team on duty.

10.2 The best answer is A. GPs are not obliged to treat patients at home if in their view a home

ANSWERS TO SINGLE BEST ANSWER QUESTIONS CONTINUED

visit is not indicated. In doing so the GP should satisfy him- or herself that this position can be justified if a complaint is made. Visiting a patient at home unnecessarily would be a waste of the valuable resource of the GP, and set a bad precedent with the patient. The GP should follow up this home visit request to ensure he or she understands the circumstances that led to the outburst and make sure there is no other health or social problem contributing to it.

10.3 The best answer is A. The provision of injectable morphine by syringe driver is widely used to control pain in terminal disease, easy to administer and relatively safe. Safety depends on the familiarity of the operator with the equipment and with the preparation of doses. For this reason it is best started by the nurse specialist. Liquid oral morphine is difficult to take in the large doses which this patient requires.

10.4 The best answer is C. This couple are clearly unable to cope with managing their home. It is possible, though unlikely, that this is their chosen lifestyle. An urgent assessment by social services should be made while the husband is in hospital to get services in place before their return, including home help and possibly meals on wheels. A reassessment of both of them together will be required when he returns home.

10.5 The best answer is E. Fever with rigors is common in respiratory infections. Fever is frequently associated with vomiting if uncontrolled, but the vomiting has been relatively minor. Blanching maculo-papular rashes are also common in viral infections and not indicative of a serious underlying cause. The GP should ensure that the mother accepts the advice and is reasonably reassured. If the mother remains anxious she could be offered a same-day consultation for her son if the paracetamol is ineffective.

11.1 The best answer is C. This enables a dialogue to be started within the short consultation time available and you can assess if his smoking concerns him or not, whether he has tried to stop or is interested. If he is not interested at present, you can easily open the dialogue again at the next visit, potentially motivating him towards contemplation for change. The doctor–patient relationship is fostered.

11.2 The best answer is E. There is minimal understanding about antenatal screening options and their purpose (i.e. to detect abnormalities). Yet 'informed' consent is required. A woman may be 'shocked' when informed of some possible problem, be unsure as to how to respond and what options there are. An otherwise well woman can be now faced with distressing information and uncertainties. If later it is confirmed that her baby has Down syndrome, it is not possible to indicate how severely this child will be affected. If amniocentesis results in a miscarriage and the tests are negative there may be a question of how well informed she actually was.

11.3 The best answer is B. You may also be tempted with C so that you can assess his knowledge and experiences about smoking cessation. Jim is likely to be disadvantaged and on low income, he has probably been told that stopping smoking will not cure COPD but may improve his condition to some degree. You can reiterate this and thus justify referral. He is compliant and 'free' during the day so he is likely to try to attend. His journey to being a non-smoker may encounter relapses but if he is in the system he can continue to get support through relapse phases. His significant other and/or carer may also be a smoker and going together will give them support. From health inequalities data, smoking prevalence is higher amongst the most vulnerable, often indicating more targeted and context-appropriate patient-centred support is needed, although evidence suggests that some GPs have been reluctant to refer people like Jim, fearing it is 'too difficult' for them to change.

11.4 The best answer is B. There is a potential to argue A, C, D and E are all relevant. However, the first answer is too risky, given the family history. Advising weight loss and more exercise can disempower patients who may already know that is needed but so far have not been able to change. The dietician may be reluctant to see

ANSWERS TO SINGLE BEST ANSWER QUESTIONS CONTINUED

patients with BMIs less than 30 and suggest he needs to learn about healthy eating, rather than specialist diets. The British Heart Foundation have good websites that enable exploration during the consultation and either printing off information or giving the link to the patient. Such intervention enables the patient to decide how much information he wants about risk factors and about approaches to behaviour modification. However, arranging the blood tests is appropriate given the history and his potential concerns. He will return for the results and you can further explore ways he can reduce risk and discuss his concerns.

11.5 The best answer is A. This may seem obvious but not all GPs or general practice teams would be proactive in this regard. Local Walking for Health schemes have had good recruitment when the local campaigns are supported by the local practices and have been shown to be useful in encouraging social engagement and active lifestyles. It further demonstrates how far general practice has engaged with the wider social determinants of health and reflects the implementation of the five domains of the Ottawa Charter.

12.1 The best answer is D. You should respect his right to know about his treatment but not leave him on his own with potentially anxiety-creating information: and the medical question might be a way of opening up a discussion about potentially embarrassing issues for him. Many older people have less sex than they did when they were younger but some still have extensive and happy sex lives, sometimes needing modification because of different abilities. The internet may be useful, but not as a way of avoiding a proper discussion between doctor and patient. It's unlikely that it is helpful to think of people having an 'absolute right' about anything, as this means there are no actual or potential conflicts that have to be taken into account.

12.2 The best answer is B. There is an extra new 'diagnosis' here: he is dying. Treatment should now be aimed at making his remaining life of as good quality as can possibly be. For some people the news should not be forced on them, but if they ask, the information should be given kindly but straightforwardly. It is this man's illness, not the relatives'. It is a mistake to try to be exact about the time left to him, as no one can tell precisely, and outliving the estimate may cause unnecessary stress.

12.3 The best answer is C. Capacity relates to the decision at the time. Drugs could be causing this, but so could an infection (such as a UTI) even in the absence of a raised temperature in the elderly. Most people in developed economies now think that the elderly should be given the same 'chances' to live as younger people: but there might be a direct competition (such as a kidney to transplant), and he might not wish to have his life prolonged and have made that clear, such as by an advance directive.

12.4 The best answer is E. This is one of those delicate situations where doing the right thing badly is almost as bad as doing the wrong thing well. It would not be a good idea to get into the habit of taking clandestine tests. The daughter has the right in current English law to request treatment off her own bat, and provided that is the best for her and that is capable of understanding and does understand all about that treatment she may also request that her parents are not informed. She has no right to demand a treatment that, in the doctor's view, may be harmful. However, she has to continue to live with her mother, we assume, and the three of you hope to remain in a positive relationship: so whatever is done should be done slowly, kindly and with as much explanation and tact as possible.

12.5 The best answer is E. For instance, do these principles apply to a dead person's kidney, a 10-week-old fetus or subsequent generations? Respect for autonomy is always to be balanced against the other principles and possibly the autonomy of others (including the people providing healthcare). Benevolence means wishing well/the best (for someone): the principle is

ANSWERS TO SINGLE BEST ANSWER QUESTIONS CONTINUED

about doing the best you can – beneficence. Medical care always risks some harm to patients, however minor and even at its best; so harm should be minimized in every way possible but cannot be excluded. The principle of justice may be both about retribution (such as in complaints or malpractice) and about fair distribution of the resources available for healthcare.

13.1 The best answer is D. Research such as that recently published by the King's Fund shows that in the main the current state of quality in general practice is good. However, there are widespread and unexplained variations, particularly in the management of patients with multiple long-term conditions. Variation in referral rates revealed that many patients are referred for secondary care when they do not need hospital treatment and as well as causing potential harm to patients and unnecessary inconvenience this does not provide the taxpayer with value for money. The King's Fund also highlighted that some patients have difficulties accessing a doctor of their choice and that there is a need for better coordination of care. The NPSA reported between 5 and 80 medical errors per 100 000 consultations, an incidence rate higher than that for lung cancer in the English population.

13.2 The best answer is A. Lord Darzi in his 2008 review of the NHS defined quality in health as having three key dimensions: patient safety, the patient experience and clinical effectiveness. By patient safety, Darzi meant that patients should not be harmed when accessing healthcare through medical error or through infection rates, for example. By the patient experience, Darzi was referring to the caring side of healthcare and in particular that patients should be treated with dignity and respect. By clinical effectiveness, Darzi meant that patients had a right to expect that they would receive the best evidence-based up-to-date treatments available to meet their needs.

13.3 The best answer is D. Donabedian argued that healthcare quality should be assessed in terms of structure, process and outcome in the belief that good structures would lead to good processes that would lead to good outcomes. *Structure* refers to the facilities and resources in healthcare settings, *process* refers to what is actually done by the doctor and by the patient, and *outcomes* refers to the effects of care on patients and populations.

13.4 The best answer is A. Quality assurance is a management process used to ensure that healthcare services that are provided by the practice are safe, meet patient's needs and expectations and improve health. For example, the Quality and Outcomes Framework introduced as part of the 2004 General Medical Services contract measures a set of structure, process and outcome criteria across the whole practice organization. Clinical audit has also been widely used across general practice as a tool to measure and improve clinical care by setting agreed standards for evidence-based criteria and making improvements where appropriate.

13.5 The best answer is B. Two definitions of clinical audit are: 'The systematic, critical analysis of the quality of medical care, including the procedures used for diagnosis and treatment, the use of resources, and the resulting outcome and quality of life for the patient' (Department of Health, 1989). Clinical audit involves 'looking at what you do in a way that allows you to see how you might do things better, making appropriate changes and then looking again to assess improvements in clinical practice' (Department of Health, 1989). The key point about clinical audit is it incorporates in a cyclical manner a process of setting standards, measuring performance, and crucially, making changes for the better and reassessment to ensure that the changes have been effective.

14.1 The best answer is C. A GMS contract is negotiated nationally. The contractor has to provide basic medical services and can also provide additional services. A PMS contract has similar terms and conditions but has more flexibility in the type of services that it can provide. The funding for a PMS contract has more flexibility in the

ANSWERS TO SINGLE BEST ANSWER QUESTIONS CONTINUED

way in which it is distributed in particular for employing GPs and nurse practitioners. The size of the practice is irrelevant when determining the type of GP contract. Contracts are negotiated and while a GP contractor would need to demonstrate that it can provide a certain level of service and is qualified to do so, the type of contract is not determined by this. Both contracts *must* provide basic medical services and both can provide additional medical services.

14.2 The best answer is B. The global sum is a payment made to the practice based on a price agreed per patient. The calculation of this sum takes into consideration money to pay for out-of-hours services and staffing costs. The total sum is determined by the number of patients on a practice's list. Income from the Quality and Outcomes Framework is linked to points earned for meeting specific clinical and organizational targets. While achieving maximum points provides a large chunk of income for the practice, it is still not the main source. QOF income is proportionate to its list size. For directed enhanced service payment the Department of Health determines priority areas and offers payment to provide certain services. The amount paid is normally based on a price per patient; however this amount is considerably lower than the amount paid per patient as part of a practice's global sum. While private income can be a good way in which to supplement a practice's income, a practice cannot earn over a certain level of private income. If this happened the reimbursement for the rent/mortgage of the practice property will be reduced. Again, local enhanced service payments are a good source of income but a practice cannot rely upon them. Contracts for local enhanced services are issued based on the needs of the local population. Those needs change over time, which can result in the termination of a locally enhanced service.

14.3 The best answer is C. Strategic planning looks at where we are now and then where we want to be in the future. The gap is the journey or actions that will be required to get there.

While you would need to ensure that a practice can raise enough funds to pay staff wages in the future, this would be part of a larger process of ensuring the practice meets future challenges. To plan for a major policy change within the NHS would be part of a larger process of planning the future for the practice, which would take into consideration a number of factors, not least planned changes to the NHS. Strategic planning is about both short- and long-term planning. It is also about determining the vision and goals for the future, not just about planning for what we know will happen but also about what we want to change. A practice will need to plan ahead when implementing a new service, although strategic planning in this context is about planning for wider and longer term changes.

14.4 The best answer is A. Option A encompasses all elements of managing a general practice and planning for changes to each. You would include the other elements within your overall plan but they would need to be linked to specific goals and take into consideration the different functions of the practice.

14.5 The best answer is B. Patient demand does not necessarily equate to patient need. Need is also determined by the population's ability to benefit from a service and this is determined by researching the incidence and prevalence of a health condition in that population, services available for the health condition and the effectiveness and quality of those services, which includes canvassing the views of patients. Gaining patient views is a positive process in order to improve services. Purely gaining patient views would not provide them with insights about the way the service is provided.

15.1 The best answer is E. The patient may need to consult with someone while you are on leave or in an emergency, and without this information whoever they see may make a flawed decision, but that is something the patient should decide, not you.

ANSWERS TO SINGLE BEST ANSWER QUESTIONS CONTINUED

15.2 Probably B is the best answer, though people will argue about it. The time sensitivity of the form and the visit are high, but you will probably do everything more quickly and with fewer errors if you have a quick snack; if you don't do the form before the collection goes, then the MSU is pointless, and it will take seconds to do, while the visit is to a nursing home close by, so the patient is probably not in danger. You should have done the letter yesterday so the embarrassment factor is high but that shouldn't push its priority unless there is some other reason. You may have sympathy with the student, but you could always share your sandwich and take them on the visit with you.

15.3 The best answer is E. This incorporates honesty, admitting that you didn't know about the new possibility, but also that you need to check the information, suitability and availability for the patient. You have not 'made a mistake' so do not need to apologize, although you can be humble about the fact that you don't know everything. D is dangerous behaviour. You are hiding, and you may forget to look it up.

15.4 C is probably the best first step. Try to contextualize the 'upset' and your own expectations of yourself. If your colleagues all know more about it than you do, then maybe a refresher course is not such a bad idea. If they say they wouldn't have let it get to them, then maybe you do need a holiday.

15.5 The best answer is probably C. Your knowledge and your tutor's insight will make for a productive conversation for both of you. The others are all rather self-indulgent: A might make the tutor feel small, B will make the tutorial boring for both of you, D is blind to the fact that your perspective on the subject is limited to what you saw in hospital, and E is disrespectful of any preparation the tutor might do in advance, and also avoids an honest discussion about your needs.

16.1 The best answer is C. Time is a valuable resource and GPs need to be sure their learning time is effective, and that education is suited to their preferred learning style and practice needs. Attending meetings or reading may be useful, if that is how they learn best, but the content may not always be relevant, and we should be selective in what we focus on for greatest value. This question emphasizes the need for careful planning of learning time – the individual GP is the best person to explore and address their learning needs, and although an appraiser can help, they cannot tell them what needs to be done.

16.2 The best answer is D. As Dr Red has a long-standing doctor–patient relationship with Mrs Smith, he is much more likely to be able to break this news to Mrs Smith in a constructive way than relative strangers. Dr Red may not always be the best person to look after Mrs Smith's diabetes in the long run, but introducing her to the diagnosis, and the practice services himself will help her to adjust to receiving care from others. Referring directly to hospital would not be appropriate without assessing the need for this and discussing with Mrs Smith.

16.3 The best answer is B. It is important for GPs to involve patients in decisions that require their cooperation. Here, weight gain may be secondary to depression or change of lifestyle since not working. The GP needs to understand the patient's perspective and how much the patient is able to influence the process in order to share options for best outcome. Giving instructions, passing them to others or dismissing the problem will likely be resented and rejected by patients.

16.4 The best answer is A. Working collaboratively with colleagues requires good communication and mutual respect. Here, direct discussion with the nurse will clarify the problem and allow discussion about management, including how best the GP can contribute to care, and whether other professionals should be involved (e.g. social care). The other responses bypass the input from the community nurse, undermining her role and risking compromising care through lack of clinical information.

ANSWERS TO SINGLE BEST ANSWER QUESTIONS CONTINUED

16.5 The best answer is B. Vacancies bring opportunity for practices to develop existing staff, recruit new skills and plan for future needs. In addition to meeting employment law requirements of equal opportunities, practices need a sound organizational structure to ensure appointments will deliver identified improvements to patient services while also protecting the interests and working conditions of existing staff.

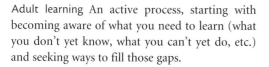

GLOSSARY

Adult learning An active process, starting with becoming aware of what you need to learn (what you don't yet know, what you can't yet do, etc.) and seeking ways to fill those gaps.

Adverse drug interaction An adverse effect on health as a result of the interaction between two or more medications.

Alcoholism or alcohol dependence An extension of normal behaviour when there is a compulsion to take alcohol. When you suspect such a problem may be present, the CAGE set of questions may be helpful: Have you ever felt you ought to cut down on your drinking? Have people annoyed you by criticizing your drinking? Have you ever felt bad or guilty about your drinking? Have you ever had a drink first thing in the morning to steady your nerves or get rid of a hangover (eye opener)?

Anorexia nervosa Self-induced weight loss, together with an intense desire to be thin, is accompanied by the view that the patient (usually, but not always, a young woman) is still too fat, whereas others clearly think she is now very thin. In its extreme form it is followed by body changes and may be fatal in 10 per cent of cases, although, with treatment, 40–50 per cent return to normal eating.

Argument In ethics this is not about a dispute but is the reasoning that justifies a particular course of action or approach.

Autonomy A person's freedom to make choices about themselves and about issues that concern them is central to the concept of autonomy, which means literally 'self-rule'. Without a justifiable reason to do otherwise, an individual's autonomous choices should be respected by healthcare staff.

Chaperone for intimate examination. Someone who accompanies a patient during an examination for the purposes of safeguarding the patient from the possibility of abuse by the examiner and safeguarding the examiner from the possibility of wrongful allegations of abuse from the patient. It usually applies to examination of intimate body areas, and the chaperone is usually a friend or relative of the patient or a member of the healthcare staff.

Chronic illness Illness which, by its impact or its duration, has implications for the health of the patient beyond the immediate presentation and usually for a period of more than three months (although this interval is arbitrary). Thirty-three per cent of illness presenting to general practice is chronic.

Classification of drug In the UK, the Medicines Control Agency is responsible for classifying drugs as Prescription only (PoM), Pharmacy only (P: sold only in pharmacies under the supervision of a registered pharmacist but without the need for a prescription) or General Sales List (GSL: available from a wide range of retailers, e.g. supermarkets).

Clinical audit The agreement and subsequent implementation of realistic plans to improve patient care.

Clinical effectiveness Clinical effectiveness and evidence-based medicine comprise a systematic quality improvement process that involves an appraisal of research evidence, the development of protocols and guidelines and their implementation into clinical practice.

Clinical iceberg Only the 'tip of the iceberg' of symptoms experienced by the general population is seen by healthcare professionals. In the UK, 79 per cent of symptoms are dealt with by self-care, 20 per cent by GPs and 1 per cent by hospitals.

Clinical reasoning Process of sorting clinical data (history, physical examination, investigations) to achieve a diagnosis and management plan.

Communication skills Proficiency in the interchange of information between people. In relation to medical practice, communication is between healthcare professionals and patients or members of the healthcare team.

Competence In medicine, this implies the broad ability of patients to make decisions about their own care. A competent person is usually thought of as someone who can be informed about the issue and make a choice, can retain the information and think about it in order to make a decision, and has a reasonably consistent, stable and personal set of values. Ultimately, the law may have to judge, in which case the word 'capacity' is usually used to cover this area.

Compliance The extent to which a patient takes or uses a medicine as intended by the prescriber.

Concordance A partnership between patient and health professional in which an agreement is reached about whether and how medicines are to be taken/used.

Consultation The meeting between a doctor and a patient at which health-related issues are presented and explored and management decisions made.

Computer-based prescribing Tools for computer-based prescribing range from existing general practice systems such as repeat prescriptions, through to computerized textbooks (e.g. the *British National Formulary*), software systems including drug interaction alerts and sophisticated decision support tools that can extract data from a patient's record and suggest a ranked list of suitable drugs with appropriate doses.

Culture The shared beliefs, values, attitudes and experiences that guide the behaviour of a group of people. Examples relate to age, gender, sexual orientation, physical difference, learning ability, educational background, ethnicity, socio-economic background and health experiences and values.

Disease protocol A set of instructions for the optimal management of a disease from its identification through the range of possible disease trajectories to its eradication or to the demise of the patient.

Disease register A list of all those affected by a particular disease for whom a doctor or an institution has clinical responsibility.

Dispensing practice In the UK, a dispensing practice acts as a pharmacy, buying drugs in, dispensing them and claiming payment from the National Health Service. Practices are allowed to dispense drugs for those patients on their practice list who live more than 1 mile from a pharmacy.

Drug formulary A document containing general information on prescribing, the choice of drugs available to treat particular conditions and detailed information on individual drugs. National formularies exist, such as the *British National Formulary*, and individual hospitals and general practices may develop their own local formularies; these usually specify a limited choice of drugs to use in any particular condition, chosen for their effectiveness, safety and cost.

Ethnic group A group of people who have certain background characteristics, such as language, culture and religion, in common, which provide the group with a distinct identity, as seen by both themselves and others.

Evidence-based medicine A process by which explicit use is made of research evidence in making medical decisions. Evidence-based medicine should integrate best research evidence with clinical expertise and take into account individual patients' circumstances and values.

Formative assessment Assessment of the development of knowledge and skills during training.

General Medical Services (GMS) The contract in the UK National Health Service under which GP principals provide medical care (or services) to patients registered with them. The patients are often referred to as 'being on the list' of the GP. Under a GMS arrangement, an individual GP contracts to deliver care to patients. Payment is through a complex system of fees and allowances aligned to nationally agreed services, without any local flexibility.

General practice An organization, also known as a family practice, providing first-contact, person-centred, comprehensive and continuing care to a patient population. The task of those who work in a general practice is to promote health and well-being and to understand and treat illness in the context of their patients' lives, belief systems and community and work with other professionals in the healthcare setting to coordinate care and make efficient use of healthcare resources.

GP cooperatives A formal business arrangement between GPs to share in the provision of services for their patients. In NHS general practice in the UK, GP cooperatives are concerned exclusively with out-of-hours general medical services.

GP principal In the UK, a GP on the list of principals of the primary care trust.

GP registrar In the UK, a qualified doctor going through a period of approved training to be eligible to become a GP principal.

Grounding Having a realistic awareness of what your peers can do, and what you should expect of yourself.

Guidelines Written statements providing 'extensive, critical and well-balanced information on the benefits and limitations of various diagnostic and therapeutic interventions'. Good-quality guidelines should consist of two components: an evidence section (based on an up-to-date literature review with the level of evidence made explicit) and a detailed instruction section (with grades of recommendations tagged to the level of evidence available).

Health belief model Individuals differ in their perception of their susceptibility and vulnerability to illness, the severity of their symptoms, and the costs and benefits of health-seeking behaviour.

Health promotion A field of study associated with informed and planned interventions to prevent disease and to maintain and improve health. There are many definitions and it is an eclectic and contested field. A working definition for those in medical education could be 'the study of, and the study of the response to, the modifiable determinants of health and disease'. Equally, there are those who advocate health promotion as an ideology, associated with addressing inequalities and poverty, about principles such as autonomy and empowerment.

Health promotion evidence This is usually related to the intervention, its aims and objectives and can relate to both the processes and the outcomes. Evidence can be qualitative and/or quantitative but is rarely conclusive or generalizable.

Health promotion specialist A professional who works in this broad field, often at a strategic level. These specialists are not regulated and come from many different academic and professional backgrounds, but are most likely to have a master's degree in health promotion. It is usually a second or third occupation for those whose previous experiences are relevant to the work area. Many health promotion specialists will be members of one or more professional bodies.

Health promotion theory The body of knowledge that informs health promotion activity is complex and incorporates both sciences and humanities. Theoretical models and approaches to practice are well established but, being a contested field, they are constantly challenged, with new models emerging.

Hospital-at-home A service that provides treatment in the home by healthcare professionals of illnesses that would otherwise require acute treatment in hospital.

Hypochondriasis The persistent preoccupation by the patient that he or she has a serious physical illness in spite of appropriate medical examination with explanation and reassurance to the contrary.

Hypothetico-deductive reasoning Ideas generated by an early phase of information gathering are tested by eliciting further data, and so on in a repeating process until decision making occurs.

Illness behaviour The ways in which given symptoms may be differentially perceived, evaluated and acted upon (or not acted upon) by different people.

Inductive reasoning Information gathering is concluded before decision making occurs.

Informed consent The process whereby a patient agrees to a procedure, care or treatment after full information has been given by the person seeking that consent.

Major illness Acute and potentially life-threatening illness – 15 per cent of illness presenting to general practice.

Medication review Structured review of the efficacy and continuing appropriateness of a patient's medication. The 'brown bag review' is a particular example of this, where patients are asked to bring in all the medication they have. This allows discussion of both prescribed and over-the-counter (OTC) medications, reveals stockpiles of particular drugs, ancient medications and the patients' degree of understanding about what they take, when and why.

Minor illness Self-limiting illness – 52 per cent of illness presenting to general practice.

Narrative approach An approach used to help people tell their stories.

Negative predictive value This expresses how likely it is that an individual with a negative test is actually clear of the disease and is calculated as the ratio of those who tested negative and do not have the disease to all those who tested negative.

Objective Structured Clinical Examination (OSCE) A standardized method for the assessment of clinical competences in which a candidate is observed and assessed in the demonstration of a range of skills. These may include history-taking and communication skills, physical examination, diagnostic ability, patient management and clinical skills. The observer uses a checklist to record the candidate's competences in the components of the skill under observation.

Out-of-hours care Healthcare provided outside office hours. In NHS general practice in the UK, out-of-hours care is usually considered to be between 7 p.m. and 9 a.m. Out-of hours organizations such as cooperatives usually only provide cover from 7 p.m. to 7 a.m.

Over-the-counter (OTC) medications Non-prescription medicines purchased from pharmacies and other outlets (including 'alternative' medications).

PACT data In England, detailed information on GPs' prescribing is available in the form of PACT (prescribing analysis and cost) data; similar systems exist in Scotland and Wales. PACT data contain information on prescribing costs, the number of items prescribed and the level of generic prescribing, at individual GP level, health authority and national level.

Paternalism Acting or deciding for someone else, supposedly in their best interests, but without regard to their choice in the matter (as a parent might do for a child) is considered paternalistic. This is not necessarily always wrong, but is to be avoided or minimized wherever possible in medical care.

Pathognomonic 'Specially or decisively characteristic of a disease; indicating with certainty a disease.' In practice, it means a sign or feature so characteristic of a particular disease that after seeing it you would entertain no other diagnosis. An example might be the Koplik's spots of measles that occur in no other situation, but not, paradoxically, the morbilliform (i.e. 'measles-like') rash seen not only in measles but also in many other viral illnesses. From the Greek *pathognomonikos*: *patho-* + *gnomonikos*, able to judge.

Patient centredness Focusing on the patient's story and taking into account the patient's desire for information and for sharing decision making.

Patient safety The process by which an organization makes patient care safer.

Personal Medical Services (PMS) A new type of UK National Health Service contract for GP practices introduced in 1998. Under a PMS arrangement, all GP principals of a general practice contract with their local primary care trust for the clinical services the practice will provide for its patients. In return, the practice is guaranteed a budget to pay for this work and the staff. This is a different contractual arrangement from the General Medical Services. PMS GPs develop their own contract. This contract is with the PCT, not with the Secretary of State for Health; it is local not national. The contract can be tailored to suit the needs of the local population and local medical service provision, focused towards locally agreed priorities. A PMS practice agrees to provide a range of primary care medical services to a defined population for an agreed sum of money.

Polypharmacy Where a patient is prescribed four or more drugs. Prescribing of four or more drugs is not necessarily bad, and indeed may be necessary. However, polypharmacy is a risk factor for potential harm from medication.

Portfolio A collection of evidence of work done, learning achieved, personal reflection, testimonials, etc.

Positive predictive value This calculates the likelihood that an individual with a positive test actually has the disease. It is a simple statistic: true positives/(true positives plus false positives)

for any test, i.e. it is the ratio of those who tested positive and who genuinely have the disease to all those who have tested positive.

Prescribing budget Budgets set by health authorities or primary care trusts (UK) for prescribing costs for individual general practices.

Primary care trust (PCT) In the UK, primary care trusts are freestanding, legally established statutory NHS bodies that are accountable to the local health authority. They are organizations that integrate primary, secondary and community health services for a locality. They have their own budget for delivering healthcare in their area; they are able to employ staff (district nurses/health visitors etc.) and to develop new integrated services for patients. They are key NHS partners for local authorities and local voluntary and community organizations. They hold a significant majority of the entire NHS budget and are responsible for GP and community health services and other primary care services such as dental, pharmaceutical and optical. In time, they may also extend to include social care and support services. PCTs commission general and acute services, invest in primary and community care and work to improve the health of their local population. GPs enter into a contract with the PCT (either GMS or PMS) to provide medical services for patients registered at the practice.

Primary healthcare That which provides healthcare in the first instance.

Primary healthcare team (PHCT) The primary healthcare team is made up of everyone who works at a general practice or primary healthcare centre: doctors, nurses, health visitors, midwives, physiotherapists, osteopaths, clinical psychologists, counsellors, dieticians, managers, secretarial staff, clerical staff, reception staff, cleaning and maintenance staff and others. The team members may be employed by the practice or by the primary care trust.

Protocol A set way of dealing with a particular condition, often based on a detailed development of existing guidelines, for use by an individual organization, e.g. general practice.

Psychosis The traditional clinical categorization of those (whom lay people might call 'mad') seriously distressed by strange beliefs and abnormal perceptions. These beliefs and perceptions often appear to lead the patients to violence or (self-) destructive behaviour.

Quality assurance Ensuring patient safety, clinical effectiveness and the quality of caring.

Quality improvement A systematic process to manage change within organizations to bring about better patient care. There are many tools and methods used for quality improvement, the most important being clinical audit.

Quality and Outcomes Framework (QOF) The QOF rewards UK general practices financially for the provision of quality care, and helps to fund further improvements in the delivery of clinical care. It measures practice achievement against a range of evidence-based clinical indicators and against a range of indicators covering practice organization and management.

Randomized controlled trial (RCT) A study in which people are allocated at random to receive one of several clinical interventions. Typically, RCTs seek to measure and compare different events that are present or absent after the participants receive the interventions. These events are called outcomes. As the outcomes are quantified (or measured), RCTs are regarded as quantitative studies.

Reflecting Thinking over what has happened and why, what this shows you, and what you need to do differently, or what you need to preserve and strengthen.

Repeat prescribing When a GP makes a decision to continue a drug long term, the patient is allowed to request further supplies without needing to see the doctor each time. Usually the system is computerized.

Research evidence The published results of clinical trials, experiments, evaluations, surveys and other projects. Research aims to answer one or more specific questions and tells us 'what we should be doing'. Research evidence is often thought of as being hierarchical and involving a five-point scale:

1. Strong evidence from at least one systematic review of multiple, well-designed, randomized controlled trials.

2. Strong evidence from at least one properly designed randomized controlled trial of appropriate size.

3. Evidence from well-designed trials such as non-randomized trials, cohort studies, time series or matched case-controlled studies.

4. Evidence from well-designed non-experimental studies from more than one centre or research group.

5. Opinions of respected authorities, based on clinical evidence, descriptive studies or reports of expert committees.

Screening The process of discovering unknown or undisclosed disease risk or actual disease with a view to intervening to prevent the occurrence or the progress of the disease.

Sensitivity A measure of how likely it is that a screening test will correctly identify individuals who really have the disease. With a highly sensitive test, there will be few 'false negatives'.

Significant event analysis A formal type of reflection, important after unusually good or bad outcomes, that is sometimes particularly useful when the event involves several people or a team, as everyone can take part in the reflection.

Skill The ability to perform a task well, usually gained by training or experience.

Skills checklist A list of the components of a specified skill that can be used as a method of ensuring consistency in the performance of a skill.

Skills competence The possession of a satisfactory level in the performance of a skill.

Skills performance The demonstration of a skill in a real-life situation.

Skills proficiency The attainment of a skill to an advanced level. (Practising a skill with adeptness.)

Specificity A measure of how likely it is that a screening test will correctly identify individuals who do not have the disease. With a highly specific test, there will be few 'false positives'.

Structured care A planned approach to disease management based on a register of those affected who can be recalled at set intervals for formal review of the disease in order to maximize the potential to control the disease, treat symptoms and prevent complications.

Suicide The taking of one's own life is still widely considered a tragedy under all circumstances and it remains the doctor's duty to detect suicidal risk and prevent the act if at all possible. In self-harm, there is a spectrum from threats or aggressive cutting/self-poisoning, which does not cause immediate loss of life (typically in the young), to the deliberate planning of a solitary death by the old and ill. However, since the best predictor of completed suicide remains an episode of self-poisoning or self-injury, all such actions should be taken equally seriously.

Summative assessment Assessment of the acquisition of and competence in knowledge, skills and attitudes at the completion of training.

Telephone consultations Consultations with patients that take place by telephone. They may be initiated by the doctor or the patient, and have medico-legal implications and obligations that differ from those of face-to-face consultations. Among these are the security of the communication line and the provision of confidential information when the identity of the other party cannot be assured.

Valuing diversity in health The appreciation of how variations in culture, background and healthcare may affect health and healthcare.